Advanced Methods and Tools
for ECG Data Analysis

This book is part of the Artech House Engineering in Medicine & Biology Series, Martin L. Yarmush and Christopher J. James, Series Editors. For a listing of recent related Artech House titles, turn to the back of this book.

Advanced Methods and Tools for ECG Data Analysis

Gari D. Clifford
Francisco Azuaje
Patrick E. McSharry

Editors

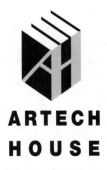

ARTECH

HOUSE

BOSTON | LONDON
artechhouse.com

Library of Congress Cataloging-in-Publication Data
A catalog record for this book is available from this U.S. Library of Congress.

British Library Cataloguing in Publication Data
A catalogue record for this book is available from the British Library.

ISBN-10: 1-58053-966-1

ISBN-13: 978-1-58053-966-1

Cover design by Michael Moretti

© 2006 ARTECH HOUSE, INC.
685 Canton Street
Norwood, MA 02062

10 9 8 7 6 5 4 3 2 1

Contents

Preface

This book is intended for graduate students collecting and/or analyzing electrocardiogram (ECG) data, industrial researchers looking to develop, test, and apply new ECG analysis tools (both hardware and software), or simply students or teachers looking for signal processing examples involving an intuitive yet complex signal. Initially, this book was conceived primarily as a vessel for collecting together current research in ECG analysis that we considered to be important guides of how to apply complex techniques to this field. However, it is not our intention to simply present a collection of colleagues' papers with an index and contents. The articles we have selected have been specifically commissioned for this book with a request to the authors that they explain how they achieved their results, why they represent a significant improvement of existing techniques, and why the particular method they used is more appropriate for the task.

Not only do we wish to present an overview of many of the most interesting and useful advanced techniques currently available (together with an analysis of the validity of the assumptions these techniques require), we also wish to provide the reader with the relevant background on where distortion, noise, and errors can creep into an experiment or analysis. This includes not only the choice of (digital) mathematical processing operations, but also the design and choice of sensors, hardware, software, data storage, data transmission methods, databases on which the techniques are evaluated, and probably most importantly of all, the metrics by which we determine one technique is superior to another. There is, of course, one other source of noise or error: the subject itself. Choosing the correct database or population, and including or excluding particular data is an essential part of experimental design. Furthermore, the quantification of a section of data in terms of noise or signal quality depends largely on the type of analysis that is being performed. For example, muscle noise can be a signal that indicates activity, whereas abnormal beats may indicate a lapse in stationarity and invalidate Fourier methods.

The analysis of the electrocardiogram as a diagnostic tool is a relatively old field and it is therefore often assumed that the ECG is a simple signal that has been fully explored. However, there remain difficult problems in this field that are being incrementally solved with advances in techniques from the fields of filtering, pattern recognition, and classification, together with the leaps in computational power and memory capacity that have occurred over the last couple of decades.

The following is a nonexhaustive list of many of the key remaining challenges in ECG signal processing today:

- *Reliable P wave identification.* P waves are usually a low-amplitude feature that can often become subsumed by the baseline noise in a signal. Detection of the onset of atrial activity at the start of the P wave is important for heart rate variability studies. However, the enormity of this problem has led to a pervasive analysis of beat-to-beat intervals based upon the QRS complex as a fiducial marker.

- *Reliable QT interval estimation.* Similarly, despite the relatively large amplitude of the QRS complex and T wave, the *onset* of the Q wave and *offset* of the T wave are difficult features to measure (even for highly trained experts). Changes in the QRS complex, ST segment, and T wave morphology due to heart rate and sympathetic nervous system changes make this problem particularly acute.

- *Distinguishing ischemic from nonischemic ST changes.* Even in subjects who are known to have myocardial ischemia, ST changes are not considered a basis for definitive diagnosis of individual episodes of ischemia. This is because the ST segment changes with a subject's body position due to the movement of the ECG electrodes relative to the heart. Recent attempts to identify such artefacts are promising (see the Computers in Cardiology Challenge 2003), but the road to a full working system (particularly for silent ischemia) is not clear.

- *Reliable beat classification in Holter monitoring.* Ambulatory monitoring presents many challenges since the data collection process is essentially unsupervised, and evolving problems in the acquisition often go undetected (or at least are not corrected). One major problem is the high level of in-band noise encountered (usually muscle- or movement-related). Another problem for ambulatory monitoring is the degradation in electrode contact over time, leading to a lower signal-to-noise ratio. Since the P wave is usually a low-amplitude feature, reliable detection of the P wave is particularly problematic in this environment.

- *Robust, reliable in-band signal filtering or source separation* (such as muscle noise removal and fetal-maternal separation). Principal and independent component analysis has shown promise in this area, but problems persist with nonstationary mixing and lead position inaccuracies/changes. Model-based filtering methods have also shown promise in this area.

- *Identification of lead position misplacements or sensor shifts.* Most classifiers assume that the label for the clinical lead being recorded is known and make assumptions about waveform morphology, amplitude, and polarity based upon the lead label. If the lead is misplaced, or shifts during recording, then misclassifications or misdetections will probably occur. In particular, the maternal-fetal signal mixing is problematic in this respect. In this case two cardiac sources are moving with respect to each other, sometimes without correlation, and sometimes entrained on one or more scales.

- *Reliable confidence measures.* The ability of an algorithm to report back a "level of trust" associated with its parameter estimates is very important, particularly if the algorithm's output is fed to another data fusion algorithm.

- *The inverse problem.* It is well known that no unique solution exists for the inverse problem in ECG mapping. Attempts to reconstruct the dipole moment in the ECG have had some degree of success, and recent models for the ECG have proved useful in this respect.

- *ECG modeling and parameter fitting.* To date there exist many accurate representations for the ECG from a cellular level up to more phenomenological models. However, at best, each of these models can accurately reproduce the ECG waveform for only a short period of time. Although models also exist for variations in the beat-to-beat timings of the heart on both short and long scales, there are no known models that can reproduce realistic dynamic activity on all scales, together with an accurate or realistic resultant ECG. Recent work in the fitting of real data to ECG and pulsatile models is certainly promising, but much work is needed in order to ascertain whether the resultant parameters will yield any more information than traditional ECG metrics.

- *The mapping of diagnostic ECG parameters to disease classifications or predictive metrics.* Neural networks have shown promise in this area due to their ability to extrapolate from small training sets. However, neural networks are highly sensitive to outliers and the size and distribution of the training set. If only a few artifacts, or mislabeled patterns, creep into the training set, the performance of the classifier is significantly reduced. Conversely, over-restricting the training set to include too few patterns from a class results in over-training. Another known problem from the use of neural networks is that it is difficult to extract meaning from the output; a classification does not obviously map back to the etiology.

- *Global context pattern analysis.* Factoring in patient-specific history (from minutes, to hours, to years) for feature recognition and classification is required if a full emulation of the clinical diagnostic procedure is to be reproduced. Hidden Markov models, extended Kalman filters, and Bayesian classifiers are likely candidates for such a problem.

- *The development of closed-loop systems.* It is always problematic for a clinician to relinquish the task of classification and intervention for personal, legal, and ethical reasons. However, with the increasing accuracy of classifiers and the decreasing costs of machines relative to human experts, it is almost inevitable that closed-loop devices will become more pervasive. To date, few such systems exist beyond the classic internal cardioverters that have been in use for several decades. Despite promising advances in atrial fibrillation detection, which may soon make the closed-loop injection of drugs for this type of condition a reality, further work is needed to ensure patient safety.

- *Sensor fusion.* Information that can be derived from the ECG is insufficient to effectively solve many of the above problems. It is likely that the combination of information derived from other sensors (such as blood pressure transducers, accelerometers, and pulse oximeters) will be required. The paradigm of multidimensional signal analysis is well known to the ECG signal analyst, and parallel analysis of the ECG (or ECG-derived parameters) almost always enhances an algorithm's performance. For instance, blood pressure waves contain information that is highly correlated with the ECG, and analysis of these changes can help reduce false arrhythmia alarms. The ECG is also highly correlated with respiration and can be used to improve respiration rate estimates or to facilitate sleep analysis. However, when the associated signals do not present in a highly correlated manner, the units of measurement are different (so that a 20-mmHg change does not mean the same as a 20-bpm change, for example) and their associated distributions differ, the task at hand is far more difficult. In fact, normalizing for these differences, and building *trust* metrics to differentiate artifactual changes from real changes in such signals, is one of the more difficult challenges in ECG signal processing today.

In order to address these issues, we have attempted to detail many of the key relevant advances in signal processing. Chapter 1 describes the physiological background and the specific autonomic mechanisms which regulate the beat-to-beat changes of timing and morphology in the ECG, together with the cause and effect of breakdowns in this mechanism. Chapter 2 presents an overview of the primary issues that should be taken into account when designing an ECG collection system. Chapter 3 presents an overview of the relevant mathematical descriptors of the ECG such as clinical metrics, spectral characteristics, and beat-to-beat variability indices. Chapter 4 presents an overview of simple, practical ECG and beat-to-beat models, together with methods for applying these models to ECG analysis. Chapter 5 describes a unified framework for linear filtering techniques including wavelets, principal component analysis, neural networks, and independent component analysis. Chapter 6 discusses methods and pitfalls of nonlinear ECG analysis, with a practical emphasis on filtering techniques.

Chapter 7 provides an overview of T wave alternan methodologies, and Chapter 8 presents a comparative study of ECG derived respiration techniques. Chapter 9 presents advanced techniques for extracting relevant features from the ECG, and Chapter 10 uses these techniques to describe a robust ST-analyzer. Chapter 11 presents a wavelet and hidden Markov model–based procedure for robust QT-analysis. Chapter 12 describes techniques for supervised classification and hybrid techniques for classifying ECG metrics, where the data labels are already known, and Chapter 13 presents unsupervised learning techniques for ECG pattern discovery and classification.

Although many of the basics of ECG analysis are presented in Chapter 1, this is simply to draw the reader's attention the etiology of many of the problems we are attempting to solve. As a thorough grounding in the basics of ECG signal processing, the reader is referred to Chapters 7 and 8 in Sörnmo and Laguna's recent book *Bioelectric Signal Processing in Cardiac and Neurological Applications* (Elsevier, 2005). The reader is assumed to be familiar with the basics of signal processing and classification techniques. Furthermore, these techniques are necessarily implemented using a knowledge of computational programming. This book follows the open-source philosophy that the development of robust signal processing algorithms is best done by making them freely available, together with the labeled data on which they were evaluated. Many of the algorithms and data sets described in this book are available from the following URLs: http://www.ecgtools.org, http://www.physionet.org, and http://alum.mit.edu/www/gari/ecgbook.

Most of these algorithms have been written either in C or Matlab. Additionally, Java applet versions of selected algorithms are also available. Libraries for reading these databases are also freely available. We hope that through these URLs this book will continue to evolve and add to the growing body of open (repeatable) biomedical research.

It is important to acknowledge the giants whose shoulders we stand upon. We would therefore like to thank the many who offered advice and help along the way, including George Moody, Roger Mark, Rachel Hall Clifford, Emmeline Skinner McSharry, Raphael Schneider, Ary Goldberger, Julie Greenberg, Lionel Tarassenko, Lenny Smith, Christopher James, Steve Roberts, Ken Barnes, and Roy Sambles. We would also like to acknowledge the many organizations that have facilitated this project, including the National Institute of Biomedical Imaging and Bioengineering (under Grant R01 EB001659), the Royal Academy of Engineering, the Engineering and Physical Sciences Research Council, United Kingdom (grants GR/N02641 and GR/S35066), the European Union's Sixth Framework Programme (Grant 502299), and, of course, Artech House Publishing for all their editorial help. Finally, and above all, we thank all the authors who have contributed their valuable knowledge, time, and energy to this book.

Gari D. Clifford
Cambridge, Massachusetts

Francisco Azuaje
Jordanstown, United Kingdom

Patrick E. McSharry
Oxford, United Kingdom
Editors
September 2006

CHAPTER 1

The Physiological Basis of the Electrocardiogram

Andrew T. Reisner, Gari D. Clifford, and Roger G. Mark

Before attempting any signal processing of the electrocardiogram it is important to first understand the physiological basis of the ECG, to review measurement conventions of the standard ECG, and to review how a clinician uses the ECG for patient care. The material and figures in this chapter are taken from [1, 2], to which the reader is referred for a more detailed overview of this subject. Further information can also be found in the reading list given at the end of this chapter.

The heart is comprised of muscle (*myocardium*) that is rhythmically driven to contract and hence drive the circulation of blood throughout the body. Before every normal heartbeat, or *systole*,[1] a wave of electrical current passes through the entire heart, which triggers myocardial contraction. The pattern of electrical propagation is not random, but spreads over the structure of the heart in a coordinated pattern which leads to an effective, coordinated systole. This results in a measurable change in potential difference on the body surface of the subject. The resultant amplified (and filtered) signal is known as an electrocardiogram (ECG, or sometimes EKG). A broad number of factors affect the ECG, including abnormalities of cardiac conducting fibers, metabolic abnormalities (including a lack of oxygen, or *ischemia*) of the myocardium, and macroscopic abnormalities of the normal geometry of the heart. ECG analysis is a routine part of any complete medical evaluation, due to the heart's essential role in human health and disease, and the relative ease of recording and analyzing the ECG in a noninvasive manner.

Understanding the basis of a normal ECG requires appreciation of four phenomena: the electrophysiology of a single cell, how the wave of electrical current propagates through myocardium, the physiology of the specific structures of the heart through which the electrical wave travels, and last how that leads to a measurable signal on the surface of the body, producing the normal ECG.

1.1 Cellular Processes That Underlie the ECG

Each mechanical heartbeat is triggered by an *action potential* which originates from a rhythmic pacemaker within the heart and is conducted rapidly throughout the organ to produce a coordinated contraction. As with other electrically active tissues

---

1. Diastole, the opposite of systole, is defined to be the period of relaxation and expansion of the heart chambers between two contractions, when the heart fills with blood.

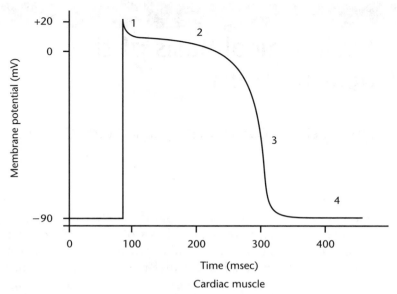

Figure 1.1 A typical action potential from a ventricular myocardial cell. Phases 0 through 4 are marked. (*From*: [2]. © 2004 MIT OCW. Reprinted with permission.)

(e.g., nerves and skeletal muscle), the myocardial cell at rest has a typical transmembrane potential, V_m, of about −80 to −90 mV with respect to surrounding extracellular fluid.[2] The cell membrane controls permeability to a number of ions, including sodium, potassium, calcium, and chloride. These ions pass across the membrane through specific ion channels that can open (become activated) and close (become inactivated). These channels are therefore said to be *gated* channels and their opening and closing can occur in response to voltage changes (voltage gated channels) or through the activation of receptors (receptor gated channels).

The variation of membrane conductance due to the opening and closing of ion channels generates changes in the transmembrane (action) potential over time. The time course of this potential as it depolarizes and repolarizes is illustrated for a ventricular cell in Figure 1.1, with the five conventional phases (0 through 4) marked. When cardiac cells are depolarized to a *threshold* voltage of about −70 mV (e.g., by another conducted action potential), there is a rapid depolarization (phase 0 — the rapid upstroke of the action potential) that is caused by a transient increase in fast sodium channel conductance. Phase 1 represents an initial repolarization that is caused by the opening of a potassium channel. During phase 2 there is an approximate balance between inward-going calcium current and outward-going potassium current, causing a plateau in the action potential and a delay in repolarization. This inward calcium movement is through long-lasting calcium channels that open up when the membrane potential depolarizes to about −40 mV. Repolarization (phase 3) is a complex process and several mechanisms are thought to be important. The potassium conductance increases, tending to repolarize the cell via a potassium-mediated outward current. In addition, there is a time-dependent

2.   Cardiac potentials may be recorded by means of microelectrodes.

decrease in calcium conductivity which also contributes to cellular repolarization. Phase 4, the resting condition, is characterized by open potassium channels and the negative transmembrane potential. After phase 0, there are a parallel set of cellular and molecular processes known as *excitation-contraction coupling*: the cell's depolarization leads to high intracellular calcium concentrations, which in turn unlocks the energy-dependent contraction apparatus of the cell (through a conformational change of the troponin protein complex).

Before the action potential is propagated, it must be initiated by *pacemakers*, cardiac cells that possess the property of *automaticity*. That is, they have the ability to spontaneously depolarize, and so function as pacemaker cells for the rest of the heart. Such cells are found in the sino-atrial node (*SA node*), in the atrio-ventricular node (*AV node*) and in certain specialized conduction systems within the atria and ventricles.[3] In automatic cells, the resting (phase 4) potential is not stable, but shows spontaneous depolarization: its transmembrane potential slowly increases toward zero due to a trickle of sodium and calcium ions entering through the pacemaker cell's specialized ion channels. When the cell's potential reaches a threshold level, the cell develops an action potential, similar to the phase 0 described above, but mediated by calcium exchange at a much slower rate. Following the action potential, the membrane potential returns to the resting level and the cycle repeats. There are graded levels of automaticity in the heart. The intrinsic rate of the SA node is highest (about 60 to 100 beats per minute), followed by the AV node (about 40 to 50 beats per minute), then the ventricular muscle (about 20 to 40 beats per minute). Under normal operating conditions, the SA node determines heart rate, the lower pacemakers being reset during each cardiac cycle. However, in some pathologic circumstances, the rate of lower pacemakers can exceed that of the SA node, and then the lower pacemakers determine overall heart rate.[4]

An action potential, once initiated in a cardiac cell, will propagate along the cell membrane until the entire cell is depolarized. Myocardial cells have the unique property of transmitting action potentials from one cell to adjacent cells by means of direct current spread (without electrochemical synapses). In fact, until about 1954 there was almost general agreement that the myocardium was an actual syncytium without separate cell boundaries. But the electron microscope identified definite cell membranes, showing that adjacent cells separate. They are tightly coupled, however, to transmit both tension and electric current from cell to cell. The low-resistance connections are known as gap junctions. Ionic currents flow from cell to cell via these intercellular connections, and the heart behaves electrically as a functional syncytium. Thus, an impulse originating anywhere in the myocardium will propagate throughout the heart, resulting in a coordinated mechanical contraction. An artificial cardiac pacemaker, for example, introduces depolarizing electrical impulses via an electrode catheter usually placed within the right ventricle. Pacemaker-induced action potentials excite the entire ventricular myocardium resulting in effective mechanical contractions.

3.   This is true for normal operating conditions. In pathological conditions, any myocardial cell may act as a pacemaker.

4.   Pacemakers other than the SA node may also take over the regulation of the heart rate when faster pacemakers are not effective, such as during episodes of *AV block*; see Section 1.3.3.

However, key structures intended to modify propagation of the action potential are interspersed throughout the heart. First, there are bands of specialized conducting fibers across which the action potential travels more rapidly compared to the conduction through the myocardium. It is by traveling across a combination of conducting fibers and myocardium that the action potential can propagate to all regions of the ventricles in less than 100 milliseconds. In subjects with conduction system disease, the propagation time is prolonged because the action potential only spreads through the myocardium itself. This unsynchronized squeezing motion of various parts of the heart can cause a mild impairment of pumping efficacy. In addition to specialized conducting fibers, there are tissues that electrically insulate the ventricles from the atria. In a normal heart, the only way the action potential passes from the atria to the ventricles is through another specialized structure called the AV node, whose function is to provide a delay in conduction, so that the atria can contract completely before the ventricles begin contracting. The function and structure of the normal heart are discussed in more detail below.

It should be noted that, through decades of investigation, much detail is available about the electrophysiologic activity of the heart and the preceding text is therefore only a highly abbreviated summary. Interested readers are referred to more detailed texts such as [2, 3].

1.2   The Physical Basis of Electrocardiography

As a result of the electrical activity of the cells, current flows within the body and potential differences are established on the surface of the skin, which can be measured using suitable equipment (see Chapter 2). The graphical recording of these body surface potentials as a function of time produces the electrocardiogram. The simplest mathematical model for relating the cardiac generator to the body surface potentials is the single *dipole model*. This simple model is extremely useful in providing a framework for the study of clinical electrocardiography and vectorcardiography, though of course much more complex treatments have been developed.[5] The descriptions in this chapter are therefore simplifications to aid the understanding of the surface potential signal that manifests as an ECG.

The dipole model has two components, a representation of the electrical activity of the heart (the dipole itself), and the geometry and electrical properties of the surrounding body. First, consider the representation of the electrical activity of the heart: as an action potential propagates through a cell (i.e., in the myocardium), there is an associated *intra*cellular current generated in the direction of propagation, at the interface of resting and depolarizing tissue. This is the elementary electrical source of the surface ECG, referred to as the current dipole. There is also an equal *extra*cellular current flowing against the direction of propagation, and so charge is conserved. All current loops in the conductive media close upon themselves, forming a dipole field (see Figure 1.2). The heart's total electrical activity at any instant of

---

5.   Models include multiple dipole models, cable models and statistical models. Further information can also be found in [3–5] and Chapter 4.

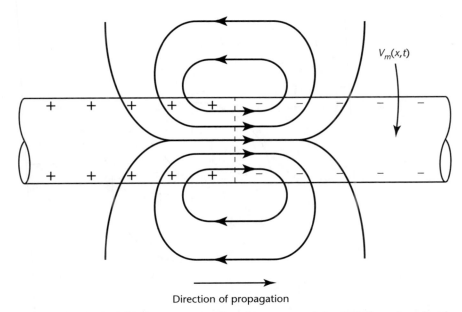

$V_m(x,t)$

Direction of propagation

Figure 1.2   The dipole field due to current flow in a myocardial cell at the advancing front of depolarization. V_m is the transmembrane potential. (*From*: [2]. © 2004 MIT OCW. Reprinted with permission.)

time may be represented by a distribution of active current dipoles. In general, they will lie on an irregular surface corresponding to the boundary between depolarized and polarized tissue.

If the heart were suspended in a homogeneous isotropic conducting medium and were observed from a distance sufficiently large compared to its size, then all of these individual current dipoles may be assumed to originate at a single point in space and the total electrical activity of the heat may be represented as a *single* equivalent dipole whose magnitude and direction is the vector summation of all the minute dipoles. The net equivalent dipole moment is commonly referred to as the (time-dependent) *heart vector* $\mathbf{M}(t)$. As each wave of depolarization spreads through the heart, the heart vector changes in magnitude and direction as a function of time.

The resulting surface distribution of currents and potentials depends on the electrical properties of the torso. As a reasonable approximation, the dipole model ignores the known anisotropy and inhomogeneity of the torso and treats the body as a linear, isotropic, homogeneous, spherical conductor of radius, R, and conductivity, σ. The source is represented as a slowly time-varying single current dipole located at the center of the sphere. The static electric field, current density, and electric potential everywhere within the torso (and on its surface) are nondynamically related to the heart vector at any given time (i.e., the model is quasi-static). The reactive terms due to the tissue impedance can be neglected. Laplace's equation (which holds within the idealized homogenous isotropic conducting spherical torso) may then be solved to give the potential distribution on the torso as

$$\Phi(t) = cos\theta(t)3|\mathbf{M}(t)|/4\pi\sigma R^2 \tag{1.1}$$

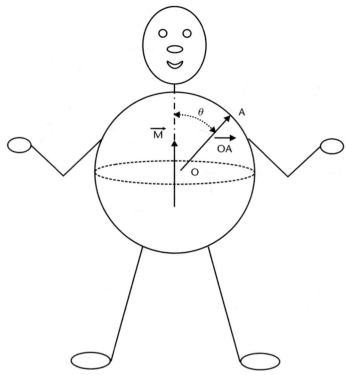

Figure 1.3 The idealized spherical torso with the centrally located cardiac source. (*From*: [2]. © 2004 MIT OCW. Reprinted with permission.)

where $\theta(t)$ is the angle between the direction of the heart vector $\mathbf{M}(t)$, and $\mathbf{OA}$ the lead vector joining the center of the sphere, O, to the point of observation, A (see Figure 1.3). $|\mathbf{M}|$ is therefore the magnitude of the heart vector. More generally, the potential difference between the two points on the surface of the torso would be

$$\mathbf{V}_{AB}(t) = \mathbf{M}(t) \cdot \mathbf{L}_{AB}(t) \tag{1.2}$$

where $\mathbf{L}_{AB}$ is known as the lead vector connecting points A and B on the torso. It is useful to define a reference central terminal (*CT*) by averaging the potentials from the three limb leads (see Section 1.2.1):

$$\Phi_{CT}(t) = \Phi_{RA}(t) + \Phi_{LA}(t) + \Phi_{LL}(t) \tag{1.3}$$

where RA indicates right arm, LA indicates left arm, and LL indicates left leg. Note that Φ_{CT} should be zero at all times. The next section describes the clinical derivation of the normal ECG.

1.2.1 The Normal Electrocardiogram

The performance of the heart as a pump is dependent primarily upon the contraction and relaxation properties of the myocardium. Other factors that must also be considered include: the geometric organization of the myocardial cells, the properties of

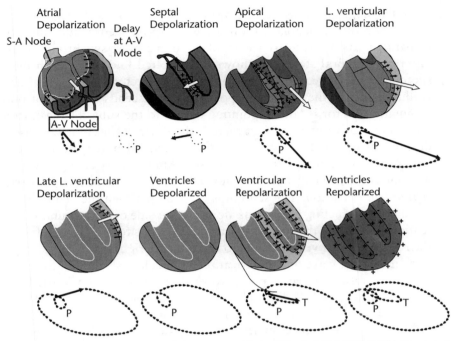

Figure 1.4 Trajectory of a normal cardiac vector. (*From*: [2]. © 2004 MIT OCW. Reprinted with permission.)

the cardiac tissue, the heart's electrical rhythm, valvular function, and the adequacy of delivery of oxygenated blood via the coronary arteries to meet the metabolic demands of the myocardium. The heart has four cavitary chambers whose walls consist of a mechanical syncytium of myocardial cells. At the exit of each chamber is a valve that closes after its contraction, preventing significant retrograde flow when the chamber relaxes and downstream pressures exceed chamber pressures. The *right heart* includes a small atrium leading into a larger right ventricle.[6] The right atrium receives blood from most of the body and feeds it into the right ventricle. When the right ventricle contracts, it propels blood to the lungs, where the blood is oxygenated and relieved of carbon dioxide.[7] The left atrium receives blood from the lungs and conducts it into the left ventricle.[8] The forceful contractions of the left ventricle propel the blood through the aorta to the rest of the body, with sufficient pressure to perfuse the brains of even the tallest humans.[9] The left atrium and left ventricle form the *left heart*. As noted earlier, under normal conditions the atria finish contracting before the ventricles begin contracting.

Figure 1.4 illustrates the normal heart's geometry and resultant instantaneous electrical heart vectors throughout the cardiac cycle. The figure shows the origination of the heart beat (at the SA node), a delay at the AV node (so that the

---

6. With a valve known as the *tricuspid* valve.
7. Its valve is the *pulmonic* valve.
8. Its valve is the *mitral* valve.
9. Its valve is the *aortic* valve.

atria, teleologically, finish contraction before the ventricles begin), and accelerated conduction of the depolarization wave via specialized conducting fibers (so that disparate parts of the heart are depolarized in a more synchronized fashion). Nine different temporal states are shown. The dotted line below each illustrated state summarizes the preceding trajectory of heart vectors. First, *atrial depolarization* is illustrated. As the wave of depolarization descends throughout both atria, the summation vector is largely pointing down (to the subject's toes), to the subject's left, and slightly anterior. Next there is the *delay at the AV node*, discussed above, during which time there is no measurable electrical activity at the body surface unless special averaging techniques are used. After activity emerges from the AV node it depolarizes the His[10] bundle, followed by the bundle branches. Next, there is the *septal depolarization*. The septum is the wall between the ventricles, and a major bundle of conducting fibers runs along the left side of the septum. As the action potential wave enters the septal myocardium it tends to propagate left to right, and so the resultant heart vector points to the subject's right. Next there is apical depolarization, and the wave of depolarization moving left is balanced by the wave moving right. The resultant vector points towards the apex of the heart, which is largely pointing down, to the subject's left, and slightly anterior. In *left ventricular depolarization* and *late left ventricular depolarization*, there is also electrical activity in the right ventricle, but since the left ventricle is much more massive its activity dominates. After the various portions of myocardium depolarize, they contract via the process of excitation-contraction coupling described above (not illustrated). There is a plateau period during which the myocardium has depolarized (*ventricles depolarized*) where no action potential propagates, and hence there is no measurable cardiac vector. Finally, the individual cells begin to repolarize and another wave of charge passes through the heart, this time originating from the dipoles generated at the interface of *depolarized* and *repolarizing* tissue (i.e., *ventricular repolarization*). The heart then returns to its resting state (such that the ventricles are repolarized), awaiting another electrical stimulus that starts the cycle anew. Note that both the polarity and the direction of propagation of the repolarizing phase are reversed from those of depolarization. As a result, repolarization waves on the ECG are generally of the same polarity as depolarization waves.

To complete the review of the basis of the surface ECG, a description of how the trajectory of the cardiac vector (detailed in Figure 1.4) results in the pattern of a normal scalar ECG is now described. The cardiac vector, which expands, contracts, and rotates in three-dimensional space, is projected onto 12 different lines of well-defined orientation (for instance, lead I is oriented directly to the patient's left). Each lead reveals the magnitude of the cardiac vector in the direction of that lead at each instant of time. The six precordial leads report activity in the *horizontal* plane. In practice, this requires that six electrodes are placed around the torso (Figure 1.5), and the ECG represents the difference *between* each of these electrodes (V1–6) and the *central terminal* [as in (1.3)].

---

10. The His bundle is a collection of heart muscle cells specialized for electrical conduction that transmits electrical impulses from the AV node, between the atria and the ventricles to the Purkinje fibers, which innervate the ventricles.

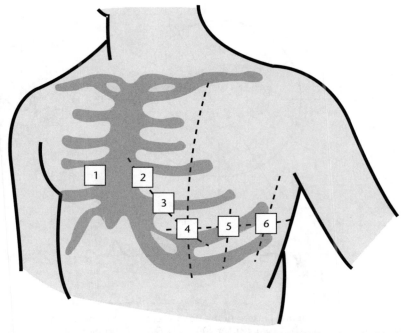

Figure 1.5 The six standard chest leads. (*From*: [2]. © 2004 MIT OCW. Reprinted with permission.)

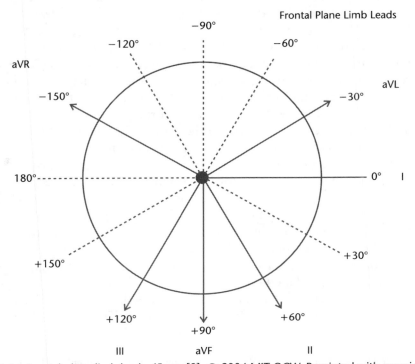

Figure 1.6 Frontal plane limb leads. (*From*: [2]. © 2004 MIT OCW. Reprinted with permission.)

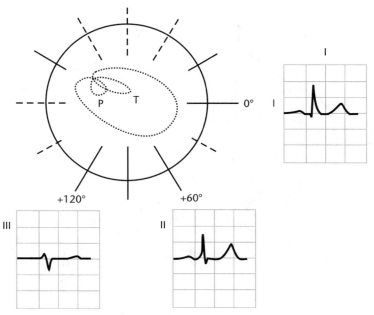

Figure 1.7 The temporal pattern of the heart vector combined with the geometry of the standard frontal plane limb leads. (*From*: [2]. © 2004 MIT OCW. Reprinted with permission.)

Additional electrodes, the *limb leads*, are placed on each of the subject's four extremities and the central terminal is the average of the potentials from the limb leads. Potential differences *between* the limb electrodes and the central terminal are the bases for the other three standard ECG leads, as illustrated (Figure 1.6): (1) Lead I, the difference between left arm (LA) and right arm (RA); (2) Lead II, the difference between the left leg (LL) and the RA; (3) Lead III, the difference between the LL and the LA. Note also that the augmented limb leads (denoted by "a") represent the potential at a given limb with respect to the average of the potentials of the other two limbs.[11] aVF is the difference between the LL and average of the arm leads; aVR is the difference between the RA and the average of LL and LA, and aVL is the difference between the LA and the average of the RA and LL. Since there are 12 leads to image three-dimensional activity, there exists considerable information redundancy in this configuration. However, this spatial "oversampling" by projecting the cardiac vector into nonorthogonal axes, tends to yield an easier representation for human interpretation and compensates for minor inconsistencies in electrode placement (after all, human forms lack geometric consistency, thus electrode placement varies with subject and with technician). Furthermore, the body is not a homogenous sphere.

The temporal pattern of the heart vector is combined with the geometry of the standard frontal plane limb leads in Figure 1.7. In black, the temporal trajectory of the heart vector, from Figure 1.4, is recreated. The frontal ECG leads are superimposed in their conventional orientation (from Figure 1.6). The resultant pattern

11. That is, the central terminal with the limb lead disconnected that corresponds to the augmented lead you are measuring. The vector is therefore longer and the signal amplitude consequently higher, hence, *augmented*.

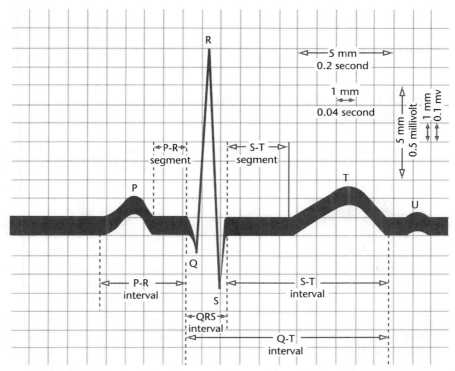

Figure 1.8   Normal features of the electrocardiogram. (*From*: [2]. © 2004 MIT OCW. Reprinted with permission.)

for three surface ECG leads, I, II, and III, are shown. Note that the QRS axis is perpendicular to the isoelectric lead (the lead with equal forces in the positive and negative direction). Significant changes in the QRS axis can be indicative of cardiac problems.

Figure 1.8 illustrates the normal clinical features of the electrocardiogram, which include wave amplitudes and interwave timings. The locations of different waves on the ECG are arbitrarily marked by the letters P, Q, R, S, and T[12] (and sometimes U, although this wave is often hard to identify, as it may be absent, have a low amplitude, or be masked by a subsequent beat). The interbeat timing (RR interval) is not marked. Note that the illustration uses the typical graph-paper presentation format, which stems from the early clinical years of electrocardiography, where analysis was done by hand measurements of hard copies. Each box is 1 mm² and the ECG paper is usually set to move at 25 mm/s. Therefore, each box represents 0.04 second in time. The amplitude scale is set to be 0.1 mV per square, although there is often a larger grid overlaid at every five squares (0.20 second/

---

12. Einthoven, who received the Nobel Prize in 1924 for his development of the first ECG, named the prominent ECG waves alphabetically, P, Q, R, S, and T. The prominent deflections were first labeled A, B, C, and D, in his preceding work with a capillary electrometer, which did not record negative deflections. The new nomenclature was to distinguish the superior signal produced by a string galvanometer. For more information, see [6].

0.5 mV).[13] The values for the clinical features indicated on the graph in Figure 1.8 are typical, although they can vary based upon gender, age, activity, and health (see Chapter 3 and [7]).

1.3 Introduction to Clinical Electrocardiography: Abnormal Patterns

The clinician who uses the electrocardiogram as a diagnostic test wishes to determine cardiac abnormalities from the body surface potentials. As a rough framework, it is worth thinking of the heart as three separate systems: a functional electrical system, a functional system of *coronary* (or cardiac) arteries to channel nourishing blood to every cell of the myocardium, and a culmination in an effective mechanical pump.

First we consider how an ECG is used to assess electrical abnormalities of the heart. The surface ECG has inherent limitations as a diagnostic tool: Given a distribution of body surface potentials, we cannot precisely specify the detailed electrophysiologic behavior of the source since this *inverse* problem does not have a unique solution (as demonstrated in 1853 by Hermann von Helmholz). It is not, in general, possible to uniquely specify the characteristics of a current generator from the external potential measurements alone. Therefore, an exacting assessment of the electrical activity of the heart involves an invasive electrode study. Despite these inherent limitations, the surface ECG is extremely useful in clinical assessments of electrical pathologies and an invasive electrophysiologic study is indicated in only a small fraction of cases.

To a first approximation, electrical problems come in two forms: those which make the heart pump too slowly or infrequently (bradycardias), and those with make the heart pump too quickly (tachycardias). If the pumping is too slow, the cardiac output of life-sustaining blood can be dangerously low. If too quick, the cardiac output can also be too low since the heart does not have time to fill, and also because the heart can suffer damage (e.g., *demand ischemia*) when it tries to pump too rapidly.

1.3.1 The Normal Determinants of Heart Rate: The Autonomic Nervous System

One class of heart rate abnormalities arises from abnormal function of the control system for heart rate. As discussed in Section 1.2.2, there are specialized cells in the SA node whose function is to act as the heart's pacemaker, rhythmically generating action potentials and triggering depolarization for the rest of the heart (recall that once any portion of the heart depolarizes, the wavefront tends to propagate throughout the entire myocardium). The SA node has an intrinsic rate of firing, but ordinarily this is modified by the *central nervous system*, specifically, the *autonomic nervous system* (ANS).[14] The decision-making for autonomic functions occurs in

---

13. In this chapter, this larger amplitude scale was used for Figures 1.9 through 1.23 and Figure 1.26.
14. The part of the nervous system that functions without conscious thought, taking care of such tasks as breathing while you sleep, thermoregulation, and optimizing heart rate.

the medulla in the brain stem and the hypothalamus. Instructions from these centers are communicated via nerves that connect the brain to the heart. There are two main sets of nerves serving the *sympathetic* and the *parasympathetic* portions of the autonomic nervous system, which both *innervate* the heart. The sympathetic nervous system is activated during stressful times. It increases the rate of SA node firing (hence raising heart rate) and also innervates the myocardium itself, increasing the propagation speed of the depolarization wavefront, mainly through the AV node, and increasing the strength of mechanical contractions. These effects are all consequences of changes to ion channels and gates that occur when the cells are exposed to the messenger chemical from the nerves. The time necessary for the sympathetic nervous system to actuate these effects is on the order of 15 seconds.

The sympathetic system works in tandem with the parasympathetic system. For the body as a whole, the parasympathetic system controls quiet-time functions like food digestion. The nerve through which the parasympathetic system communicates with the heart is named the *vagus*.[15] The parasympathetic branch's major effect is on heart rate and the velocity of propagation of the action potential through the AV node.[16] Furthermore, in contrast with the sympathetic system, the parasympathetic nerves act quickly, decreasing the velocity through the AV node and slowing the heart rate within a second when they activate. Most organs are innervated by both the sympathetic and the parasympathetic branches of the ANS and the balance between these competing effects determines function.

The sympathetic and parasympathetic systems are rarely totally off or on; instead, the body adjusts their levels of activation, known as *tone*, as is appropriate to its needs. If a medication that inactivates the sympathetic system (e.g., propranolol) is used on a healthy resting subject with a heart rate of 60 bpm, the classic response is to slow the heart rate to about 50 bpm. If a medication that inactivates the parasympathetic system (e.g., atropine) is used, the classic response is an elevation of the heart rate to about 120 bpm. If you administer both medications and inactivate both systems (parasympathetic and sympathetic withdrawal), the heart rate rises to 100 bpm. Therefore, in this instance for normal subjects at rest, the effects of the heart rate's "brake" are greater than the effects of the "accelerator," although it is the balance of both systems that dictates the heart rate. The body's normal reaction when vagal tone is increased (the brake) is to simultaneously reduce sympathetic tone (the accelerator). Similarly, when sympathetic tone is increased, parasympathetic tone is usually withdrawn. Indeed, if a person is suddenly startled, the earliest increase in heart rate will simply be due to parasympathetic withdrawal rather than the slower-acting sympathetic activation.

On what basis does the autonomic system make heart rate adjustments? There are a series of sensors throughout the body sending information back to the brain (*afferent nerves*, bringing information to the central nervous system). Those parameters sensed by afferent nerves include the blood pressure in the arteries (baroreceptors), the acid-base conditions in the blood (chemoreceptors), and the pressure within the heart's walls (mechanoreceptors). Based on this feedback, the brain unconsciously adjusts heart rate. The system is predicated on the fact that,

---

15. Parasympathetic activity is therefore sometimes termed *vagal* activity.
16. It has little effect on cardiac contractility.

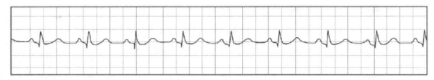

Figure 1.9   Normal sinus rhythm. (*From*: [2]. © 2004 MIT OCW. Reprinted with permission.)

as heart rate increases, cardiac pumping and blood output should increase, and so increase arterial blood pressure, blood flow and oxygen delivery to the peripheral tissues, carbon dioxide clearance from the peripheral tissues, and so on.

When the heart rate is controlled by the SA node's rate of firing, the sequence of beats is known as a *sinus rhythm* (see Figure 1.9). When the SA node fires more quickly than usual (for instance, as a normal physiologic response to fear, or an abnormal response due to a cocaine intoxication), the rhythm is termed *sinus tachycardia* (see Figure 1.10). When the SA node fires more slowly than usual (for instance, either as a normal physiologic response in a very well-conditioned athlete, or an abnormal response in an older patient taking too much heart-slowing medication), the rhythm is known as *sinus bradycardia* (see Figure 1.11). There may be cyclic variations in heart rate due to breathing, known as *sinus arrhythmia* (see Figure 1.12). This nonpathologic pattern is caused by activity of the parasympathetic system (the sympathetic system responds too slowly to alter heart rate on this time scale), which is responding to subtle changes in arterial blood pressure, cardiac filling pressure, and the lungs themselves, during the respiratory cycle.

Sinus Tachycardia—Rate 122

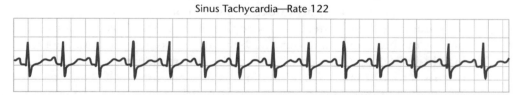

Figure 1.10   Sinus tachycardia. (*From*: [2]. © 2004 MIT OCW. Reprinted with permission.)

Sinus Bradycardia—Rate 48

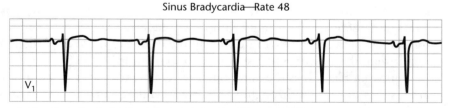

Figure 1.11   Sinus bradycardia. (*From*: [2]. © 2004 MIT OCW. Reprinted with permission.)

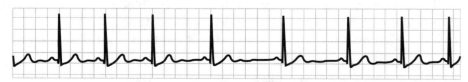

Figure 1.12   Sinus arrhythmia. (*From*: [2]. © 2004 MIT OCW. Reprinted with permission.)

1.3.2   Ectopy, Tachycardia, and Fibrillation

An *arrhythmia* is any abnormal cardiac rhythm. One category of arrhythmias occurs when the trigger to depolarize originates outside of the SA node, in another part of the myocardium (known as *ectopic depolarization*, leading to *ectopic beats*). Common causes of ectopy include a drug effect (e.g., caffeine) or a viral infection of the myocardium, or other inflammation or damage of part of the heart (e.g., ischemia). When the ectopic beat originates in the atria, it leads to a *premature atrial beat*, also known as an *atrial premature contraction* (APC) (see Figure 1.13). When it originates in the ventricles, it leads to a *premature ventricular beat* or *ventricular premature contraction* (VPC); see Figure 1.14.

Note in Figure 1.14 that the ectopic ventricular beat looks very different from the other sinus beats. The spread of the wavefront for a VPC can be backwards, such as when the action potential starts at the apex of the heart rather than the septum. The depolarization wavefront can move in very different directions than the typical sinus-driven heart vector. Compare Figure 1.15 with the wavefront trajectory in

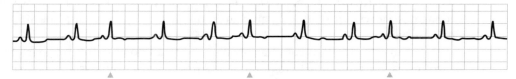

Figure 1.13   Atrial premature contractions (indicated by arrowheads). (*From*: [2]. © 2004 MIT OCW. Reprinted with permission.)

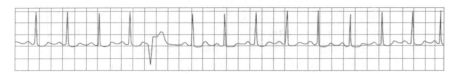

Figure 1.14   Ventricular premature contractions. (*From*: [2]. © 2004 MIT OCW. Reprinted with permission.)

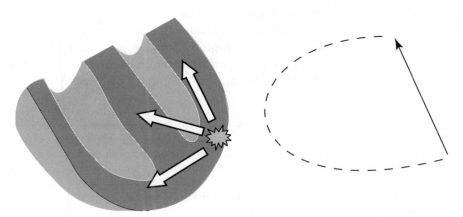

Figure 1.15   Wavefront trajectory in a ventricular premature contraction. (*From*: [2]. © 2004 MIT OCW. Reprinted with permission.)

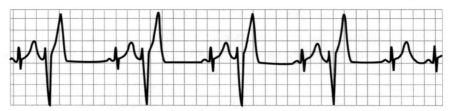

Figure 1.16   Ventricular bigeminy. (*From*: [2]. © 2004 MIT OCW. Reprinted with permission.)

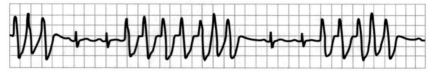

Figure 1.17   Three episodes of nonsustained ventricular tachycardia. There are two normal sinus beats in between each episode of VT. (*From*: [2]. © 2004 MIT OCW. Reprinted with permission.)

Figure 1.4. Furthermore, the ectopic beat is typically wider because its wavefront propagates slowly through the myocardium rather than through the high-speed Purkinji system.

After an ectopic wavefront has propagated to all portions of the heart, the myocardium is left temporarily depolarized. After a pause, the tissue repolarizes and the regular sinus mechanism can instigate a subsequent beat. The conditions that caused the ectopic beat might persist (e.g., still too much caffeine leading to an excitable myocardium), but the ectopic beat itself is left behind in the past. Sometimes, a semistable pattern of sinus beats and ectopic beats develops. For instance, a repeating pattern of "sinus beat – VPC – sinus beat – VPC – and so forth." can occur, termed *ventricular bigeminy* (see Figure 1.16). There can be so many ectopic beats ongoing that the overall heart rate is driven much higher than normal.[17]

The potential for serious problems is higher for those less common conditions in which a wavefront continues to propagate in a quasi-stable state, circulating repeatedly through the heart leading to repeated waves of tissue depolarization at an abnormally high rate.[18] When this cyclic, quasi-stable phenomenon occurs in the heart, it is called a *reentrant* arrhythmia. A classic example often caused by a reentrant pattern is *ventricular tachycardia* (VT) (see Figure 1.17). These states are extremely pathologic and can be rapidly fatal, because the rate of depolarization can be incompatible with effective cardiac pumping. At one extreme (rapid VT in an older frail heart) VT can be fatal in seconds to minutes. At the other extreme

17. For instance, *multifocal atrial tachycardia* (MAT) is an arrhythmia in which two or more ectopic atrial sites generate ectopic beats leading to heart rates greater than 100 bpm. The classic MAT finding on ECG is three or more P wave morphologies, due to the normal sinus beats plus two or more atrial ectopic foci.
18. To understand this, it is useful to describe the process in terms of "excitable media" models [4, 5]. Consider the analogy of the wavefront acting like a wildfire propagating through a landscape. If the vegetation grew back quickly (in a matter of minutes), one could envision a state in which the fire rotated through the forest in a large circle in a sustained fashion, and continued to "burn" vegetation just as it grew back. It might also be intuitive that this state would be more stable if there was a large fire barrier at the center of this rotation.

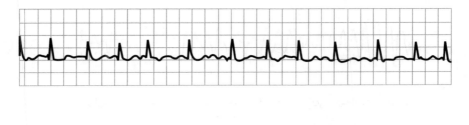

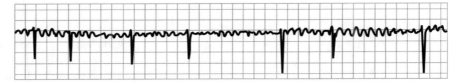

Figure 1.18   Atrial fibrillation—two examples. (*From*: [2]. © 2004 MIT OCW. Reprinted with permission.)

(slow VT in a younger healthy heart) the cardiac output[19] can remain at a life-sustaining level. The ECG criteria for VT are three or more consecutive ectopic ventricular beats at a rate over 100 bpm. If the VT terminates within 15 seconds (or 30 seconds, by some conventions) it is known as *nonsustained VT*; otherwise it is *sustained VT*. Because of the grave medical consequences of VT and related reentrant arrhythmias, they have been well investigated experimentally, clinically, and theoretically.

In some cases, the unified wavefront of depolarization can break down into countless smaller wavefronts which circulate quasi-randomly over the myocardium. This leads to a total breakdown of coordinated contraction, and the myocardium will appear to quiver. This is termed *fibrillation*. In *atrial fibrillation* (see Figure 1.18) the AV node will still act as a gatekeeper for these disorganized atrial wavefronts, maintaining organized ventricular depolarization distal to the AV node with normal QRS complexes. The ventricular rhythm is generally quite irregular and the rate will often be elevated. Often atrial fibrillation is well tolerated, provided the consequent ventricular rate is not excessive. AF can lead to a minor impairment in cardiac output due to reduced ventricular filling. In the long term, there can be regions in a fibrillating atrium where, because of the absence of contractions, the blood sits in stasis, and this can lead to blood clot formation within the heart. These clots can reenter the circulation and cause acute arterial blockages (e.g., cerebrovascular strokes) and therefore patients with atrial fibrillation are often anticoagulated. In contrast to atrial fibrillation, untreated *ventricular fibrillation* (see Figure 1.19) is fatal in seconds to minutes: The appearance of fibrillating ventricles has been likened to a "bag of worms" and this causes *circulatory arrest*, the termination of blood flow through the cardiovascular circuit.

---

19. The volume of blood pumped by the heart per minute, calculated as the product of the stroke volume (SV) and the heart rate. The SV is the amount of blood pushed into the aorta with each heart beat. Stroke volume = end-diastolic volume (EDV) minus end-systolic volume (ESV).

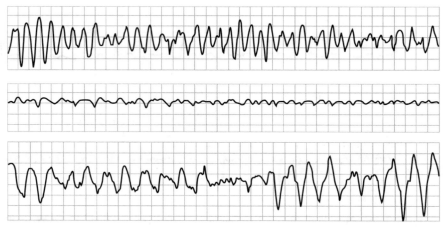

Figure 1.19 Ventricular fibrillation—three examples. (*From*: [2]. © 2004 MIT OCW. Reprinted with permission.)

1.3.3 Conduction Blocks, Bradycardia, and Escape Rhythms

The other category of arrhythmias is related to excessively slow rhythms, and ab-normal blockages of wavefront propagation. For instance, an aging SA node may pace the heart too slowly, leading to low blood pressure and weakness or fainting. Assuming this is not a result of excessive medication, these symptoms might require that an artificial pacemaker be implanted. The AV node may also develop conduc-tion pathologies which slow the ventricular heart rate: It may fail to conduct *some* atrial wavefronts (termed *second-degree AV block*; see Figure 1.20), or it may fail to conduct *all* atrial wavefronts (termed *third-degree AV block*; see Figure 1.21). Assuming this is not a result of excessive medication, most third-degree AV block, and some second-degree AV block, require pacemaker therapy. In first-degree AV block, the AV node conducts atrial wavefronts with an abnormal delay, but because the atrial wavefronts are eventually propagated to the ventricles, first-degree AV block does not slow the overall ventricular rate.

Sections of the specialized conducting fibers in the ventricles can also fail, such that depolarization waves must reach some portions of the ventricles via slower

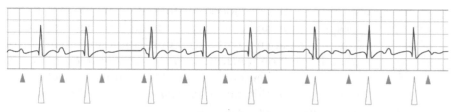

Figure 1.20 Second-degree AV block. In this subtype of second-degree AV block, termed *Wencke-bach*, also termed *Mobitz Type I*, there is a characteristic lengthening of the delay between the atrial P wave and the ventricular QRS, and ultimately there is a failure to conduct a P wave. Then this cycle repeats. In the example illustrated, there are three P waves (indicated by small gray arrowheads) followed by ventricular beats (indicated by large white arrowheads), and then the AV node fails to conduct the fourth P wave in each cycle (small gray arrowheads without a subsequent large white arrowheads). (*From*: [2]. © 2004 MIT OCW. Reprinted with permission.)

Complete A-V Block with Junctional Escape Rhythm

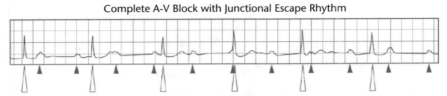

Figure 1.21 Third-degree AV block. There is a failure of the AV node to conduct any wavefronts from the atria to the ventricles. The ventricular beats are escape beats, originating electrically from the specialized conducting fibers just below the AV node. The ability to generate escape beats is the heart's fail-safe mechanism for what would otherwise cause fatal cardiac (e.g., ventricular) arrest. Notice there is no relationship between the atrial P waves (indicated by small gray arrowheads) and the junctional escape beats (indicated by large white arrowheads). Also see Figure 1.23 for an example of a ventricular escape beat. (*From*: [2]. © 2004 MIT OCW. Reprinted with permission.)

muscle-to-muscle propagation. There are a classic set of changes associated with failures of different conduction bundles (e.g., *right bundle branch block* and *left bundle branch block*; see Figure 1.22). These blocks usually have a minimal effect on pumping efficacy. However, they can dramatically change the cardiac vector's trajectory and hence the surface ECG. They can mask other ECG changes indicative of disease (e.g., ischemia). In some cases, these conduction abnormalities indicate some other underlying pathology of great importance (for instance, a pulmonary embolism can cause a new right bundle branch block, and acute anterior ischemia can cause a new left bundle branch block).

The topic of bradyarrhythmias and heart blocks leads to the topic of *escape beats* (see Figures 1.21 and 1.23). An escape beat is similar to an ectopic beat, in that it is the initiation of a depolarization wavefront outside of the SA node. However, the difference is that the escape beat is a normal, compensatory response, a normal fail-safe functionality of the heart: There is a network of cardiac cells able to initiate

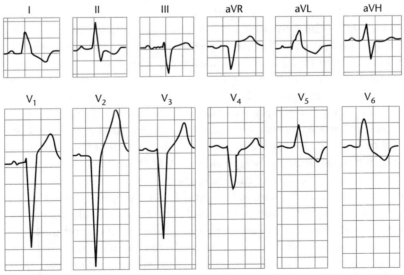

Figure 1.22 Classic ECG pattern of left bundle branch block. (*From*: [2]. © 2004 MIT OCW. Reprinted with permission.)

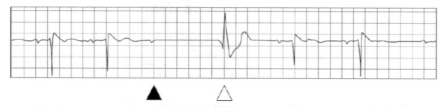

Figure 1.23 Ventricular escape beat. Note the atrial P wave (black arrowhead) followed by an evident pause, indicating a failure to conduct through the AV node. The ventricular escape beat (white arrowhead) is a fail-safe mechanism so that conduction blocks do not cause ventricular cardiac arrest. Also see Figure 1.21. (*From*: [2]. © 2004 MIT OCW. Reprinted with permission.)

heart beats, so that a key life-sustaining function (e.g., pacing the heart) is not exclusively relegated to a microscopic collection cells in the SA node. The cells in the backup system have intrinsic rates of firing that are slower than the SA node. So while the SA node is given the opportunity to pace the heart, the other regions will initiate heart beats if there has been an excessively long pause in the SA node. Therefore, a ventricular beat which occurs in the setting of third-degree heart block is termed a ventricular escape beat, and it represents an appropriate healthy response to the lack of any other pacemaker trigger. When nonsinus beats appear on the ECG, it is important to differentiate ectopic beats (where the pathology is aberrant automaticity) from escape beats (where the pathology is abnormal conduction), because the treatments are quite different. Note that ectopic beats are generally premature, and escape beats terminate a prolonged RR interval.

1.3.4 Cardiac Ischemia, Other Metabolic Disturbances, and Structural Abnormalities

The ECG can reveal metabolic abnormalities of the myocardium. The most medically significant abnormality is *ischemia*, when part of the myocardium is not receiving enough blood flow, often caused by disease of the coronary arteries (ischemia will ultimately progress to myocardial cell death). Recording a 12-lead ECG is a standard-of-care diagnostic test in any evaluation of possible cardiac ischemia. Ischemia often changes the appearance of the T wave and the ST interval. This is because of a current of injury between the ischemic and nonischemic myocardium, which alters the main cardiac vector. There are classic patterns of ischemia, which are seen in only a minority of ischemic events (see Figure 1.24). In most ischemic events, there are "nonspecific" ECG changes, such as changes in the T wave that may or may not be caused by ischemia. In a small percentage of cases, there can be ischemia without any grossly evident ECG changes. Overall, the ECG is not highly sensitive nor specific for cardiac ischemia, but larger regions of cardiac ischemia are associated with more substantial ECG changes (as well as a higher mortality rate), so this information is very useful in decision-making. For example, a patient with classic changes of acute ischemia is often a good candidate for powerful thrombolytic (clot dissolving) medication. Whereas patients without those classic changes are not considered good candidates for these drugs because, on average, the risks of the therapy, including intracranial hemorrhage and internal bleeding, outweigh the benefits.

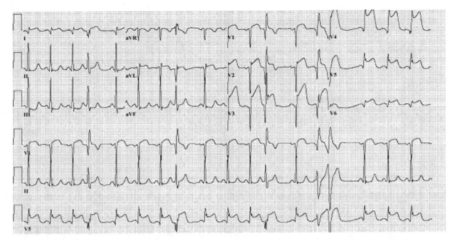

Figure 1.24 Acute myocardial infarction. Large areas of ischemic anterior myocardium often produce ST-segment elevation in multiple contiguous precordial ECG leads (or in *all* the precordial leads, in this dramatic example). Also note there is minor ST-segment depression in the inferior lead III, which in this context is referred to as a "reciprocal change." (*From*: [9]. © 2001–2006 Beth Israel Deaconess Medical Center. Reprinted with permission.)

Other metabolic abnormalities which cause characteristic changes in the ECG include electrolyte abnormalities. The classic indicators of high serum potassium levels (*hyperkalemia*) include a high, pointed T wave, and ultimately, loss of the P wave and distortion of the QRS (see Figure 1.25). *Hypokalemia* causes an undulation after the T wave called a U wave. Calcium and magnesium disturbances, and

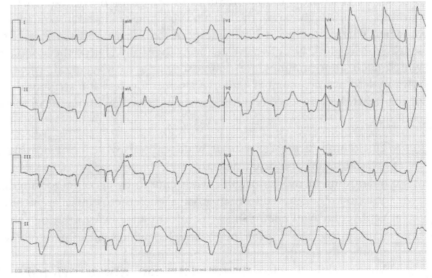

Figure 1.25 Hyperkalemia (moderate/severe). The K$^+$ was 10.5 mEq/L in a patient with renal failure. Note the loss of P waves and the widening of the QRS complex. There are numerous classic ECG morphologies associated with hyperkalemia. This example shows what Marriott [8] has termed a "dumping pattern" because "it looks as though a rotund body has been dumped in the hammock of the ST segment ... making the ST segment sag horizontally ... and verticalizing the proximal limb of the upright T wave." (*From*: [9]. © 2001–2006 Beth Israel Deaconess Medical Center. Reprinted with permission.)

R-on-T VPB Initiates Ventricular Flutter

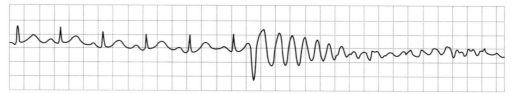

Figure 1.26 An R-on-T ventricular premature beat initiations polymorphic ventricular tachycardia. (*From*: [2]. © MIT OCW. Reprinted with permission.)

also extreme cold body temperature, are other causes of ST–T wave abnormalities. Therapeutic drugs can also alter the appearance of the ECG. One alteration of significance is a delay in the T wave relative to the QRS, so-called *QT prolongation*. A prolonged[20] QT indicates a myocardium at risk for *triggered activity*, in which a cardiac cell will rapidly and repeatedly depolarize, associated with a kind of dangerous ventricular tachycardia called *torsades des pointes*. In the so-called R-on-T phenomenon, the heart depolarizes in the midst of its repolarization and can trigger a life-threatening tachyarrhythmia (see Figure 1.26). R-on-T can occur because the QT interval is abnormally long. It also can occur because of a mechanical blow to the chest during repolarization (e.g., a young hockey player struck in the chest). And relevant to signal processors, it can occur if a patient receives electrical cardioversion in the middle of repolarization when the T wave occurs (hence these devices are imbued with a synchronization mode in which the QRS complex is automatically identified, and the device is prevented from discharging in the temporal vicinity of the following T wave).

The ECG can reveal abnormalities of the geometry of the heart. This refers to pathologies in which part of the heart has become enlarged (too much myocardium), or when part of the heart has undergone cell death and scarring (electrically absent myocardium). Noninvasive echocardiography is now the standard method by which such abnormalities are diagnosed, and so in general, the ECG has been relegated to a convenient if imperfect screening test for structural abnormalities of the heart. Examples of conditions which are often apparent in the surface ECG include:

- Thickening of the ventricular walls caused by years of beating against high arterial blood pressure (hypertrophy);
- Ballooning of the ventricular walls caused by accommodating large volumes of blood regurgitated from upstream when there is a leaky, incompetent valve;
- Ventricular wall aneurysms which form after heart attacks;
- Scars in the heart (after heart attacks) which cause part of the heart to be electrically silent;
- Abnormal fluid collecting around the heart (termed an *effusion*) which can impair the heart's ability to fill and hence pump effectively (*cardiac tamponade*).

---

20. It is important to allow for the shortening of the QT interval due to increases in heart rate, and so a *corrected* QT interval, QTc, is usually used. See Chapter 3 for more details.

These conditions change the trajectory and/or magnitude of the normal heart vector, which can distort the normal ECG morphology. A review of all these conditions and their resultant ECG appearance is beyond the scope of this chapter, and introductory or advanced textbooks focused solely on the clinical interpretation of the ECG are plentiful. However, in the following section a brief overview of how clinicians analyze the ECG is presented. This should not be taken as a definitive guide, but as a general strategy that may prove useful in designing an ECG analysis algorithm.

1.3.5 A Basic Approach to ECG Analysis

In analyzing the clinical electrocardiogram, it is important to use a systematic approach. The following overview, which illustrates a clinical approach, should not be considered completely thorough, but simply a guide to understanding how clinicians identify abnormalities in the ECG.

1. *Identify the QRS complexes.* The following observations should be made:
   - What is the ventricular rate?
   - Are the QRS complexes spaced at regular intervals? If not, what is the nature of the irregularity?
   - Are the QRS complexes identical in shape in a given lead? Are they of normal size and morphology?
2. *Identify the P waves.* In some cases this will require careful observation, and more than one lead axis may be necessary. The following questions should be explored:
   - Is there a one-to-one relationship between P-waves and QRS complexes? If not, is there a definable pattern?
   - Is the PR interval of normal duration?
   - What is the atrial rate?
   - Are the P waves identical in shape in a given lead? Are they of normal size and shape?

   Based on the above analysis, it should be possible to identify the mechanism of the rhythm in most cases. See Chapter 3 for more information.
3. *Examine the QRS complex in each lead.* Is the QRS axis normal? Overall, are the QRS widths and amplitudes normal? Often, the QRS complexes are viewed in several "groups" that are specific to a particular region of the heart.[21] The waveform patterns should also be checked for signs of intra-ventricular conduction block, significant amplitude Q waves and precordial R-wave pattern normality.
4. *Examine the ST-T segments.* Are there abnormalities (such as elevation or depression; see Chapter 10)? Is the abnormality suggestive of ischemia, infarction, or hypothermia?

---

21. The basic lead groups are: the *inferior* leads (II, III, and aVF), the *anterior* leads (V2, V3, and V4), the *lateral* precordial leads (V4, V5, and V6), and the *high lateral* leads (I and aVL).

5. *Examine the T waves.* Are their shapes normal? In each lead, are they oriented in the same direction as the QRS complex? If not, is it suggestive of ischemia or ventricular conduction abnormalities, or a potassium abnormality?

6. *Examine the QT interval.* Is it over half the RR interval? (See Chapters 3 and 11.)

Once an abnormality is identified, there are often several potential explanations, many of which lead to several ECG pathologies and it may not be possible to determine the significance of the abnormality with certainty. To confirm a potential diagnosis from the ECG, other characteristic abnormalities are often sought. For a given individual, comparing a new ECG with a prior ECG provides an invaluable reference, particularly if trying to ascertain when ECG abnormalities are acute or not. For instance, for a patient with chest pain, abnormal ST-T wave patterns are much more concerning for ischemia when they are new (e.g., not present in an ECG recorded 1 year earlier). If the ST-T wave patterns existed long before the new symptoms, one may deduce that these patterns are not directly related to the acute pathology.

1.4 Summary

This chapter has presented a brief summary of the etiology of the electrocardiogram, together with an overview of the mechanisms that lead to the manifestation of both normal and abnormal morphologies on the many different vectors that constitute the clinical ECG leads. After an overview of the variables to be considered in any ECG data collection exercise (Chapter 2), Chapters 3 and 4 provide a more mathematical analysis of the normal and abnormal waveforms that may be encountered, and some empirical models available for describing these waveforms (or their underlying processes). It is hoped that these introductory chapters will provide the reader with the relevant framework in which to apply numerical analysis techniques to the ECG.

References

[1]   Mark, R. G., "Biological Measurement: Electrical Characteristics of the Heart," in *Systems & Control Encyclopedia*, Singh, M. G., (ed.), Oxford, U.K.: Permagon Press, 1990, pp. 450–456.

[2]   Mark, R. G., *HST.542J/2.792J/BE.371J/6.022J Quantitative Physiology: Organ Transport Systems*, Lecture notes from HST/MIT Open Courseware 2004, available at http://ocw.mit.edu/OcwWeb/Health-Sciences-and-Technology/HST-542JSpring-2004/Course Home/.

[3]   Malmivuo, J., and R. Plonsey, *Bioelectromagnetism: Principles and Applications of Bioelectric and Biomagnetic Fields*, Oxford, U.K.: Oxford University Press, 1995, available at http://butler.cc.tut.fi/~malmivuo/bem/bembook/.

[4]   Barkley, D., M. Kress, and S. Tucherman, "Spiral-Wave Dynamics in a Simple Model of Excitable Media: Transition from Simple to Compound Rotation," *Phys. Rev. A.*, Vol. 42, 1990, pp. 2489–2491.

[5]   Ito, H., and L. Glass, "Spiral Breakup in a New Model of Discrete Excitable Media," *Phys. Rev. Lett.*, Vol. 66, No. 5, 1991, pp. 671–674.

[6]   Katz, A. M., *Physiology of the Heart*, 4th ed., Philadelphia, PA: Lippincott Williams & Wilkins, 2006.

[7]   Fletcher, G. F., et al., "Exercise Standards; A Statement for Healthcare Professionals from the American Heart Association," *Circulation*, Vol. 91, 2001, p. 580.

[8]   Marriott, H. J. L., *Emergency Electrocardiography*, Naples: Trinity Press, 1997.

[9]   Nathanson, L. A., et al., "ECG Wave-Maven: Self-Assessment Program for Students and Clinicians," http://ecg.bidmc.harvard.edu.

Selected Bibliography

Alexander, R. W., R. C. Schlant, and V. Fuster, (eds.), *Hurst's The Heart*, 9th ed., Vol. 1, *Arteries and Veins*, New York: McGraw-Hill, Health Professions Division, 1998.

El-Sherif, N., and P. Samet, *Cardiac Pacing and Electrophysiology*, 3rd ed., Philadelphia, PA: Harcourt Brace Jovanovich, Inc., W. B. Saunders Company, 1991.

Gima, K., and Y. Rudy, "Ionic Current Basis of Electrocardiographic Waveforms: A Model Study," *Circulation*, Vol. 90, 2002, pp. 889–896.

Katz, E., *Willem Einthoven; A Biography*, 2005, available at http://chem.ch.huji.ac.il/~eugeniik/history/einthoven.html.

Lilly, L. S., *Pathophysiology of Heart Disease*, 3rd ed., Philadelphia, PA: Lippincott Williams & Wilkins, 2002.

Marriott, H. J., *Rhythm Quizlets: Self Assessment*, 2nd ed., Baltimore, MD: Williams & Wilkins, 1996.

Massie, E., and T. J. Walsh, *Clinical Vectorcardiography and Electrocardiography*, Chicago, IL: The Year Book Publishers, Inc., 1960.

Netter, F. H., *A Compilation of Paintings on the Normal and Pathologic Anatomy and Physiology, Embryology, and Diseases of the Heart*, edited by Fredrick F. Yonkman, Volume 5 of The Ciba Collection of Medical Illustrations, Summit, NJ: Ciba Pharmaceutical Company, 1969.

Wagner, G. W., *Marriott's Practical Electrocardiography*, 9th ed., Baltimore, MD: Williams & Wilkins, 1994.

Wellens, H. J., K. I. Lie, and M. J. Janse, (eds.), *The Conduction System of the Heart*, The Hague: Martinus Nijhoff Medical Division, 1978.

Zipes, D. P., and J. Jalife, (eds.), *Cardiac Electrophysiology: From Cell to Bedside*, 4th ed., Philadelphia, PA: W.B. Saunders and Company, 2004.

Zipes, D. P., et al., (eds.), *Braunwald's Heart Disease*, 7th ed., Oxford, U.K.: Elsevier, 2004.

CHAPTER 2

ECG Acquisition, Storage, Transmission, and Representation

Gari D. Clifford and Matt B. Oefinger

2.1 Introduction

This chapter is intended as a brief introduction to methods for acquiring and storing data. Although it may be tempting for the signal analyst to skip ahead to the chapters concerning the processing of the digital ECG, it is important to understand the etiology of a signal as far as possible. In particular, it is essential to know whether an observed anomaly in the ECG is due to a signal processing step (in either the hardware or software), an electronic artifact, an error in the storage of data, a disturbance on the sensor, or due to a pertinent physiological phenomenon. Furthermore, despite the diligence of the engineer concerning these issues, the error (or success/failure of a particular technique) may simply be due to the selection of the source of data itself.

Toward this end, the present chapter provides an overview of many of issues that should be considered before designing an ECG-based project, from the selection of the patient population, through hardware choices, to the the final signal processing techniques employed. These issues are intricately linked, and choices of one can restrict the analysis at another stage. For instance, choosing (either implicitly or explicitly) a population with low heart rate variability will mean that a higher acquisition sampling frequency is required to study such variability, and certain postprocessing interpolation techniques should be avoided (see Chapter 3). Apart from obvious confounding factors such as age, gender, and medication, variables such as lead configuration and patient activity are also considered.

Errors may creep into an analysis at any and every stage. Therefore, it is important to carefully design not only the hardware acquisition system, but also the transmission, storage, and processing libraries to be used. Although issues such as hardware specification, and relevant data formats are discussed, this chapter is not intended as a definitive or thorough exploration of these fields. However, it is intended to provide sufficient information to enable readers to design their own ECG data collection and storage program with the facility for easy analysis.

Freely available hardware designs and the software to utilize the hardware are discussed, and the electronic form of these designs are available from [1]. This design, although fully functional, cannot be used in a plug-and-play sense due to the serious design and test requirements that are required when attaching a live electrical circuit to any animal, particularly humans. Furthermore, regulations differ from country to country and change over time. It is, therefore, unwise (and impractical) to list all the required steps to ensure the safety (and legality) of attaching this hardware to any living entity. This chapter does attempt, however, to discuss the major issues connected with ECG acquisition, provide the background to facilitate the design of a useful system, and ensure the associated patient safety issues and regulations can be addressed.

For relevant background reading on hardware and software issues, Mohan et al. [2] and Oppenheim et al. [3] are suitable texts. The reader should also be familiar with the clinical terminology described in Chapter 1.

2.2 Initial Design Considerations

Before describing an example of a hardware configuration for an ECG acquisition system, it is important to consider many issues that may impact the overall design and individual components. Often each choice in the design process impacts on a previously made (perhaps ideal) choice, necessitating an iterative sequence of trade-offs until a suitable compromise is found.

2.2.1 Selecting a Patient Population

Before deciding to collect data, it is important to consider the population demographic and the confounding factors that may complicate subsequent analysis of the ECG. The following issues should be considered when selecting a patient population:

1. *Drugs:* Medication regimens can cause significant differences in baseline cardiovascular behavior. Rapid administration of some drugs can lead to changes in stationarity and confound short-term analysis.
2. *Age:* Significant differences in the ECG are observed between pediatric, young adult, and elderly adult populations.
3. *Gender:* Subtle but important differences in men and women's physiology lead to significant differences. If a study is attempting to identify small variations in a particular metric, the intergender difference may mask these variations.
4. *Preexisting conditions:* A person's past is often the best indicator of what may happen in the future. Using prior probabilities can significantly improve a model's predictive power.
5. *Genetics/family history:* Genetic markers can predispose a subject to certain medical problems, and therefore, genetic information can be considered another method of adding priors to a model.
6. *Numbers of patients in each category:* In terms of learning algorithms, a balanced learning set is often required. Furthermore, to perform statistically accurate tests, sufficient samples are required in each category.

7. *Activity:* Certain medical problems only become apparent at certain activity
    levels (see Chapter 3). Some patient populations are incapable of certain
    activities or may experience certain states infrequently. Furthermore, a pop-
    ulation should be controlled for individual activity differences, including
    circadian rhythms.

In clinical investigations it is common to control for items 1 to 4 (and sometimes 5)
above, but it is rare that a researcher has the luxury to control for the number of
patients. Statistical techniques must therefore be employed to correct for unbalanced
data sets or low numbers, such as bootstrap methods.

2.2.2 Data Collection Location and Length

When collecting ECG data from subjects, it is important to consider what the subject pool will easily tolerate. Although hospitalized patients will tolerate numerous
recording devices and electrodes, as they recover there is an expectation to reduce
the intensity of the recording situation. Ambulatory patients are unlikely to tolerate
anything that impedes their normal activity.

Although joining with an existing clinical protocol to fast-track data collection may seem an attractive option (not least because of the extra information and
clinical expertise that may be available), it can often be more beneficial to develop
experimental recording conditions that allow for greater control and for the adjustment of noise and recording times.

Unrealistic expectations about the quality of data to be collected may lead to
a large and expensive data set with low quality ECG information, which requires
significant postprocessing. Recommendations for the minimum time for monitoring patients to produce clinically useful data do exist. For instance, Per Johanson
et al. [4] indicate that at least 60 minutes of data should be recorded for effective
ST analysis. However, if the ST changes are thought to be infrequent (such as in
silent ischemia), it is important to perform data collection over longer periods, such
as overnight.

In fact, the miniaturization of Holter monitors, coupled with the increasing body
of literature connecting cardiac problems with sleep, indicates that home Holter
monitoring is a promising option. Recent studies on the ECG during sleep indicate
that segmenting ECG data on a per sleep stage basis can significantly increase patient
class separation [5, 6]. This approach is essentially the opposite of conventional
perturbative experiments such as the Valsalva or stress test, where the patient is
forced to an extreme of the cardiovascular system in order to help identify cardiac
anomalies under stress. Monitoring during sleep not only provides a low-noise,
long-term ECG to analyze but also helps identify cardiac anomalies that manifest
infrequently during quiescent activity periods.

Changes in the cardiovascular system due to biological rhythms that extend
over days, weeks, and months suggest that long term monitoring may be helpful
in preventing these changes confounding an analysis. However, when analyzing
extensive ECG records, it is important to develop efficient and reliable algorithms
that can easily process such data as well as reliable signal quality indexes to identify
and discard noisy segments of data.

2.2.3 Energy and Data Transmission Routes

One additional factor that often influences the population choice is the environment in which the equipment will operate. An ambulatory design means that one must carefully consider power consumption issues, both in terms of how much energy the processor requires to acquire (and process) data and how much energy is required to store or transmit data. Although recent advances in battery technology have made long-term ECG monitoring more feasible, battery technology is still limited, and techniques for reducing power consumption remain important. These include recording infrequent ECG segments (triggered by simple, but not overly sensitive algorithms) and minimizing the number of physical moving parts or the time they are in operation (such as by recording to flash memory rather than removable media, or using *sleep* operations). Furthermore, the addition of new technology, such as wireless data transmission modules, increases power consumption rates.

Sedentary or immobile patients may be more amenable to fixed-location power sources. Therefore, power consumption issues may not be important for this type of population (except for temporary power loss battery back-up considerations). The size of the battery obviously depends on the response time for power restoration. Typically, less mobile patient groups are found within a clinical setting, and therefore, electronic interference issues become more important (see Section 2.5.10).

2.2.4 Electrode Type and Configuration

The interface between an ECG signal source (the patient) and any acquisition device is a system of two or more electrodes from which a differential voltage is recorded. Two electrodes comprise a single lead of ECG. The electrodes may be surface electrodes, which are noninvasive and utilize a conductive gel to reduce skin-electrode impedance. The electrodes may be implanted and therefore have excellent contact (low impedance) and lower susceptibility to motion artifact. The electrodes may also be noncontact, and may sense electromagnetic activity through capacitive coupling. The terminology in this section refers to the clinical lead configuration descriptions given in Chapter 1.

In addition to determining the type of electrodes, one must consider the quantity of electrodes to be used. In diagnostic quality ECG, for example, 12 leads of ECG are acquired simultaneously. Each lead represents a different electrical axis onto which the electrical activity of the heart is projected. One may consider each lead to represent a different spatial perspective of the heart's electrical activity (if we ignore the dispersive effects of the torso upon the signal). If leads are appropriately placed in a multilead ECG, the ensemble of the different waveforms provides a robust understanding of the electrical activity throughout the heart, allowing the clinician to determine pathologies through spatial correlation of events on specific leads.

A variety of lead configurations should be considered, from a full 12-lead setup (with a possible augmentation of the perpendicular Frank leads [7]), a six-lead montage, the reduced Frank or EASI configurations, a simple hospital two- or three-lead configuration (often just lead II and V5), or perhaps just a single lead. Although one would expect that three perpendicular leads should be sufficient to obtain all the electrocardiographic information, the presence of capacitive agents in the torso mean that an overcomplete set of leads is required. Various studies have been performed to assess the accuracy of diagnoses when using a reduced set of leads and the ability to reconstruct 12-lead information from a lower number of leads.

The standard 12-lead ECG may be derived from the orthogonal Frank lead configuration by the inverse Dower transform [8], and can be useful in many circumstances [9]. Furthermore, the six chest leads (V1 to V6) can be derived from leads I and II by Einthoven's Law [10]. However, the quality of derived leads may not be sufficient for analyzing subtle morphologic changes in the ECG (such as the ST segment). For instance, significant differences in QT dispersion between the Frank leads and the standard 12-lead ECG have been reported [11]. Kligfield [12] points out, there is no consensus regarding which lead or set of leads should be routinely used in QT analysis, in part due to the varying definitions of the end of the T wave,[1] which produce differing results on differing leads.

In general, it seems sensible to assume that we should use as many maximally orthogonal leads as possible.[2] Above this, as many extra leads as possible should be used, to increase the signal-to-noise ratio, noise rejection, and redundancy. However, the anisotropic and nonstationary dielectric properties of the human torso (due to respiratory and cardiovascular activity) mean that spatial oversampling is often required to give an accurate evaluation of clinical features. In other words, multiple leads in similar locations (such as V1 though V6) are often required.

For example, the ST Segment Monitoring Practice Guideline Working Group [13, 14] recommends that if only two leads are available for ST segment monitoring (for patients with acute coronary syndromes), leads III and V3 should be used. If information from a patient's prior 12-lead ECG recorded during an ischemic event indicates that another lead is more sensitive, then this should be used instead of lead III or V3. The working group also states that the best three-lead combination is III-V3-V5. However, many bedside cardiac monitors are capable of monitoring only a single precordial (V) lead because the monitors provide only a single chest electrode. In addition, these two- and three-lead combinations for ischemia exclude lead V1, which is considered the best lead to monitor for detection of cardiac arrhythmias. Furthermore, the use of at least three chest leads (V3, V4, V5) is recommended for ST analysis, to allow noise reduction and artifact identification (although four- or five-lead configurations give better results). In particular, the addition of V2 (which is orthogonal to V5), V6 (which had been shown to be predictive of ischemia), and Y (which is also orthogonal to V5 and V2 [15]) are recommended. A six-lead configuration, and sometimes just a two-lead configuration, can be substituted for the standard 12-lead ECG in certain limited clinical and research applications.[3] It should also be noted that attempts to augment the Frank system with additional leads have led to improved methods for deriving 12-lead

1.   Including estimation of the T wave's apparent baseline termination, the nadir of T-U fusion, and extrapolation to baseline from its steepest descending point.
2.   There is another approach to lead selection. When there are grounds for suspecting a particular condition with a localized problem, one can choose to use a set of leads that represents a localized area of the heart (clinically known as *lead groups*; see Chapter 1).
3.   In particular, where the amplitude of QRS complex is the most important feature, such as in ECG-derived respiration [10, 16].

representations; for example, the EASI lead system, which like the Frank system, is based on the dipole hypothesis of vectorcardiography. The EASI system uses only four electrode sites, the Frank E, A, and I electrode locations, and a fourth electrode location (S) at the manubrium (plus one reference electrode) [17]. Since different leads exhibit different levels of noise under different activity conditions, the choice of lead configuration should be adapted to the type of activity a patient is expected to experience. Electrode configurations that are suitable for sedated hospital patients may not be suitable for ambulatory monitoring. A statement from the American Heart Association (AHA) on exercise standards [18] points out that CM5 is the most sensitive lead for ST segment changes during exercise. CC5 excludes the vertical component included in CM5 and decreases the influence of atrial repolarization, thus reducing false-positive responses. For comparison of the resting 12-lead recording, arm and leg electrodes should be moved to the wrists and ankles with the subject in the supine position.

In 1966, Mason and Likar [19] introduced a variation on the positioning of the standard limb electrodes specifically designed for 12-lead ECG exercise stress testing. To avoid excessive movement in the lead wires attached to the four recording points on the limbs, they suggested shifting the right and left arm (RA and LA) electrodes together with the right and left leg (RL and LL) electrodes. Welinder et al. [20] compared the susceptibility of the EASI and Mason-Likar systems to noise during physical activity. Although they found that the two systems have similar susceptibilities to baseline wander, the EASI system was found to be less susceptible to myoelectric noise than the Mason-Likar system. However, the low number of electrodes used in the EASI system indicates that caution should be used when adopting such a system.

An excellent overview of lead configuration issues and alternative schemes for different recording environments can be found in Drew et al. [14]. Furthermore, they point out the importance of careful electrode preparation and placement. Careful skin preparation that includes shaving electrode sites and removing skin oils and cutaneous debris with alcohol and a rough cloth or preparation gel. This reduces contact impedance and reduces noise in the recording (which can be especially important when attempting to identify subtle morphology changes such as ST elevation/depression).

Electrodes located in close proximity to the heart (i.e., precordial leads) are especially prone to waveform changes when electrodes are relocated as little as 10 mm away from their original location. This can be particularly important for studies which need to be repeated or when electrodes need to be replaced because of signal quality issues or skin irritation.

One method for reducing increasing noise due to electrode degradation and skin irritation is to use noncontact electrodes [21, 22]. These high input impedance electrodes have typical noise levels of $2 \mu V\ Hz^{-1}$ at 1 Hz, down to $0.1 \mu V\ Hz^{-1}$ at 1 kHz, and an operational bandwidth from 0.01 Hz to 100 kHz. Hence, they are well suited to the recording of ECGs. However, the lack of a need for direct skin contact can result in other problems, including artifacts due to movement of the electrode position relative to the body (and heart).

2.2.5 ECG-Related Signals

Recording several ECG leads simultaneously obviously adds extra information to a study, and allows a more robust estimate of noise, artifacts, and features within the ECG. Furthermore, the ECG is strongly related to the respiratory and blood pressure signals (see Chapter 4). It can be advantageous, therefore, to either derive surrogates for these coupled signals from the ECG or to make direct simultaneous recordings of related signals.

A nonexhaustive list of the major information sources related to the ECG that one should consider is as follows:

- *Respiration:* This can be derived from the ECG (see Chapter 8) or measured directly from strain-bands around the torso, nasal flow-meters, or impedance pneumography. Impedance pneumography involves measuring the differential impedance changes (at kilohertz frequencies) across two of the ECG electrodes that have been altered to inject a small current through the patient at this frequency. For ECG-derived respiration (EDR) [16], the best set of electrodes for deriving respiration depends on whether you breathe from the chest or from the diaphragm. Furthermore, if respiratory sinus arrhythmia is present, respiration can also be derived from the dominant high-frequency component of the RR interval time series (see Chapter 3), although this is less reliable than morphology-based EDR.
- *Blood pressure (BP):* This can be measured invasively via an arterial line or noninvasively through periodic pressure cuff inflations. Relative BP measures include the Finapres and pulse transit time (the time from the R-peak on the ECG to a peak on a pulsatile pressure-related waveform).
- *Activity:* Often studies attempt to control for the intersubject and intrasubject variability due to activity and circadian rhythms a patient experiences. Unfortunately, the activity due to the uncontrollable variable of mental activity can often lead to a larger interpatient and intrapatient variability than between patient groups and activities [5]. A good method to control for both mental and physical activity is to use some form of objective measure of level of consciousness. Although none exists for conscious subjects, electroencephalogram (EEG)-based scales do exist for sleep [23] and sedation [24]. Recent studies have shown that controlling for mental and physical activity in this manner leads to a more sensitive measure of difference between cardiovascular metrics [5]. Studies that attempt to stage sleep from heart rate variability (HRV) have proved inconclusive. Conversely, although heart rate artifacts can be observed in the EEG, the broadness of the artifact (and its origin from an arterial pressure movement) are such that accurate HRV cannot be accurately assessed from the EEG. However, recent work on cardiorespiratory coupling in sleep has shown that sleep staging from the ECG is possible.
- *Human-scored scales:* It is important to consider whether a human (such as a nurse or clinician) should be present during some or all of the experiments to make annotations using semiobjective scales (such as the Riker Sedation/Agitation Scale [24]).

2.2.6   Issues When Collecting Data from Humans

When collecting data from humans, not only should the patient population demographics be considered, but also the entire process of data collection, through each intermediate step, to the final storage location (presumably on a mirrored server in some secure location). The following major issues should be seriously considered, and in many cases, thoroughly documented for legal protection:

1. *IRB/ethics board approval:* Before any data can be collected, most institutions require that the experimental protocol and subsequent data use be preapproved by the institutional review board (IRB) or institutional ethics committee.

2. *Device safety:* If the device is not a commercially FDA/EC (or equivalent) approved device, it must be tested for electrical safety (including electrical isolation), even if the design is already approved. The institution at which data are being collected may require further electrical tests on each unit to be used within the institution. (See Section 2.5.10.)

3. *Patient consent:* If collecting data from humans, it is important to investigate whether data being collected is covered under an existing IRB approval (and there is no conflict with another study) and whether explicit consent must be collected from each patient.

4. *Future uses of data:* It is important to consider whether data may be used in other studies, by other groups, or posted for open dissemination. It is often easier to build in relevant clauses to the IRB at the onset of the project rather than later on.

5. *Traceability and verification:* When collecting data from multiple sources, (even if this is simply ECG plus patient demographics) it is important to ensure that the paired data can be unambiguously associated with relevant "twin(s)." Integrity checks must be made at each storage and transfer step (e.g., by running the Unix tool *MD5SUM* on each file and comparing it to the result of the same check before and after the transfer).

6. *Protected health information (PHI):* It is essential, however, that the individuals being monitored should have their identity thoroughly protected. This means removing all PHI that can allow someone using public resources to identify the individual to whom the ECG (and any associated data) belongs. This includes pacemaker serial numbers, names of relatives, and any other personal identifiers (such as vehicle license numbers). Date-shifting that preserves the day of the week and season of the year is also required.

7. *Data synchronicity:* When collecting data over a network, or from multiple sources, it is important that some central clock is used (which is constantly being adjusted for clock drift, if absolute times are required). It is also important to consider that most conventional operating systems are not intended for real-time data acquisition and storage. (In fact, for life-critical applications, only certain processors and operating systems are allowable.) Although there are methods for adjusting for clock drift (such as averaging independent clocks), standard OS distributions such as Linux or Windows are inadvisable. Rather, one should choose a real-time operating systems (RTOS) such as LynxOS, which is used in the GE/Marquette patient

monitors, or a real-time kernel such as Allegro. Care should also be taken to mitigate for time differences caused by daylight savings.

8. *Data integrity:* The collected data must be stored securely (in case any PHI was not removed) and safely. In other words, data should be backed up in two geographically separate locations using a RAID storage system, which is regularly checked for disk integrity. This is particularly important for long-term data storage (on the order of a year or more) since individual hard disks, CDs, and DVDs have a short shelf life. Magnetic tape can also be used, but data access can be slow.

9. *Storage capacity and file size limits:* If certain file size limits are exceeded, then problems may result, not only in the online writing of the file to disk but in subsequent transfers to disk or over a network. In particular, upper limits of 500 MB and 2 GB exist for single files on DOS-based disks and DVD storage, respectively. Furthermore, the larger the file, the more likely there will be errors when transferring data over networks or writing to other media. It should also be noted that, currently, none of the writable DVD formats are fully compatible with all drive types.

10. *Resolution, dynamic range, and saturation:* Sufficient frequency resolution and dynamic range in the amplification (or digital storage) of ECG data should be specified. For example, if the data storage format is limited to 12 bits, a 2-mV signal on the input should correspond to 10 bits or less in the digital recording. It is important not to be too conservative, however, in order to ensure that the amplitude resolution is sufficient for the signal processing tasks.

11. *Data formats:* When storing data, it is important to use an accurate and verifiable data format (at each step). If data are to be converted to another format, the method of conversion should be checked thoroughly to ensure that it does not introduce errors or remove valuable information. Furthermore, a (final) data format should be chosen that allows the maximum flexibility for data storage, transmission, access, and processing.

12. *Electronic security:* In the United States, new legislation requires that any researchers transmitting or storing data should do so in a secure manner, enabling the correct security mechanisms at each step and keeping an access log of all use. Users should be required to sign a data use/privacy contract in which they agree not to pass on any data or store it in an nonsecure manner. The latter phrase refers in particular to removable media, laptops, and unencrypted hard drives (and even swap space).

13. *Availability of data:* It is also important to consider how frequently data can be collected and at what rate to ensure that sufficient transmission bandwidth is guaranteed and storage capacity is available.

2.3   Choice of Data Libraries

The choice of libraries to store the ECG data may at first glance seem like a peripheral subject of little importance. However, poor choices of storage format can often lead to enormous time-sinks that cause significant delays on a project. Important questions to ask when choosing a data format and access libraries include:

- What are the data going to be used for?
- Are the data format and libraries extensible?
- Is the data format compact?
- Are the libraries open-source?
- Do the libraries and format support annotations?
- Is the format widely accepted (and well tested)?
- Can I easily (and verifiably) de-identify my data using this format?
- Are the libraries for reading and writing data available for all the operating systems on which the ECG will be analyzed?
- Are there additional associated libraries for signal processing freely available?
- Can the libraries be used in conjunction with all the programming languages you are likely to use (C, Java, Matlab, Perl)?
- Are there libraries that allow the transmission of the data over the Internet?
- Are there libraries that allow me to protect access to the data over the Internet?
- Can the data format be easily converted into other data formats that colleagues might require for viewing or analysis?

Clinical formats that are in general use include: the extended European Data Format (EDF+) [25], which is commonly used for electroencephalograms (and more increasingly is becoming the standard for ECGs); HL7 [26, 27] (an XML-based format for the exchange of data in hospitals); and WaveForm DataBase (WFDB), a set of libraries developed at MIT [28, 29]. HL7 is by nature a very noncompact data format that is better suited to the exchange of small packets of data, such as for billing. Despite this, the FDA recently introduced an XML-based file standard for submitting clinical trails data [30, 31]. The main rationale behind the move was to unify the submission format (previously PDF) for what are essentially small amounts of data.

A recent attempt to improve on this format and integrate it with other existing waveform reading libraries, such as WFDB, is ecgML [32]. Although EDF+ solves some of problems of EDF (such as the lack of annotations), it is still restrictive on many levels and is not well supported under many different languages. Furthermore, it is not easily extensible, and does not cope well with sudden changes in the data format. In contrast, WFDB is a suite of libraries for accessing many different data formats and allows positive answers to the above questions. WFDB records have three main components; an ASCII header file, a binary data file, and a binary annotation file. The header file contains information about the binary file format variety, the number and type of channels, the lengths, gains, and offsets of the signals, and any other clinical information that is available for the subject. The separate header file allows for rapid querying. Similarly, any number of annotation files can be associated with the main binary file just by using the same name (with a different extension). Again, rapid reading of the annotations is then possible, without the need to seek around in a large binary file. Furthermore, WFDB allows the virtual concatenation of any number of separate files, without the need to actually merge them.

Past and recent developments that set WFDB apart from other data reading and writing libraries include:

- The ability to read data over HTTP protocols;
- The extensibility of the annotations format to allow the use of defined labels and links to external documents, including the use of hypertext links;
- The inclusion of *libcurl* libraries to allow access to secure data behind password protected sites;
- The ability to seamlessly cope with changes in signal gain, sampling frequency, lead configuration, data dimensionality, and arbitrary noncontiguous breaks in the record;
- The flexibility to work with many data formats (arbitrary dynamic ranges, resolutions, byte order, and so forth);
- The development of open-source signal processing libraries that have been well tested and documented;
- Supported libraries for multiple programming languages, such as C, Java, Matlab, and Python (using *SWIG* wrappers), on multiple platforms;
- Conversion tools between other standard formats (EDF, ASCII) and between sampling frequencies.

WFDB, therefore, is an excellent (if not the best) current choice for storing ECG data. Another parallel resource development, intricately connected with WFDB, is libRASCH [33]. This is a set of cross-platform C-based libraries that provides a common interface to access biomedical signals, almost regardless of the format in which they are stored. Many proprietary biomedical signal formats are accessible through this set of libraries, which work with a wide variety of languages (Perl, Python, Matlab, Octave, and SciLab). The libraries are modular, based upon an Application Programming Interface (API), that allows the easy addition of *plug-ins*. Therefore, it is easily extensible for any new data formats, programming languages, viewing tools, or signal processing libraries. A set of signal processing plugins are available for this tool, including fetal heart rate analysis, heart rate turbulence, and other more standard heart rate variability metrics. See Schneider [33] for more information on libRASCH.

2.4   Database Analysis—An Example Using WFDB

Before performing any data collection, or more frequently during data collection, it is important to test proposed algorithms on freely available (annotated) data, using standard tools and metrics. Without such data and tools, it is impossible to judge the scientific merit of a particular approach, without reimplementing the research completely.[4]

Over recent years, advances in hardware technology have made the acquisition of large databases of multichannel ECGs possible. The most extensive and freely available collection of ECG (and related) waveforms can be found on PhysioNet [28] (the MIT Laboratory for Computation Physiology's Web site) or one of its many

---

4.   Furthermore, since it is extremely difficult and time-consuming to reproduce an algorithm in its entirety from a short paper, the posting of the code used to generate the quoted results is essential.

mirrors. This collection of databases comprises hundreds of multilead ECGs recorded from patients who suffer from various known heart conditions, as well as examples of healthy ECGs, for periods from 30 minutes to more than a day. These records have been annotated by expert clinicians and, in some cases, verified by automatic algorithms to facilitate the further evolution of diagnostic software.

Tools, available from the same location, enable the researcher to call libraries that read and compare the clinician-annotated or verified files for each patient with a number of freely available clinically relevant algorithms (such as QRS detection, ECG-segmentation, wave onset location, and signal quality) or any self-created algorithm, using the WFDB data reading libraries. The database and libraries of comparative tests conform to the relevant American National Standards Institute (ANSI) guidelines [34] developed by the Association for the Advancement of Medical Instrumentation (AAMI) [35]. Furthermore, medical devices that use a QRS and arrhythmia detection algorithm must quote performance statistics on the MIT-BIH database.

Each patient record in the MIT-BIH database, labeled 100 to 124 and 200 to 234, consists of 30 minutes of ECGs sampled at 360 Hz with 16 bit accuracy and labeled by experts. These records can be antialias upsampled or downsampled using the WFDB tools[5] to any required frequency and resolution. The WFDB tools account for any changes caused by the downsampling (such as aliasing and annotation timing differences) and generate header files to allow synchronization of the labels with the new data files. The clinicians' annotations consist of the following labels for each beat[6]:

- V—Ventricular Ectopic Beat (VEB): a ventricular premature beat, (such as an R-on-T[7]), or a ventricular escape beat.
- F—Fusion Beat: a fusion of a ventricular and a normal beat.
- Q—Paced Beat: a fusion of a paced (artificially induced) and a normal beat or a beat that cannot be classified.
- S—Supraventricular Ectopic Beat (SVEB): an atrial or nodal (junctional) premature or escape beat, or an aberrant atrial premature beat.
- N—Normal: any beat that does not fall into the S, V, F, or Q categories. This category also includes Bundle Branch Block Beats (BBBB) which give a widened QRS complex and can be indicative of myocardial infarction.[8] However, the broadening is very hard to detect.
- X: a pseudo-beat label generated during a segment marked as unreadable.
- U: marks the center of unreadable data segments, beginning 150 ms after the last beat label and 150 ms before the next.

---

5. The *xform* executable.
6. A full list, including arrhythmia onsets and noise labels, can be found at [36].
7. A potentially dangerous condition is induced when a premature ventricular contraction occurs during the T wave of the preceding QRS-T complex. R-on-T phenomenon can induce ventricular tachycardia or ventricular fibrillation.
8. A blockage in the normal conduction paths of the heart that leads to permanent damage to the heart muscle.

- [and]: Rhythm labels marking the onset and cessation of ventricular fibrillation or flutter (VF), respectively.

Note that beat labels are never paired with rhythm labels, and beat labeling is
discontinued between these labels. Incorporation of the WFDB libraries into an
algorithm that a user wishes to test enables the generation of a test annotation file
of time-stamped event labels in a comparable format to the clinician annotation
files. When the WFDB tools are run on these files a beat-by-beat comparison is
performed, and an output file is created that compares the time-scoring of events.
Two events are held to be simultaneous (by the ANSI standards [35]) if they occur
within ±150 ms of each other. Thus, in order to perform beat-by-beat comparisons,
a pseudo-beat label 'O' is generated any time the test algorithm labels a point in the
ECG as a beat and there is no clinician scored label within 150 ms.

Table 2.1 is a typical file generated by these tools[9] for scoring the results from a
standard, freely available, QRS detector,[10] that was applied to the MIT-BIH arrhythmia database. Columns 2 to 12 refer to the beat-by-beat scoring with a capitalized
label denoting the actual event (as labeled by the clinicians) and the lower-case let-
ter denoting the labeling provided by the algorithm under test. Nn', Vn', and Fn'
are thus the number of normals, VEBs, and fusion beats that the test algorithm
labeled as normals, respectively. On' is the number of normal pseudo-beats that
the algorithm generated (a "normal" label being generated when there was no beat
there). Nv' and Vv' are, respectively, the numbers of normals and VEBs that have
been labeled as VEBs. Fv' is the number of fusion beats labeled as VEBs, and Ov'
is the number of pseudo-VEB labels (a VEB label being generated by the algorithm
when no beat at all occurred in the original).[11] No', Vo', and Fo' are the number
of pseudo-beats generated in the test annotation file for the cases when there was a
normal, VEB, or fusion beat in the original ECG, but the algorithm failed to detect
such a beat.

Thus, the records are scored with the number of false positives (FP; beats identified by the algorithm when the clinician has not scored one), false negatives (FN;
beats missed by the algorithm when the clinician has scored one), and true positives (TP; both annotations agree on the time of the event). These are defined as[12]
$TP = Nn' + Vn' + Fn'$, $FN = No' + Vo' + Fo'$, and $FP = On'$. The second-to-
last column in Table 2.1 is Q Se, which gives the sensitivity of the algorithm, or
the number of TPs as a percentage of the total that really exist. The last column
gives the positive predictivity, Q + P, or the number of TPs as a percentage of the
number detected by the algorithm. These two parameters are therefore calculated

---

9.   The "bxb," beat-by-beat comparison algorithm in particular.
10. These results were generated using the author's own C-code version of the Pat Hamilton's QRS detector
     [37, 38]. The latter has now been improved and is freely available [39]. There is also a Matlab version
     which works in a batch manner, available from this book's accompanying Web site [1].
11. Note that these latter four columns are zero in this example since the example algorithm was not designed
     to classify, and all beats are assumed to be normal sinus beats.
12. Beat type classification is detailed in the output file, but incorrect classification (such as labeling a VEB as a
     normal) does not affect the statistics; they are based on how many QRS complexes are detected regardless
     of their classification.

Table 2.1 Standard Output of PhysioNet's *bxb* Algorithm for a Typical QRS Detector (Subjects 109 Through 222 Omitted)

Record	Nn'	Vn'	Fn'	On'	Nv'	Vv'	Fv'	Ov'	No'	Vo'	Fo'	Q Se	Q+P
100	1901	1	0	0	0	0	0	0	0	0	0	100.00	100.00
101	1521	0	1	4	0	0	0	0	0	0	1	99.93	99.74
103	1725	0	0	1	0	0	0	0	4	0	0	99.77	99.94
105	2117	29	4	133	0	0	0	0	4	0	1	99.77	94.17
106	1236	459	0	1	0	0	0	0	0	1	0	99.94	99.94
108	1461	13	2	257	0	0	0	0	4	0	0	99.73	85.17
...	...	...	...	...	...	...	...	...	...	...	...	...	...
...	...	...	...	...	...	...	...	...	...	...	...	...	...
...	...	...	...	...	...	...	...	...	...	...	...	...	...
223	1736	447	8	1	0	0	0	0	0	8	0	99.64	99.95
228	1225	300	0	49	0	0	0	0	176	2	0	89.55	96.89
230	1858	1	0	1	0	0	0	0	0	0	0	100.00	99.95
231	1278	0	0	1	0	0	0	0	0	0	0	100.00	99.92
232	1485	0	0	5	0	0	0	0	0	0	0	100.00	99.66
233	1862	688	6	1	0	0	0	0	1	4	0	99.80	99.96
234	2288	0	0	1	0	0	0	0	0	3	0	99.87	99.96
Sum	77011	5822	623	774	0	0	0	0	427	78	15		
Gross												99.38	99.08
Average												99.33	99.06

Note that all beats detected have been assumed to be normals, since no beat classification has been performed.

as follows:

$$Q \, Se = \frac{TP}{TP + FN} = \frac{Nn' + Vn' + Fn'}{Nn' + Vn' + Fn' + No' + Vo' + Fo'} \qquad (2.1)$$

$$Q + P = \frac{TP}{TP + FP} = \frac{Nn' + Vn' + Fn'}{Nn' + Vn' + Fn' + On'} \qquad (2.2)$$

From Table 2.1 one can see that patient 100's heart beat 1,902 times over the 30-minute period, an average heart rate of 63.4 bpm. All the beats were classified as normals by the algorithm (nonzero entries in the second, third, and fourth columns), although one of these beats was actually a VEB. For this record, the Q Se and Q + P are therefore both 100% for the algorithm under test.

Note that the algorithm labeled patient 101's ECG as containing 1,522 normals. All the beats were actually normal except one fusion beat. However, four normals were detected by the algorithm when there were no actual beats present. Thus, the sensitivity is $\frac{1521+1}{1521+1+4} = 0.9974$ or 99.74%. Furthermore, one fusion beat was missed since a pseudo-beat was generated from the WFDB annotation file (Fo' = 1). Thus, positive predictivity is reduced to $\frac{1521+1}{1521+1+1} = 0.9993$ or 99.93%. Patient 103 has a total of 1,729 beats. All these beats were normal, but four were missed by the algorithm. Only one beat was labeled as a normal and did not actually occur. It is important to note that the ANSI standards [34] allow 5 minutes of adjustment and adaptation for any algorithm being tested, and therefore, the first 5 minutes of data are not included in the results generated by the WFDB tools. The average performance over all the files is usually quoted as the *gross* or average (Av). Note

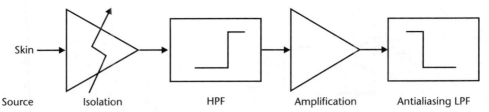

Skin →

Source   Isolation   HPF   Amplification   Antialiasing LPF

Figure 2.1   Simplified diagram of hardware setup. The fluctuations in PD between the differential ECG leads on the skin's surface (or sometimes inside the body) are amplified with an optically isolated instrumentation amplifier. The signal is then passed through a HP filter, a second amplification stage, then a lowpass antialiasing filter. The signal is finally sampled by an A/D card (not shown). The opto-isolation can also be moved so it occurs after the final A/D stage.

that the values of 99.33% sensitivity and 99.06% positive predictivity for this implementation of this algorithm is comparable to that of the original Hamilton, Pan, and Tompkins algorithm [37, 38]. The latest version of their algorithm [39] reports average Q Se and Q + P values of 0.9977 and 0.9979, respectively, which compare well to state-of-the-art QRS detectors. Excellent surveys and comparative analyses are available on this topic [40–42].

2.5   ECG Acquisition Hardware

In this section, the issues surrounding the design and fabrication of a hardware unit for ECG signal conditioning are discussed. More detailed information is available from the book's companion Web site [1], together with example schematics and PCB layouts. The reader is also referred to Mohan et al. [2] and Oppenheim et al. [3] for more detailed theory.

2.5.1   Single-Channel Architecture

Figure 2.1 illustrates the general process for recording an ECG from a subject. The (millivolt) fluctuations in potential difference (PD) between the differential ECG leads on the skin's surface (or sometimes inside the body) are amplified with an optically isolated instrumentation amplifier (see Figure 2.2). Note that, in general, three leads are required for one differential signal from the subject since a ground electrode (Input C) is also required.[13] The voltage difference between the other electrodes (Inputs A and B) serves as the signal input that is amplified through the op-amps U1A and U1B. These signals are then differentially amplified and passed through a highpass filter (such as an eighth order Bessel filter).

By using a suitable design tool (such as Orcad/PSpice [43]) or free software (such as PCB123 [44]), this schematic can be converted into a printed circuit board (PCB) schematic with all the relevant microchip dimensions specified. Fabrication services

---

13. In fact, there are two basic lead types: bipolar and unipolar. Bipolar leads (the *standard limb leads*) use one positive and a one negative electrode. Unipolar leads (the *augmented leads* and *chest leads*) have a single positive electrode and use a combination of the other electrodes to serve as a composite negative electrode.

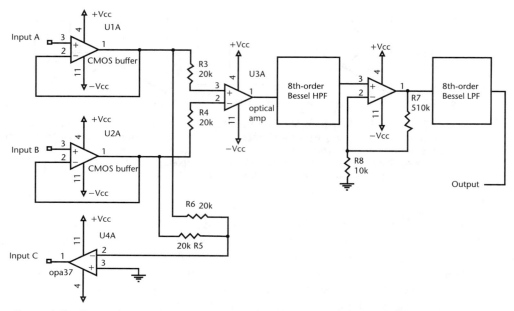

Figure 2.2 Circuit diagram for acquiring a single lead ECG signal. One electrode (Input C) serves as ground while the voltage difference between the other electrodes (Inputs A and B) serves as the signal input. Eighth-order Bessel (HP) filters are used to minimize noise, with minimal distortion.

for a PCB are cheap and rapid, therefore alleviating the need for in-house production. An example of a PCB design can be found on this book's accompanying Web site [1].

2.5.2   Isolation and Protection

For any circuit that uses a significant power source (such as mains electricity) and that comes into contact with a human, the board must be segmented into isolated and nonisolated sections. These sections must be separated by approximately 10 mm (or more) of free space or circuit board from each other (depending on the dielectric constant of the board). Even tiny amounts of current leakage (less than $100 \, \mu A$ [45]) through the subject can induce lethal ventricular fibrillation in catheterized human subjects.

The power from the directly (mains) powered nonisolated section of the board is transferred to the isolated section of the board using DC-to-DC converters. The use of a transformer to use magnetic induction to transfer the power results in only the transfer of photons, rather than electrons (and hence current) to the isolated region of the board. There is, therefore, no current path to the monitored subject from the mains power. The voltages in the figures in this chapter are denoted ±Vcc regardless of whether they are on the isolated or nonisolated side of the board. However, ±Vcc on the isolated side is not connected to ±Vcc on the nonisolated side.

Similarly, information is transmitted back from the isolated (patient) side of the circuitry to the nonisolated side via light in the opto-isolators. Opto-isolators convert electrons (current) into photons and back into electrons, thereby transmitting only light (and not current) across the isolation gap. The opto-isolators are placed such that they span the 10-mm gap between the isolated and nonisolated sections of the board and are powered on either side by either the isolated output of the DC-to-DC converters or the live mains power, respectively. See [2] for more information.

After the opto-isolation stage, the signal is then passed through a highpass (HP) filter, a second amplification stage, then a lowpass (LP) antialiasing filter. The signal is finally sampled by an analog-to-digital (A/D) conversion card.[14] The details of each of these stages are discussed below.

Note that resistors with extremely high values should also be placed between each input and ground for static/defibrillation voltage protection. Furthermore, a current limiting resistor at output is required in case the op-amps fail. These components are not shown in the diagrams in this chapter. It should also be noted that optical isolation in an early stage of amplification can introduce significant noise. It is, therefore, often preferable to isolate directly after digitizing the signal.

2.5.3   Primary Common-Mode Noise Reduction: Active Grounding Circuit

Power-line, or mains, electromagnetic noise (and to a lesser extent harmonics thereof) is ubiquitous indoors, since electrical systems in buildings utilize AC power delivered at these frequencies. The spectrum of some ECGs (murine, for example) can span from DC to 1 kHz, and therefore, using a 50-Hz to 60-Hz notch filter to remove mains noise will invariably remove at least some signal content.[15] An active ground circuit (illustrated in Figure 2.3) is the preferred means of removing such common-mode noise.

The active grounding circuit, shown in Figure 2.3, works by taking the average (common mode) of the voltages at the two input terminals of the preamplification stage. It then amplifies and inverts the signal, and then feeds the resultant signal back as the ground, or reference voltage, for the circuit. The circuit does not remove differential signal content but mitigates common-mode noise. That is, it removes the part of the signal that is simultaneously present on both electrodes.

2.5.4   Increasing Input Impedance: CMOS Buffer Stage

High input impedance is requisite in a biomedical instrumentation design, as the signals of interest (particularly electro-physiological signals) are extremely weak (on the order of several hundred microvolts) and, consequently, cannot supply substantial current. An extremely high input impedance and corresponding power amplification is an inherent property of a CMOS circuit. A CMOS preamplifier op-amp circuit, therefore, serves as an ideal decoupling stage between the weak electro-physiological signal and subsequent analog signal processing circuitry.

---

14. The A/D card is not shown in Figure 2.1. Recommendations for possible cards can be found on this book's accompanying Web site [1].
15. The width of the notch must be at least 2 Hz since the frequency of the interference is not constant.

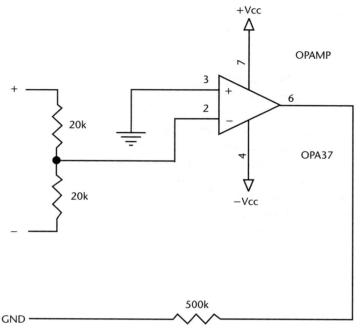

Figure 2.3 Active ground circuit used for common-mode noise reduction. The common-mode signal at the input electrodes is inverted and fed back through a current-limiting resistor (for subject projection). This circuit is particularly useful in reducing prevalent mains noise, which is capacitively coupled into both signal input wires. GND indicates ground. (*After:* [46].)

2.5.5 Preamplification and Isolation

Although it is preferable to place the isolation step after the amplifiers, this means that the user must write their own drivers for the A/D controllers. If subtleties in the ECG, such as late potentials, are not important, then it is possible to provide optical isolation at the preamplification stage. This ensures that an electrical surge within the instrumentation circuitry cannot electrocute the subject, and conversely, a surge at the input terminals will not damage instrumentation circuitry beyond the preamplifier. The strongest source of such currents originates from capacitive coupling through the power supply to the grounded instrumentation chassis. However, if the chassis that houses the ECG hardware is properly grounded, the minimal resistance of the case to ground will lead most of the current to sink to ground through this pathway. The optical isolation amplifier discussed in this section provides a very high dielectric interruption, or equivalently a very small capacitance, in series between the lead wire and instrumentation, protecting the subject from acting as a pathway for leakage current to ground.

The physiological voltages produced by mammal hearts are on the order of 100 μV to several microvolts, and the dynamic range of the preamplifier is usually ±12V DC. Accounting for different half-cell potentials in the electrodes that could produce a differential DC voltage as high as 100 mV, an expected a gain of 25 is appropriate for the preamplification stage provides an adequate SNR and, upon reaching steady-state, does not saturate. However, care must be taken as higher

PDs might be encountered in some situations (such as extreme baseline wander in exercise, for example), and a lower gain may be appropriate.

2.5.6 Highpass Filtering

The output signal from the instrumentation amplifier is input to an eighth-order Bessel HP filter with a cutoff frequency of 0.1 Hz. Note that for ST analysis, a cutoff of 0.05 Hz is required (see Chapter 10), and other evidence indicates that useful information exists down to 0.02 Hz [47]. This HP filter serves to remove the DC offset due to half-cell potential differences in the electrodes as well as other low-frequency signal noise (mostly baseline wander). The choice of a Bessel transfer function is motivated by the fact that it has optimal phase response. That is, it has the desirable property of near-constant group delay, and negligible phase distortion. This optimality in phase response comes at the price of decreased roll-off steepness in the transition band relative to other transfer functions.

2.5.7 Secondary Amplification

After passing through the HP filter, the signal is again amplified; this time by a gain of 52 in the arrangement illustrated in Figure 2.4. This is the final amplification stage in the signal conditioning pipeline. This second amplification stage further increases the SNR of the signal and boosts the signal voltage to a range appropriate for sampling with an A/D converter with a dynamic range of ± 10V. The amplification circuit (Figure 2.4) is a simple feedback op-amp network utilizing the familiar gain equation $1 + Rf/R_{in}$, where in this system $Rf = 510\,\mathrm{k\Omega}$ and $R_{in} = 10\,\mathrm{k\Omega}$, to provide the gain factor of 52. The signal entering this amplification stage, in contrast with that entering the preamplification stage, is not offset due to half-cell potential differences and baseline drift because of the preceding HP filter stage. As such, this amplification stage can comfortably amplify the signal by the rather sizable factor of 52 without saturating the amplifiers.

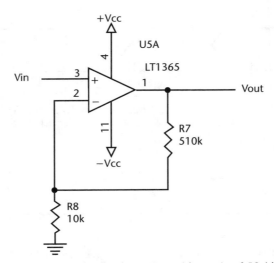

Figure 2.4 A noninverting negative-feedback op-amp with a gain of 52 (determined by the ratio of the 510 kΩ to 10 kΩ resistors).

2.5.8　Lowpass Filtering and Oversampling

Since the ECG spectrum may occupy the DC to 1 kHz [48], the Nyquist sampling criterion mandates that, with an *ideal* LP filter with a passband of 0 to 1 kHz one should sample the signal at 2 kHz to avoid aliasing. Since a circuit filter implementation is never ideal, one must enforce a relationship between the filter type, the filter's cutoff frequency, and the A/D sampling rate that produces an acceptably small amount of aliasing. The filter transfer function for the LP filter, as for the HP filter, was chosen to have a Bessel transfer characteristic to minimize phase distortion. This optimization for phase response comes at the expense of a slow roll-off in the transition region.

Oversampling is a technique often employed in systems using an antialiasing filter with relatively slow roll-off. It can be shown that sampling of an analog signal produces spectral copies of the analog spectrum at multiples of the sampling frequency, f_s, in the discrete-time frequency domain [3]. Consider the example in which a signal is filtered in the analog domain with a nonideal LP filter of cutoff 1 kHz, then sampled at 2 kHz. The result is an aliased signal, which is manifested in overlapping spectral regions in Figure 2.5. One might consider building a higher-order analog filter to reduce the transition band, which would prove costly and time-consuming, to mitigate the effects of aliasing. Alternatively, one could sample the signal at a faster rate, thereby spreading the spectral copies further apart, as Figure 2.6 illustrates. Of course, a high-order digital filter, which is cheap and relatively simple to implement, can be used to LP filter the digitized signal, followed by simple decimation. This achieves the same effect as with a high-order antialiasing filter, without the hardware complexity.

Such a technique, known as oversampling, is often employed in data-sampling systems to minimize the complexity and cost of analog circuitry and harness the power of fast digital processing power. In the case of this system, a high-order antialiasing filter is used. However, since the filter is optimized for minimal phase distortion, its roll-off is similar to that of a lower-order filter. A reasonable

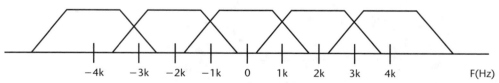

Figure 2.5　A signal band-limited to approximately 1.75 kHz (due to slow roll-off of 1 kHz cutoff Bessel antialiasing analog filter) sampled at 2 kHz has spectral copies at multiples of 2 kHz and suffers aliasing (overlapping regions).

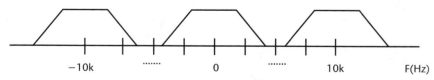

Figure 2.6　The same signal, band-limited to approximately 1.75 kHz (due to slow roll-off of 1 kHz cutoff Bessel antialiasing analog filter) sampled at 10 kHz (5× oversampling) has spectral copies repeating at multiples of 10 kHz and does not suffer aliasing.

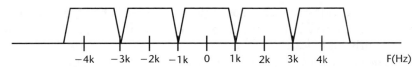

Figure 2.7 After applying a high-order digital lowpass filter then decimating by a factor of 5, the spectra are spaced by multiples of 2 kHz but with no aliasing. This combination of digital LP filtering and decimation prevents the need for an expensive analog antialiasing filter.

approach for this type of signal is to employ five-times oversampling, so that the signal is sampled at five times the Nyquist rate of 2 kHz. After being sampled at this high rate, the signal can then be digitally LP filtered and decimated[16] by a factor of five to give an effective sampling rate of 2 kHz. A symmetric digital LP FIR filter preceding the decimation avoids aliasing. The initial use of oversampling also minimizes aliasing, and subsequent downsampling (after LP filtering) provides the minimum allowable lossless data storage requirement without resorting to compression. Figure 2.7 shows the spectral content of a signal after it has been oversampled (five times), digitally LP-filtered, then decimated by a factor of five. The spectral copies do not overlap, indicating that no aliasing has occurred. However, the spectra are closely spaced, indicating that the signal is not oversampled, and disk storage space is minimized.

2.5.9 Hardware Design Issues: Sampling Frequency Choice

The hardware implementation described so far is an example of how one might choose to design an ECG acquisition system. Of course, variants of this design are likely to be more useful to a specific application. Some general guidelines in designing such a system should be followed. First, when selecting filter components, ensure that they are functional over the entire frequency range (particularly down to 0.05 Hz or lower if you are designing an application that requires ST analysis or apnea detection; see Section 2.5.6). Second, it is important to consider the resonant frequencies of the components chosen for the design. Third, the cable shielding should be terminated at an isolated ground or, preferably, to the board enclosure. If the cable shield is terminated to an isolated ground using a small capacitor from the isolated ground to the enclosure ground, CM interference is reduced. Finally, the circuit board layout should be such that the coupling between components is minimized.

The designs illustrating this chapter provide for a sampling frequency of 2 kHz. Although this sampling rate might seem to be rather high, (except for high-frequency ECG applications analysis such as late potentials [49–52]), it has been shown that a sampling rate of at least 500 Hz (and sometimes 1 kHz) is required for applications such as heart rate variability and PR interval variability analysis [53–55]. In general, when recording the ECG of an animal smaller than a human, the ECG may extend to even higher frequencies. Therefore, a sampling rate of 2 kHz may be too low for

---

16. Really this is semidecimation, since decimation strictly means keeping every tenth item; here we twist the meaning slightly and keep every fifth sample.

some applications, and changes to the hardware (in the oversampling stage) may be required. However, even in murine studies, a sampling rate of 2 kHz is considered sufficiently high [48].

The system design described above is available from the Web site that accompanies this book [1]. However, this circuit should not be used on living entities without further tests. The next section outlines many of the issues that must be addressed before live subject data acquisition can commence.

2.5.10   Hardware Testing, Patient Safety, and Standards

Once fabricated and tested for basic functionality, it is important to test that a wide range of ECG signals will not be distorted by the acquisition system. There are several ways to achieve this. For instance, the transfer function for the system can be experimentally derived by using a signal generator to pump a range of frequencies with known amplitudes into the input electrodes and compared with the output response. However, the inevitable imperfections in this derived transfer function do not give a direct understanding of how significantly distorted clinical metrics derived from the ECG may be. In order to test such a system, one may choose to drive the inputs with either a database of representative signals or an artificial ECG-like signal. Although the former approach provides a realistic range of data (using a variety of known databases), there is an inherent noise component in the signal which confounds any measure of fidelity. The difficulty in measuring the clinical parameters in such data further confounds the problem. Furthermore, the use of a particular database may bias the performance results. Unrepresentative, yet perhaps critical, waveform types may remain untested.

Conversely, an artificial signal is noise-free and (in theory) has well-known properties. Conventional *phantom* ECG generators exist in the commercial domain which provide a noise-free wide range of lead configurations, heart rates, and arrhythmias. Unfortunately the details of the hardware used to generate these artificial signals are not available and so one can never know what the *ideal* input signal is, and what the clinical parameters in the signal are exactly. Another alternative is to generate the input signal by using an open-source algorithm (such as [56, 57]) which has completely known signal qualities, with markers for each clinical parameter. By varying the model over all possible heart rates, leads, and rhythms, and measuring the difference in all the clinical parameters, it is possible to rapidly determine under what circumstances the acquisition hardware causes significant distortions in the clinical parameters measured from the ECG. Of course, this method assumes that hardware to generate such as signal (with no significant distortions) already exists.

By far the most important step in the process of acquiring ECG is to ensure the safety of the subject being recorded. The standards that govern this evolve over time and differ from region to region, so no attempt is made in this chapter to give a definitive list of steps, and it is up to the reader to ensure that these steps are adhered to. At the time of this writing, the current international parent standard that addresses the many safety risks associated with electrical medical equipment (such as fire, mechanical hazards, and electric shock) is the International Electrotechnical Commission (IEC) Standard IEC 60601-1. This standard also forms the basis for standards in many other countries including UL 60601-1 for the United States, CAN/CSA C22.2 No. 601.1 for Canada, and EN 60601-1 for the European Union.

However, the common issues that arise in testing electrical circuits that are connected to living subjects tend to be centered around how energy can be transmitted from or absorbed into the device. The ECG acquisition system not only has to be of no significant danger to the subject for which it is intended, but it must also not interfere with any other devices either directly or through radio frequency (RF) energy. Therefore, each device fabricated must be tested (and documented) for:

- *Isolation:* Power transfer must be limited between the nonisolated and isolated parts of the circuit (both through the DC-to-DC converters and opto-isolators).
- *Leakage currents:* The human body has a finite resistance (or rather reactance) and therefore conducts (and stores) electricity. Any powered device that is physically connected to the body (or comes within a certain physical range) can lead to the conduction of electricity from the device to the body.
- *RF emissions:* There are strict upper limits of the RF energy that a device may emit (within individual frequency bands) so that it does not interfere with other electronic devices in close proximity.
- *RF shielding*: Similarly, there are strict lower limits on the amount of RF energy that a device must be shielded against. That is, one must test a device to determine that all its modes of operation are unaffected when bombarded with RF energy across a wide frequency spectrum.
- *Surge protection:* In some environments, massive electrical surges are possible, such as in hospital, when a patient is defibrillated. If the equipment is to be used in such environments, it must be capable of returning to a normal mode of operation within a few seconds (depending on the device's exact function).

The exact acceptable limits often depend on a device's classification (which usually depends on its intended use, intended environment, power source, and electronic configuration). Such testing and adherence to regulations are particularly important when the device is to be used in clinical (or aviation) environments. Furthermore, the rapid progress of RF technology and the subsequent evolution in RF shielding requirements, indicates that a forward-thinking policy should be adopted when designing ECG acquisition systems (particularly for ambulatory or uncontrolled environments). Even in 1998, the IEEE Committee on Man and Radiation (COMAR)[17] [58] released a statement expressing concern about the growing number of RF emitting devices becoming available and what this would mean for medical device safety. COMAR recommended that RF interference-prone medical devices should be reevaluated and redesigned to to avoid serious safety-related RF interference problems. Of particular concern is the growing use of cellular phone technology. For a more detailed discussion of these issues and the latest IEEE standards information, see [58–63].

---

17. A group of experts on health and safety issues related to electromagnetic fields.

2.6 Summary

One of the most often overlooked issues when dealing with ECG analysis, is the path of the recorded signal between the sensor and the signal processing algorithm, and hence any possible biases the collection and storage methods may have caused in the subsequent analysis. These include the activity of the patient, the resolution and quality of the ECG, the lack of sufficient information (either from too few leads, or too few related signals such as blood pressure or activity annotations), and the selection of the population itself. Furthermore, the safe and secure storage of the ECG in a format that is easily read and annotated leads to an efficient and verifiable analysis.

In this chapter the main steps for designing and implementing an ECG acquisition system have been described with attention to the possible sources of error, particularly from signal acquisition, transmission, and storage. It is hoped that these discussions will not only provide the reader with sufficient background to design their own ECG collection system, but will also provide food for thought during the analysis stage. Being able to identify systematic anomalies in signals, that appear to have a physiological origin, is of great importance. Without experience or knowledge of the hardware used to acquire the ECG, it is often difficult, and sometimes impossible, to make this distinction.

References

[1]   Clifford, G. D., F. Azuaje, and P. E. McSharry, "Advanced Tools for ECG Analysis," http://www.ecgtools.org/, September 2006.

[2]   Mohan, T. M., N. abd Undeland, and W. P. Robbins, *Power Electronics: Converters, Applications and Design*, New York: Wiley, 1989.

[3]   Oppenheim, A. V., and R. W. Schafer, *Discrete-Time Signal Processing*, Englewood Cliffs, NJ: Prentice-Hall, 1999.

[4]   Johanson, P., et al., "Prognostic Value of ST-Segment Resolution—When and What to Measure," *Eur. Heart J.*, Vol. 24, No. 4, 2003, pp. 337–345.

[5]   Clifford, G. D., and L. Tarassenko, "Segmenting Cardiac-Related Data Using Sleep Stages Increases Separation Between Normal Subjects and Apnoeic Patients," *IOP Physiol. Meas.*, Vol. 25, 2004, pp. N27–N35.

[6]   Clifford, G. D., and L. Tarassenko, "Quantifying Errors in Spectral Estimates of HRV Due to Beat Replacement and Resampling," *IEEE Trans. Biomed. Eng.*, Vol. 52, No. 4, April 2005, pp. 630–638.

[7]   Frank, E., "An Accurate, Clinically Practical System for Spatial Vectorcardiography," *Circulation*, Vol. 13, No. 5, 1956, pp. 737–749.

[8]   Edenbrandt, L., A. Houston, and P. W. Macfarlane, "Vectorcardiograms Synthesized from 12-Lead ECGs: A New Method Applied in 1792 Healthy Children," *Pediatr. Cardiol.*, Vol. 15, 1994, pp. 21–26.

[9]   Riekkinen, H., and P. Rautaharju, "Body Position, Electrode Level and Respiration Effects on the Frank Lead Electrocardiogram," *Circulation*, Vol. 53, 1976, pp. 40–45.

[10] Madias, J. E., "A Comparison of 2-Lead, 6-Lead, and 12-Lead ECGs in Patients with Changing Edematous States: Implications for the Employment of Quantitative Electrocardiography in Research and Clinical Applications," *Chest*, Vol. 124, No. 6, 2003, pp. 2057–2063.

[11]   Macfarlane, P. W., S. C. McLaughlin, and J. C. Rodger, "Influence of Lead Selection and Population on Automated Measurement of QT Dispersion," *Circulation*, Vol. 98, No. 20, 1998, pp. 2160–2167.

[12]   Kligfield, P., "QT Analysis: Problems and Prospects," *International Journal of Bioelectromagnetism*, Vol. 5, No. 1, 2003, pp. 205–206.

[13]   Drew, B. J., and M. W. Krucoff, "Multilead ST-Segment Monitoring in Patients with Acute Coronary Syndromes: A Consensus Statement for Healthcare Professionals," *ST-Segment Monitoring Practice Guideline International Working Group*, Am. J. Crit. Care, Vol. 8, 1999, pp. 372–388.

[14]   Drew, B. J., et al., "Practice Standards for Electrocardiographic Monitoring in Hospital Settings: An American Heart Association Scientific Statement from the Councils on Cardiovascular Nursing, Clinical Cardiology, and Cardiovascular Disease in the Young: Endorsed by the International Society of Computerized Electrocardiology and the American Association of Critical-Care Nurses," *Circulation*, Vol. 110, No. 17, 2004, pp. 2721–2746.

[15]   Weyne, A. E., et al., "Assessment of Myocardial Ischemia by 12-Lead Electrocardiography and Frank Vector System During Coronary Angioplasty: Value of a New Orthogonal Lead System for Quantitative ST Segment Monitoring," *J. Am. Coll. Cardiol.*, Vol. 18, No. 7, December 1991, pp. 1704–1710.

[16]   Moody, G. B., et al., "Clinical Validation of the ECG-Derived Respiration (EDR) Technique," *Computers in Cardiology*, Vol. 13, 1986, pp. 507–510.

[17]   Feild, D. Q., C. L. Feldman, and B. M. Horacek, "Improved EASI Coefficients: Their Derivation, Values, and Performance," *Journal of Electrocardiology*, Vol. 35, No. 4(2), October 2002, pp. 23–33.

[18]   Fletcher, G. F., et al., "Exercise Standards: A Statement for Healthcare Professionals from the American Heart Association," *Circulation*, Vol. 91, No. 2, 2001, pp. 580–615.

[19]   Mason, R. E., and I. Likar, "A New System of Multiple-Lead Exercise Electrocardiography," *Am. J. Heart*, Vol. 71, 1966, pp. 196–205.

[20]   Welinder, A., et al., "Comparison of Signal Quality Between EASI and Mason-Likar 12-Lead Electrocardiograms During Physical Activity," *Am. J. Crit. Care.*, Vol. 13, No. 3, 2004, pp. 228–234.

[21]   Prance, R. J., et al., "An Ultra-Low-Noise Electrical-Potential Probe for Human-Body Scanning," *Measurement Science and Technology*, Vol. 11, No. 3, 2000, pp. 291–297.

[22]   Harland, C. J., T. D. Clark, and R. J. Prance, "Electric Potential Probes—New Directions in the Remote Sensing of the Human Body," *Measurement Science and Technology*, Vol. 13, No. 2, 2002, pp. 163–169.

[23]   Rechtschaffen, A., and A. Kales, *A Manual of Standardized Terminology, Techniques and Scoring System for Sleep Stages of Human Subjects*, Washington, D.C.: Public Health Service, U.S. Government Printing Office, 1968.

[24]   Riker, R. R., J. T. Picard, and G. L. Fraser, "Prospective Evaluation of the Sedation-Agitation Scale for Adult Critically Ill Patients," *Crit. Care. Med.*, Vol. 27, 1999, pp. 1325–1329.

[25]   Kemp, J., and B. Olivan, "European Data Format 'Plus' (EDF+), an EDF Alike Standard Format for the Exchange of Physiological Data," *Clinical Neurophysiology*, Vol. 114, 2003, pp. 1755–1761, http://www.hsr.nl/edf/specs/edfplus.html.

[26]   Fischer, R., et al., "Communication and Retrieval of ECG Data: How Many Standards Do We Need?" *Computers in Cardiology*, Vol. 30, 2003, pp. 21–24.

[27]   Yoo, S., et al., "Design and Implementation of HL7 Based Real-Time Clinical Data Integration System," *METMBS*, 2003, pp. 222–230.

[28]   Goldberger, A. L., R. G. Mark, and G. B. Moody, "PhysioNet: The Research Resource for Complex Physiologic Signals," http://www.physionet.org.

[29]   Goldberger, A. L., et al., "Physiobank, Physiotoolkit, and Physionet: Components of a New Research Resource for Complex Physiologic Signals," *Circulations*, Vol. 101, No. 23, 2000, pp. e215–e220.

[30]   FDA XML Data Format Design Specification, Draft C. "Technical Report," FDA, April 2002.

[31]   Specification for the CDISC operational data model (ODM), version 1.1., "Technical Report, The Clinical Data Interchange Standards Consortium (CDISC)," May 2002.

[32]   Wang, H., et al., "Methods and Tools for Generating and Managing ecgML-Based Information," *Computers in Cardiology*, Vol. 31, 2004, pp. 573–576.

[33]   Schneider, R., libRASCH, http://www.librasch.org/.

[34]   ANSI/AAMI-EC38, *Ambulatory Electrocardiographs*, technical report, American National Standard Institute, August 1994.

[35]   AAMI-ECAR, *Recommended Practice for Testing and Reporting Performance Results of Ventricular Arrhythmia Detection Algorithms*, technical report, Association for the Advancement of Medical Instrumentation, April 1987.

[36]   Moody, G. B., "PhysioNet: The Research Resource for Complex Physiologic Signals: Physiobank Annotations," http://www.physionet.org/physiobank/annotations.shtml.

[37]   Hamilton, P., and W. Tompkins, "Quantitative Investigation of QRS Detection Rules Using the Mit/Bih Arrythmia Database," *IEEE Trans. Biomed. Eng.*, Vol. 33, No. 12, 1986.

[38]   Pan, J., and W. J. Tompkins, "A Real-Time QRS Detection Algorithm," *IEEE Trans. Biomed. Eng.*, Vol. 32, No. 3, 1985, pp. 220–236.

[39]   Hamilton, P., and M. Curley, "EP Limited: Open Source Arrhythmia Detection Software," http://www.eplimited.com/.

[40]   Sörnmo, L., and P. Laguna, *Bioelectric Signal Processing in Cardiac and Neurological Applications*, Amsterdam: Elsevier Academic Press, 2005.

[41]   Khöler, B.-U., C. Hennig, and R. Orglmeister, "The Principles of Software QRS Detection," *IEEE Eng. in Med. and Biol. Mag.*, Vol. 21, No. 1, January/February 2002, pp. 42–57.

[42]   Martínez, J. P., et al., "A Wavelet-Based ECG Delineator: Evaluation on Standard Database," *IEEE Trans. on Biomed. Eng.*, Vol. 51, No. 4, 2004, pp. 558–570.

[43]   OrCAD, "PCB Design Software," http://www.orcad.com/.

[44]   PCB123, "PCB Design Software," http://www.pcb123.com/.

[45]   Feinberg, B. N., *Applied Clinical Engineering*, Englewood Cliffs, NJ: Prentice-Hall, 1986.

[46]   Webster, J. G., "Interference and Motion Artifact in Biopotential," *IEEE Region 6 Conference Record*, May 25–27, 1977, pp. 53–64, http://ieeexplore.ieee.org/ie14/5782/15429/00721100.pdf.

[47]   Jarvis, M. R., and P. P. Mitra, "Apnea Patients Characterized by 0.02 Hz Peak in the Multitaper Spectrogram of Electrocardiogram Signals," *Computers in Cardiology*, Vol. 27, 2000, pp. 769–772.

[48]   Ai, H. B., et al., "Studies on the Time Domain and Power Spectrum of High Frequency ECG in Normal Mice," *Sheng Li Xue Bao (Acta physiologica Sinica)*, Vol. 48, No. 8, October 1996, pp. 512–516.

[49]   Hunt, A. C., "T Wave Alternans in High Arrhythmic Risk Patients: Analysis in Time and Frequency Domains: A Pilot Study," *BMC Cardiovasc. Disord.*, Vol. 2, No. 6, March 2002.

[50]   Pettersson, J., O. Pahlm, and E. Carro, "Changes in High-Frequency QRS Components Are More Sensitive Than ST-Segment Deviation for Detecting Acute Coronary Artery Occlusion," *J. Am. Coll. Cardiol.*, Vol. 36, 2000 pp. 1827–1834.

[51]   Schlegel, T. T., et al., "Real-Time 12-Lead High-Frequency QRS Electrocardiography for Enhanced Detection of Myocardial Ischemia and Coronary Artery Disease," *Mayo Clin. Proc.*, Vol. 79, 2004, pp. 339–350.

[52]   Spackman, T. N., M. D. Abel, and T. T. Schlegel, "Twelve-Lead High-Frequency QRS Electrocardiography During Anesthesia in Healthy Subjects," *Anesth. Analg.*, Vol. 100, No. 4, 2005, pp. 1043–1047.

[53]   Abboud, S., and O. Barnea, "Errors Due to Sampling Frequency of Electrocardiogram in Spectral Analysis of Heart Rate Signals with Low Variability," *Computers in Cardiology*, Vol. 22, September 1995, pp. 461–463.

[54]   Ward, S., et al., "Electrocardiogram Sampling Frequency Errors in PR Interval Spectral Analysis," *Proc. IEEE PGBIOMED'04*, Southampton, U.K., August 2004.

[55]   Clifford, G. D., and P. E. McSharry, "Method to Filter ECGs and Evaluate Clinical Parameter Distortion Using Realistic ECG Model Parameter Fitting," *Computers in Cardiology*, Vol. 32, 2005.

[56]   McSharry, P. E., G. D. Clifford, and L. Tarassenko, "A Dynamical Model for Generating Synthetic Electrocardiogram Signals," *IEEE Trans. Biomed. Eng.*, Vol. 50, No. 3, 2003, pp. 289–294.

[57]   McSharry, P. E., and G. D. Clifford, "ECGSYN—A Realistic ECG Waveform Generator," http://www.physionet.org/physiotools/ecgsyn/.

[58]   The IEEE Committee on Man and Radiation (COMAR) Technical Information Statement, "Radiofrequency Interference with Medical Devices," *IEEE Eng. in Med. and Biol. Mag.*, Vol. 17, No. 3, May/June 1998, pp. 111–114.

[59]   "IEC1000-4-3, International Electrotechnical Commission: Electromagnetic Compatibility, Part 4: Testing and Measurement Techniques—Section 3: Radiated Radio Frequency, Electromagnetic Field Immunity Test," IEEE Standard C95.1–1991, 1995.

[60]   U.S. Food and Drug Administration, "Medical Device User Facility and Manufacturer Reporting, Certification, and Registration: Delegations of Authority; Medical Device Reporting Procedures; Final Rules, 21 CFR Part 803," USFDA, December 1995.

[61]   IEEE C95.1-1991, "Standard for Safety Levels with Respect to Human Exposure to Radio Frequency Electromagnetic Fields, 3 kHz to 300 GHz, Updated 1999," IEEE Standard C95.1–1991, 1999.

[62]   COMAR Technical Information Statement, "The IEEE Exposure Limits for Radiofrequency and Microwave Energy," *IEEE Eng. in Med. and Biol. Mag.*, Vol. 24, No. 2, March/April 2005, pp. 114–121.

[63]   Petersen, R. C., et al., "International Committee on Electromagnetic Safety," http://grouper.ieee.org/groups/scc28/.

CHAPTER 3

ECG Statistics, Noise, Artifacts, and Missing Data

Gari D. Clifford

3.1 Introduction

Chapter 1 presented a description of the ECG in terms of its etiology and clinical features, and Chapter 2 an overview of the possible sources of error introduced in the hardware collection and data archiving stages. With this groundwork in mind, this chapter is intended to introduce the reader to the ECG using a signal processing approach. The ECG typically exhibits both persistent features (such as the average P-QRS-T morphology and the short-term average heart rate, or average RR interval), and nonstationary features (such as the individual RR and QT intervals, and long-term heart rate trends). Since changes in the ECG are quasi-periodic (on a beat-to-beat, daily, and perhaps even monthly basis), the frequency can be quantified in both statistical terms (mean, variance) and via spectral estimation methods. In essence, all these statistics quantify the power or degree to which an oscillation is present in a particular frequency band (or at a particular scale), often expressed as a ratio to power in another band. Even for scale-free approaches (such as wavelets), the process of feature extraction tends to have a bias for a particular scale which is appropriate for the particular data set being analyzed. ECG statistics can be evaluated directly on the ECG signal, or on features extracted from the ECG. The latter category can be broken down into either morphology-based features (such as ST level) or timing-based statistics (such as heart rate variability). Before discussing these derived statistics, an overview of the ECG itself is given.

3.2 Spectral and Cross-Spectral Analysis of the ECG

The short-term spectral content for a lead II configuration and the source ECG segment are shown in Figure 3.1. Note the peaks in the power spectral density (PSD) at 1, 4, 7, and 10 Hz, corresponding approximately to the heart rate (60 bpm), T wave, P wave, and the QRS complex, respectively. The spectral content for each lead is highly similar regardless of the lead configuration, although the actual energy at each frequency may differ.

55

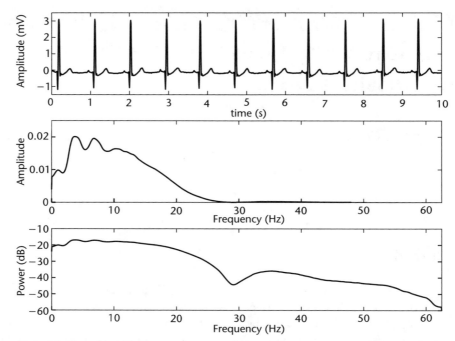

Figure 3.1   Ten seconds of 125-Hz typical ECG in sinus rhythm recorded with a lead II placement (upper plot) and associated linear and log-linear periodograms (middle and lower plots, respectively). A 256-point Welch periodogram was used with a hamming window and a 64-point overlap for the PSD calculation.

Figure 3.2 illustrates the PSDs for a typical full (12-lead) 10-second recording.[1] To estimate the spectral similarity between pairs of leads, the cross spectral coherence (CSC) can be calculated. The magnitude squared coherence estimate between two signals x and y, is

$$C_{xy} = \left| P_{xy}^2 \right| / (P_x P_y) \tag{3.1}$$

where P_x is the power spectral estimate of x, P_y is the power spectral estimate of y, and P_{xy} is the cross power spectral estimate[2] of x and y. Coherence is a function of frequency with C_{xy} ranging between 0 and 1 and indicates how well signal x corresponds to signal y at each frequency.

The CSC between any pair of leads will give values greater than 0.9 at most physiologically significant frequencies (1 to 10 Hz); see Figure 3.3. Note also that there is a significant coherent component between 12 and 50 Hz. By comparing this with the CSC between two adjacent 10-second segments of the same ECG lead, we can see that this higher frequency component is absent, indicating that it is due to some transient or incoherent phenomena, such as observation or muscle noise. Note that there is still a significant amount of coherence within the spectral band

---

1.   [Px, Fx] = PWELCH(ECG,HAMMING(512),256,512,1000); in Matlab.
2.   This operation can be achieved by using Matlab's MSCOHERE.M which uses Welch's averaged periodogram method [1], or by using COHERE.C from PhysioNet [2].

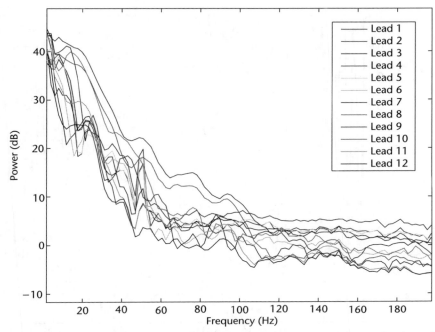

Figure 3.2 PSD (dB/Hz) of all 12 standard leads of 10 seconds of an ECG in sinus rhythm. A 512-point Welch periodogram was used with a hamming window and with a 256-point overlap. Note that the leads are numbered arbitrarily, rather than using their clinical labels.

corresponding to the heart rate (HR), T wave, P wave, and QRS complex (1 to 10 Hz). Changing heart rates (which lead to changing morphology; see Section 3.3) and varying the FFT window size and overlap will change the relative magnitude of this cross-coherence. Furthermore, different pairs of leads may show differing degrees of CSC due to dispersion effects (see Section 3.3).

3.2.1 Extreme Low- and High-Frequency ECG

Although the accepted range of the diagnostic ECG is often quoted to be from 0.05 Hz (for ST analysis) to 40 or 100 Hz, information does exist beyond these limits. Ventricular late potentials (VLPs) are microvolt fluctuations that manifest in the terminal portion of the QRS complex and can persist into the ST-T segment. They represent areas of delayed ventricular activation which are manifestations of slowed conduction velocity (resulting from ischemia or deposition of collagens after an acute myocardial infarction). VLPs, therefore, are interesting for heart disease diagnosis [3–5]. The upper frequency limit of VLPs can be as high as 500 Hz [6].

On the low frequency end of the spectrum, Jarvis and Mitra [7] have demonstrated that sleep apnea may be diagnosed by observing power changes in the ECG at 0.02 Hz.

3.2.2 The Spectral Nature of Arrhythmias

Arrhythmias, which manifest due to abnormalities in the conduction pathways of the heart, can generally be grouped into either atrial or ventricular arrhythmias. Ventricular arrhythmias manifest as gross distortions of the beat morphology since

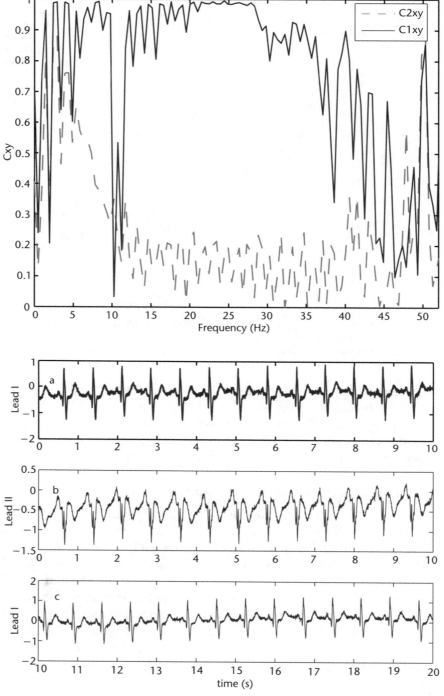

Figure 3.3 Cross-spectral coherence of two ECG sections in sinus rhythm. $C1_{xy}$ (solid line) is the CSC between two simultaneous lead I and lead II sections of ECG (plot *a* and plot *b* in the lower half of the figure). Note the significant coherence between 3 Hz and 35 Hz. $C2_{xy}$ (dashed line) is the CSC between two adjacent 10-second sections of lead I ECG (plot *a* and plot *c* in the lower half of the figure). Note that there is significantly less coherence between the adjacent signals except at 50 Hz (mains noise) and between 1 and 10 Hz.

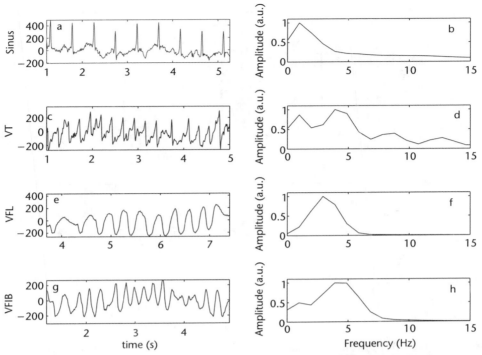

Figure 3.4   (a) Sinus rhythm and (b) corresponding PSD. (c) Ventricular tachycardia (VT) and (d) corresponding PSD. (e) Ventricular flutter (VFL) and (f) corresponding PSD. (g) Ventricular fibrillation (VFIB) and (h) corresponding PSD. Note that ventricular beats exhibit broader QRS complexes and therefore a shift in QRS energy to lower frequencies. Note also that higher frequencies (than normal) also manifest. VFL destroys many of the subtle ECG features and manifests as a sinusoidal-like oscillation around the frequency of the (rapid) heart rate. VFIB manifests as a less organized and more rapid oscillation, and therefore the spectrum is broader with more energy at higher frequencies. (All PSDs were calculated on 5-second segments with the same parameters as in Figure 3.1, but linear scales are used for clarity.)

the depolarization begins in the ventricles rather than the atria. The QRS complex becomes broader due to the depolarization occurring along an abnormal conduction path and therefore progressing more slowly, masking the latent P wave from delayed atrial depolarization. Figure 3.4(a) illustrates a 5-second segment of ventricular tachycardia (VT) with a high heart rate of around 180 bpm or 3 Hz, and the accompanying power spectral density [Figure 3.4(b)]. Although the broadening of the QRS complexes during VT causes a shift in the QRS spectral peak to slightly lower frequencies, the overall peaks are similar to the spectrum of a sinus rhythm[3] (see Figure 3.1), and therefore, spectral separation between sinus and VT rhythms is difficult. Figure 3.4(a) shows a 5-second segment of sinus rhythm ECG for the same patient before the episode of VT, with a relatively high heart rate (108 bpm). Note that although the P waves, QRS complexes, and T waves are discernible above the noise, the main spectral component is the 1- to 2-Hz baseline noise.

3.   Below 60 bpm sinus rhythm is known as sinus bradycardia, and between 100 to 150 bpm it is known as sinus tachycardia. Note also that sinus rhythm is sometimes known as sinus arrhythmia if the heart rate rises and falls periodically, such as in RSA; see Section 3.7.

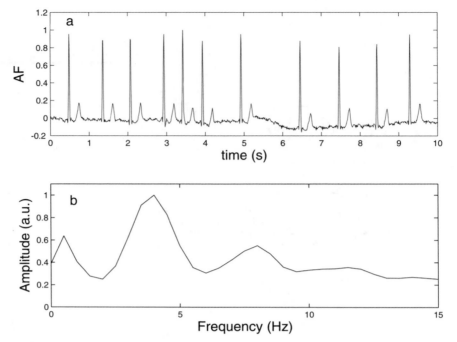

Figure 3.5   (a) Atrial fibrillation (AF) and (b) corresponding PSD. Note the similarity to sinus rhythm in Figure 3.4(a, b). (All PSDs were calculated with the same parameters as in Figure 3.4.)

When the ventricular activation time slows sufficiently, QRS complexes become severely broadened and ventricular flutter (VFL) is possible. This arrhythmia manifests as sinusoidal-like disturbances in the ECG, and is therefore relatively easy to detect through spectral methods. Figure 3.4(e) illustrates a 4-second segment of transient VFL and the corresponding power spectrum [Figure 3.4(f)]. If the ventricular arrhythmia is more erratic and manifests with a higher frequency of oscillation, then it is known as the extreme condition ventricular fibrillation (VFIB). Colloquially, the heart is said to be *squirming* "like a bag of worms," with little or no coherent activity. At this point, the heart is virtually useless as a pump and immediate physical or electrical intervention is required to encourage the cardiac cells to depolarize/repolarize in a coherent manner.

Atrial arrhythmias, in contrast to ventricular arrhythmias, manifest as small disturbances in the timing and relative position of the (relatively low amplitude) P wave and are therefore difficult to detect through spectral methods. Figure 3.5 illustrates the ECG and its corresponding power spectrum for an atrial arrhythmia. Atrial arrhythmias do, however, manifest significantly different changes in the beat-to-beat timing and can therefore be detected by collecting and analyzing statistics on such intervals [8] (see Section 3.5.3).

3.3   Standard Clinical ECG Features

Clinical assessment of the ECG mostly relies on relatively simple measurements of the intrabeat timings and amplitudes. Averaging over several beats is common to

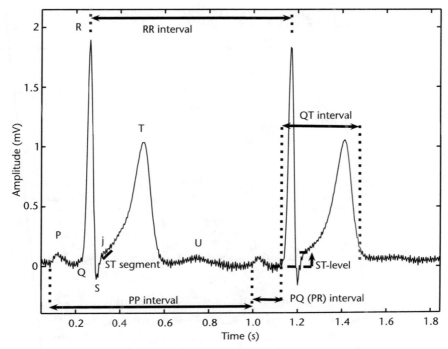

Figure 3.6 Standard fiducial points in the ECG (P, Q, R, S, T, and U) together with clinical features (listed in Table 3.1).

either reduce noise or average out short-term beat-to-beat interval-related changes. The complex heart rate-related changes in the ECG morphology (such as QT hysteresis[4]) can themselves be indicative of problems. However, a clinician can extract enough diagnostic information to make a useful assessment of cardiac abnormality from just a few simple measurements.

Figure 3.6 illustrates the most common clinical features, and Table 3.1 illustrates typical normal values for these standard clinical ECG features in healthy adult males in sinus rhythm, together with their upper and lower limits of normality. Note that these figures are given for a particular heart rate. It should also be noted that the heart rate is calculated as the number of P-QRS-T complexes per minute, but is often calculated over shorter segments of 15 and sometimes 30 seconds. In terms of modeling we can think of this heart rate as our *operating point* around which the local interbeat interval rises and falls. Of course, we can calculate a heart rate over any scale, up to a single beat. In the latter case, the heart rate is termed the instantaneous (or beat-to-beat) heart rate, $HR_i = 60/RR_n$, of the nth beat. Each consecutive beat-to-beat, or RR, interval[5] will be of a different length (unless the patient is paced), and a correlated change in ECG morphology is seen on a beat-to-beat basis.

---

4. See Section 3.4 and Chapter 11.
5. The beat-to-beat interval is usually measured between consecutive R-peaks and hence termed the RR interval. See Section 3.7.

Table 3.1 Typical Lead II ECG Features and Their Normal Values in Sinus Rhythm at a Heart Rate of 60 bpm for a Healthy Male Adult (see text and Figure 3.6 for definitions of intervals)

Feature	Normal Value	Normal Limit
P width	110 ms	±20 ms
PQ/PR interval	160 ms	±40 ms
QRS width	100 ms	±20 ms
QTc interval	400 ms	±40 ms
P amplitude	0.15 mV	±0.05 mV
QRS height	1.5 mV	±0.5 mV
ST level	0 mV	±0.1 mV
T amplitude	0.3 mV	±0.2 mV

Note: There is some variation between lead configurations. Heart rate, respiration patterns, drugs, gender, diseases, and ANS activity also change the values. $QTc = \alpha QT$ where $\alpha = (RR)^{-\frac{1}{2}}$. About 95% of (normal healthy adult) people have a QTc between 360 ms and 440 ms. Female durations tend to be approximately 1% to 5% shorter except for the QT/QTc, which tends to be approximately 3% to 6% longer than for males. Intervals tend to elongate with age, at a rate of approximately 10% per decade for healthy adults.

Often, the RR interval will oscillate periodically, shortening with inspiration (and lengthening with expiration). This phenomenon, known as respiratory sinus arrhythmia (RSA) is partly due to the Bainbridge reflex, the expansion and contraction of the lungs and the cardiac filling volume caused by variations of intrathoracic pressure [9]. During inspiration, the pressure within the thorax decreases and venous return increases, which stretches the right atrium resulting in a reflex that increases the local heart rate (i.e., shortens the RR intervals). During expiration, the reverse of this process results in a slowing of the local heart rate. In general, the normal beat-to-beat changes in morphology are ignored, except for derivations of respiration, although the phase between the respiratory RR interval oscillations and respiratory-related changes in ECG morphology is not static; see Section 3.8.2.2 and Chapter 8. The reason for this is that the mechanisms which alter amplitude and timing on the ECG are not exactly the same (although they are coupled either mechanically or neurally with a phase delay which may change from beat to beat; see Chapter 8). Changes in the features in Table 3.1 and Figure 3.6, therefore, occur on a beat-to-beat basis as well as because of shifts in the operating point (average heart rate), although this is a second order effect.

The PR interval extends from the start of the P wave to the end of the PQ-junction at the very start of the QRS complex (that is, to the start of the R or Q wave). Therefore, this interval is sometimes known as the PQ interval. This interval represents the time required for the electrical impulse to travel from the SA node to the ventricle and normal values range between 120 and 200 ms. The PR interval has been shown to lengthen and shorten with respiration in a similar manner to the RR interval, but is less pronounced and is not fully correlated with the RR interval oscillations [10].

The global point of reference for the ECG's amplitude is the isoelectric level, measured over the short period on the ECG between the atrial depolarization (P wave) and the ventricular depolarization (QRS complex). In general, this point is thought to be the most stable marker of 0V for the surface ECG since there is a short pause before the current is conducted between the atria and the ventricles.

Interbeat segments are not usually used as a reference point because activity before the P wave can often be dominated by preceding T-wave activity.

The QRS width is representative of the time for the ventricles to depolarize, typically lasting 80 to 120 ms. The lower the heart rate, the wider the QRS complex, due to decreases in conduction speed through the ventricle. The QRS width also changes from beat-to-beat based upon the QRS axis (see Chapter 1), which is correlated with the phase of respiration (see Chapter 8) and with changes in RR interval and therefore the local heart rate. The RS segment of the QRS complex is known as the ventricular activation time (VAT) and is usually shorter (lasting around 40 ms) than the QR segment. This asymmetry in the QRS complex is not a constant and varies based upon changes in the autonomic nervous system (ANS) axis, lead position, respiration and heart rate (see Chapter 8).

The QRS complex usually rises (for positive leads) or falls to about 1 to 2 mV from the isoelectric line for normal beats. Artifacts (such as electrode movements) and abnormal beats (such as ventricular ectopic beats) can be several times larger in amplitude. In particular, baseline wander can often be the largest amplitude signal on the ECG, with the QRS complexes appearing as almost indistinguishable periodic anomalies. For this reason, it is important to allow sufficient dynamic range in the amplification (or digital storage) of ECG data; see Chapter 2.

The point of inflection after the S wave is known as the j-point, and is often used to define the beginning of the ST segment. In normals, it is expected to be isoelectric since it is the pause between ventricular depolarization and repolarization. The ST level is generally measured around 60 to 80 ms after the j-point, with adjustments for local heart rates (see Chapters 9 and 10). Abnormal changes in the ECG, defined by the Sheffield criteria [11], are ST level shifts ≥ 0.1 mV (or about 5% to 10% of the QRS amplitude for a sinus beat on a V5 lead). Since only small deviations form the isoelectric level are significant markers of cardiac abnormality (such as ischemia), the correct measurement of the isoelectric line is crucial. The interbeat segments between the end of the P wave and start of the Q wave are so short (less than 10 samples at 125 Hz), that the isoelectric baseline measurement is prone to noise. Multiple-beat averaging is therefore often employed. ST segment and j-point elevation, common in athletes, has been reported to normalize with exercise [12] and therefore j-point elevations may be difficult to distinguish from other changes seen in ECG.

The QT interval is measured between the onset of the QRS complex and the end of the T wave. It is considered to represent the time between the start of ventricular depolarization and the end of ventricular repolarization and is therefore useful as a measure of the duration of repolarization (see Chapter 11). The QT interval varies depending on heart rate, age, and gender. As with some other parameters in the ECG, it is possible to approximate the (average) heart rate dependency of the QT interval by multiplying it by a factor $\alpha = (\hat{R}R)^{-\frac{1}{2}}$ where $\hat{R}R$ is the local average RR interval. The resultant QT interval is called the *corrected* QT interval, QTc [13]. However, this factor works over a limited range and is subject dependent to some degree, over and above the usual confounding variables of age, gender, and drug regime; see Section 3.4.1.

Furthermore, ANS activity shifts can also change α. In general, the last RR interval duration affects the action potential (see Chapter 1) and hence the QT interval. It is also known that the QT-RR dependence is both a function of the average heart rate and the instantaneous interval, RR_i [14]. Note that there is some variation in these parameters between lead configurations. Although inter-lead differences are sometimes used as cardiovascular markers themselves (such as in QT dispersion [15]), it is unclear whether there is a specific physiological origin to such differences, or whether such metrics are just measuring an artifact which correlates with a clinical marker [16, 17].

One of the problems in measuring the QT interval correctly (apart from the noise in the ECG and the resultant onset and offset ambiguities) is due to the changes in the j-point and T wave morphology with heart rate. It has been observed that as the heart rate increases, the T wave increases in height and becomes more symmetrical [18]. Furthermore, in some subject groups (such as athletes), the T wave is often observed to be inverted [12].

To summarize, the following changes are typically observed with increasing heart rate [12, 18, 19]:

- The average RR interval decreases.
- The PR segment shortens and slopes downward (in the inferior leads).
- The P wave height increases.
- The Q wave becomes slightly more negative (at very high heart rates).
- The QRS width decreases.
- The R wave amplitude decreases in the lateral leads (e.g., V5) at and just after high heart rates.
- The S wave becomes more negative in the lateral and vertical leads (e.g., V5 and aVF). As the R wave decreases in amplitude, the S wave increases in depth.
- The j-point often becomes depressed in lateral leads. However, subjects with a normal or resting j-point elevation may develop an isoelectric j-point with higher heart rates.
- The ST level changes (depressed in inferior leads).
- The T wave amplitude increases and becomes more symmetrical (although it can initially drop at the onset of a heart rate increase).
- The QT interval shortens (depending on the autonomic tone).
- The U wave does appear to change significantly. However, U waves may be difficult to identify due to the short interval between the T and following beat's P waves at high heart rates.

It should be noted however, that this simple description is insufficient to describe the complex changes that take place in the ECG as the heart rate increases and decreases. These dynamics are further explored in the following section.

3.4 Nonstationarities in the ECG

Nonstationarities in the ECG manifest both in an interbeat basis (as RR interval timing changes) and on an intrabeat basis (as morphological changes). Although the former changes are often thought of as rhythm disturbances and the latter as beat abnormalities, the etiology of the changes are often intricately connected. To be clear, although we could categorize the beat-to-beat changes in the RR interval timing and ECG morphology as nonstationary, they can actually be well represented by nonlinear models (see Section 3.7 and Chapter 4). This chapter therefore refers to these changes as stationary (but nonlinear). The transitions between rhythms is a nonstationary process (although some nonlinear models exist for limited changes). In this chapter, abnormal changes in beat morphology or rhythm that suggest a rapid change in the underlying physiology are referred to as nonstationary.

3.4.1   Heart Rate Hysteresis

So far we have not considered the dynamic effects of heart rate on the ECG morphology. Sympathetic or parasympathetic changes in the ANS which lead to changes in the heart rate and ECG morphology are asymmetric. That is, the dynamic changes that occur as the heart rate increases, are not matched (in a time symmetric manner) when the heart rate reduces and there is a (several beat) lag in the response between the RR interval change and the subsequent morphology change. One well-known form of heart rate-related hysteresis is that of *QT hysteresis*. In the context of QT interval changes, this means that the standard QT interval correction factors[6] are a gross simplification of the relationship, and that a more dynamic model is required. Furthermore, it has been shown that the relationship between the QT and RR interval is highly individual-specific [20], perhaps because of the dynamic nature of the system. In the QT-RR phase plane, the trajectory is therefore not confined to a single line and *hysteresis* is observed. That is, changes in RR interval do not cause immediate changes in the QT interval and ellipsoid-like trajectories manifest in the QT-RR plane. Figure 3.7 illustrates this point, with each of the central contours indicating a response of either tachycardia (RT) and bradycardia (RB) or normal resting. From the top right of each contour, moving counterclockwise (or anticlockwise); as the heart rate increases (the RR interval drops) the QT interval remains constant for a few beats, and then begins to shorten, approximately in an inverse square manner. When the heart rate drops (RR interval lengthens) a similar time delay is observed before the QT interval begins to lengthen and the subject returns to approximately the original point in the QT-RR phase plane. The difference between the two trajectories (caused by RR acceleration and deceleration) is the QT hysteresis, and depends not only on the individual's physiological condition, but also on the specific activity in the ANS. Although the central contour defines the limits of normality for a resting subject, active subjects exhibit an extended QT-RR contour. The 95% limits of normal activity are defined by the large, asymmetric dotted contour, and activity outside of this region can be considered abnormal.

The standard QT-RR relationship for low heart rates (defined by the Fridericia correction factor $QTc = QT/RR^{1/3}$) is shown by the line cutting the phase plane from lower left to upper right. It can be seen that this factor, when applied to the resting QT-RR interval relationship, overcorrects the dynamic responses in the normal range (illustrated by the striped area above the correction line and below the normal dynamic range) or underestimates QT prolongation at low heart rates

---

6.   Many QT correction factors have been considered that improve upon Bazett's formula ($QTc = QT/\sqrt{RR}$), including linear regression fitting ($QTc = QT + 0.154(1 - RR)$), which works well at high heart rates, and the Fridericia correction ($QTc = QT/RR^{1/3}$), which works well at low heart rates.

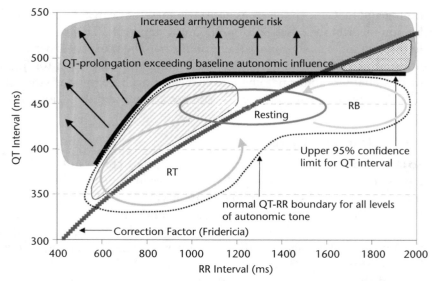

Figure 3.7 Normal dynamic QT-RR interval relationship (dotted-line forming asymmetric contour) encompasses autonomic reflex responses such as tachycardia (RT) and bradycardia (RB) with hysteresis. The statistical outer boundary of the normal contour is defined as the upper 95% confidence bounds. The Fridericia correction factor applied to the resting QT-RR interval relationship overcorrects dynamic responses in the normal range (striped area above correction line and below 95% confidence bounds) or underestimates QT prolongation at slow heart rates (shaded area above 95% confidence bounds but below Fridericia correction). QT prolongation of undefined arrhythmogenic risk (dark shaded area) occurs when exceeding the 95% confidence bounds of QT intervals during unstressed autonomic influence. (*From:* [21]. © 2005 ASPET: American Society for Pharmacology and Experimental Therapeutics. Reprinted with permission.)

(shaded area above normal range but below Fridericia correction) [21]. Abnormal QT prolongation is illustrated by the upper dark shaded area, and is defined to be when the QT-RR vector exceeds the 95% normal boundary (dotted line) during unstressed autonomic influence [21].

Another, more recently documented heart rate-related hysteresis is that of ST/HR [22], which is a measure of the ischemic reaction of the heart to exercise. If ST depression is plotted vertically so that negative values represent ST elevation, and heart rate is plotted along the horizontal axis typical ST/HR diagrams for a clinically normal subject display a negative hysteresis in ST depression against HR, (a clockwise hysteresis loop in the ST-HR phase plane during postexercise recovery). Coronary artery disease patients, on the other hand, display a positive hysteresis in ST depression against HR (a counterclockwise movement in the hysteresis loop during recovery) [23].

It is also known that the PR interval changes with heart rate, exhibiting a (mostly) respiration-modulated dynamic, similar to (but not as strong as) the modulation observed in the associated RR interval sequence [24]. This activity is described in more detail in Section 3.7.

3.4.2 Arrhythmias

The normal nonstationary changes are induced, in part, by changes in the sympathetic and parasympathetic branches of the autonomic nervous system. However, sudden (abnormal) changes in the ECG can occur as a result of malfunctions in the normal conduction pathways of the heart. These disturbances manifest on the ECG as, sometimes subtle, and sometimes gross distortions of the normal beat (depending on the observation lead or the physiological origin of the abnormality). Such beats are traditionally labeled by their etiology, into ventricular beats, supraventricular and atrial.[7]

Since ventricular beats are due to the excitation of the ventricles before the atria, the P wave is absent or obscured. The QRS complex also broadens significantly since conduction through the myocardium is consequently slowed (see Chapter 1). The overall amplitude and duration (energy) of such a beat is thus generally higher. QRS detectors can easily pick up such high energy beats and the distinct differences in morphology make classifying such beats a fairly straightforward task. Furthermore, ventricular beats usually occur much earlier or later than one would expect for a normal sinus beat and are therefore known as VEBs, ventricular *ectopic* beats (from the Greek, meaning out of place).

Abnormal atrial beats exhibit more subtle changes in morphology than ventricular beats, often resulting in a reduced or absent P wave. The significant changes for an atrial beat come from the differences in interbeat timings (see Section 3.2.2). Unfortunately, from a classification point of view, abnormal beats are sometimes more frequent when artifact increases (such as during stress tests). Furthermore, artifacts can often resemble abnormal beats, and therefore extra information from multiple leads and beat context are often required to make an accurate classification.

3.5   Arrhythmia Detection

If conduction abnormalities are transient, then an abnormal beat manifests. If conduction problems persist, then the abnormal morphology repeats and an arrhythmia is manifest, or the ECG degenerates into an almost unrecognizable pattern. There are three general approaches to arrhythmia analysis. One method is to perform QRS detection and beat classification, labeling an arrhythmia as a quorum of a series of beats of a particular type. The common alternative approach is to analyze a section of the ECG that spans several beat intervals, calculate a statistic (such as variance or a ratio of power at different frequencies) on which the arrhythmia classification is performed. A third option is to construct a model of the expected dynamics for different rhythms and compare the observed signal (or derived features) to this model. Such model-based approaches can be divided down into ECG-based methods or RR interval statistics-based methods. Linear ECG-modeling techniques [26] are essentially equivalent to spectral analysis. Nonlinear state-space model reconstructions have also been used [27], but with varying results. This may be partly due to the sensitivity of nonlinear metrics to noise. See Chapter 6 for a more detailed description of this technique together with a discussion of the problems associated with applying nonlinear techniques to noisy data.

---

7.   The table in [25], which lists all the beat classifications labeled in the PhysioNet databases [2] together with their alphanumeric labels, provides an excellent detailed list of beat types and rhythms.

3.5.1 Arrhythmia Classification from Beat Typing

A run of abnormal beats can be classified as an arrhythmia. Therefore, as long as consistent fiducial points can be located on a series of beats, simple postprocessing of a beat classifier's output together with a threshold on the heart rate can be sufficient for correctly identifying many arrhythmias. For example, supraventricular tachycardia is the sustained presence of supraventricular ectopic beats, at a rate over 100 bpm. Many more complex classification schemes have been proposed, including the use of principal component analysis [28, 29] (see Chapters 9 and 10) hidden Markov models [30], interlead comparisons [31], cluster analysis [32], and a variety of supervised and unsupervised neural learning techniques [33–35]. Further details of the latter category can be found in Chapters 12 and 13.

3.5.2 Arrhythmia Classification from Power-Frequency Analysis

Sometimes there is no consistently identifiable fiducial point in the ECG, and analysis of the normal clinical features is not possible. In such cases, it is usual to exploit the changes in frequency characteristics that are present during arrhythmias [36, 37]. More recently, joint time-frequency analysis techniques have been applied [38–40], to take advantage of the nonstationary nature of the cardiac cycle.

   Other interesting methods that make use of interchannel correlation techniques have been proposed [31], but results from using a decision tree and linear classifier on just three AR coefficients (effectively performing a multiple frequency band thresholding) give some of the most promising results. Dingfei et al. [26] report classification performance statistics (sensitivity, specificity) on the MIT-BIH database [2] of 93.2%, 94.4% for sinus rhythm, 100%, 96.2% for superventricular tachycardia, 97.7%, 98.6% for VT, and 98.6%, 97.7% for VFIB. They also report classification statistics (sensitivity, specificity) of 96.4%, 96.7% for atrial premature contractions (APCs), and 94.8%, 96.8% for premature ventricular contractions (PVCs).[8] Sensitivity and specificity figures in the mid to upper 90s can be considered state of the art. However, these results pertain to only one database and the (sensitive) window size is prechosen based upon the prior expectation of the rhythm. Despite this, this approach is extremely promising, and may be improved by developing a method for adapting the window size and/or using a nonlinear classifier such as a neural network.

3.5.3 Arrhythmia Classification from Beat-to-Beat Statistics

Zeng and Glass [8] described a model for AV node conduction which was able to accurately model many observations of the statistical distribution of the beat-to-beat intervals during atrial arrhythmias (see Chapter 4 for a more details on this model). This model-based approach was further extended in [41] to produce a method of classifying beats based upon their statistical distribution. Later, Schulte-Frohlinde et al. [42] produced a variant of this technique that includes a dimension of time and allows the researcher to observe the temporal statistical changes. Software for this technique (known as *heartprints*) is freely available from [43].

   More recent algorithms have attempted to combine both the spectral characteristics and time domain features of the ECG (including RR intervals) [44].

---

8.   Sometimes called VPCs (ventricular premature contractions).

The integration of such techniques can help improve arrhythmia classification, but only if the learning set is expanded in size and complexity in a manner that is sufficient to provide enough training examples to account for the increased dimensionality of the input feature space. See Chapters 12 and 13 for further discussions of training, test, and validation data sets.

3.6 Noise and Artifact in the ECG

3.6.1 Noise and Artifact Sources

Unfortunately, the ECG is often contaminated by noise and artifacts[9] that can be within the frequency band of interest and can manifest with similar morphologies as the ECG itself. Broadly speaking, ECG contaminants can be classified as [45]:

1. *Power line interference:* 50 ± 0.2 Hz mains noise (or 60 Hz in many data sets[10]) with an amplitude of up to 50% of full scale deflection (FSD), the peak-to-peak ECG amplitude;

2. *Electrode pop or contact noise:* Loss of contact between the electrode and the skin manifesting as sharp changes with saturation at FSD levels for periods of around 1 second on the ECG (usually due to an electrode being nearly or completely pulled off);

3. *Patient–electrode motion artifacts:* Movement of the electrode away from the contact area on the skin, leading to variations in the impedance between the electrode and skin causing potential variations in the ECG and usually manifesting themselves as rapid (but continuous) baseline jumps or complete saturation for up to 0.5 second;

4. *Electromyographic (EMG) noise:* Electrical activity due to muscle contractions lasting around 50 ms between dc and 10,000 Hz with an average amplitude of 10% FSD level;

5. *Baseline drift:* Usually from respiration with an amplitude of around 15% FSD at frequencies drifting between 0.15 and 0.3 Hz;

6. *Data collecting device noise:* Artifacts generated by the signal processing hardware, such as signal saturation;

7. *Electrosurgical noise:* Noise generated by other medical equipment present in the patient care environment at frequencies between 100 kHz and 1 MHz, lasting for approximately 1 and 10 seconds;

8. *Quantization noise and aliasing;*

9. *Signal processing artifacts* (e.g., Gibbs oscillations).

Although each of these contaminants can be reduced by judicious use of hardware and experimental setup, it is impossible to remove all contaminants. Therefore, it is important to quantify the nature of the noise in a particular data set and

---

9. It should be noted that the terms *noise* and *artifact* are often used interchangeably. In this book *artifact* is used to indicate the presence of a transient interruption (such as electrode motion) and *noise* is used to describe a persistent contaminant (such as mains interference).

10. Including recordings made in North and Central America, western Japan, South Korea, Taiwan, Liberia, Saudi Arabia, and parts of the Caribbean, South America, and some South Pacific islands.

choose an appropriate algorithm suited to the contaminants as well as the intended application.

3.6.2 Measuring Noise in the ECG

The ECG contains very distinctive features, and automatic identification of these features is, to some extent, a tractable problem. However, quantifying the nonsignal (noise) element in the ECG is not as straightforward. This is partially due to the fact that there are so many different types of noises and artifacts (see above) that can occur simultaneously, and partially because these noises and artifacts are often transient, and largely unpredictable in terms of their onset and duration. Standard measures of noise-power assume stationarity in the dynamics and coloration of the noise. These include:

- Route mean square (RMS) power in the isoelectric region;
- Ratio of the R-peak amplitude to the noise amplitude in the isoelectric region;
- Crest factor / peak-to-RMS ratio (the ratio of the peak value of a signal to its RMS value);
- Ratio between in-band (5 to 40 Hz) and out-of-band spectral power;
- Power in the residual after a filtering process.

Except for (16.6, 50, or 60 Hz) mains interference and sudden abrupt baseline changes, the assumption that most noise is Gaussian in nature is approximately correct (due to the central limit theorem). However, the coloration of the noise can significantly affect any interpretation of the value of the noise power, since the more colored a signal is, the larger the amplitude for a given power. This means that a signal-to-noise ratio (SNR) for a brown noise contaminated ECG (such as movement artifact) equates to a much cleaner ECG than the same SNR for an ECG contaminated by pink noise (typical for observation noise). Figure 3.8 illustrates this point by comparing a zero-mean unit-variance clean ECG (upper plot) with the same signal with additive noise of decreasing coloration (lower autocorrelation). In each case, the noise is set to be zero-mean with unit variance, and therefore has the same power as the ECG (SNR = 1). Note that the whiter the noise, the more significant the distortion for a given SNR. It is obvious that ECG analysis algorithms will perform differently on each of these signals, and therefore it is important to record the coloration of the noise in the signal as well as the SNR.

Determining the color of the noise in the ECG is a two-stage process which first involves locating and removing the P-QRS-T features. Moody et al. [28, 29] have shown that the QRS complex can be encoded in the first five principal components (PCs). Therefore, a good approximate method for removing the signal component from an ECG is to use all but the first five PCs to reconstruct the ECG. Principal component analysis (PCA) involves the projection of N-dimensional data onto a set of N orthogonal axes that represent the maximum directions of variance in the data. If the data can be well represented by such a projection, the p axes along which the variance is largest are good descriptors of the data. The $N - p$ remaining components are therefore projections of the noise. A more in-depth analysis of PCA can be found in Chapters 5 and 9.

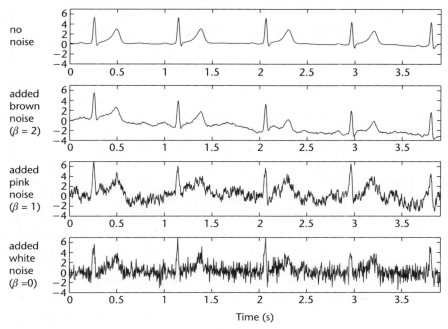

no noise

added brown noise ($\beta = 2$)

added pink noise ($\beta = 1$)

added white noise ($\beta = 0$)

Time (s)

Figure 3.8 Zero-mean unit-variance clean ECG with additive brown, pink, and white noise (also zero-mean and unit-variance, and hence SNR = 1 in all cases).

Practically, this involves segmenting each beat in the given analysis window[11] such that the start of each P wave and the end of each T wave (or U wave if present) are captured in each segmentation with m-samples. The N beats are then aligned so that they form an $N \times m$ matrix denoted, X. If singular value decomposition (SVD) is then performed to determine the PCs, the five most significant components are discarded (by setting the corresponding eigenvalues to zero), and the SVD inverted, X becomes a matrix of only noise. The data can then be transformed back into a 1-D signal using the original segmentation indices.

The second stage involves calculating the log power-spectrum of this noise signal and determine its slope. The resultant spectrum has a $1/f^{\beta}$ form. That is, the slope β determines the color of the signal with the higher the value of β, the higher the auto-correlation. If $\beta = 0$, the signal is white (since the spectrum is flat) and is completely uncorrelated. If $\beta = 1$, the spectrum has a $1/f$ spectrum and is known as *pink* noise, typical of the observation noise on the ECG. Electrode movement noise has a Brownian motion-like form (with $\beta = 2$), and is therefore known as *brown* noise.

3.7 Heart Rate Variability

The baseline variability of the heart rate time series is determined by many factors including age, gender, activity, medications, and health [46]. However, not only

---

11. The window must contain at least five beats, and preferably at least 30 to capture respiration and ANS-induced changes in the ECG morphology; see Section 3.3.

does the mean beat-to-beat interval (the heart rate) change on many scales, but the variance of this sequence of each heartbeat interval does so too. On the shortest scale, the time between each heartbeat is irregular (unless the heart is paced by an artificial electrical source such as a pacemaker, or a patient is in a coma). These short-term oscillations reflect changes in the relative balance between the sympathetic and parasympathetic branches of the ANS, the *sympathovagal balance*. This heart rate irregularity is a well-studied effect known as *heart rate variability* (HRV) [47]. HRV metric values are often considered to reflect the competing actions of these different branches of the ANS on the sinoatrial (SA) node.[12] Therefore, RR intervals associated with abnormal beats (that do not originate from the SA node) should not be included in a HRV metric calculation and the series of consecutive normal-to-normal (NN) beat intervals should be analyzed.[13]

It is important to note that, the fiducial marker of each beat should be the onset of the P wave, since this is a more accurate marker than the R peak of the SA node stimulation (atrial depolarization onset) for each beat. Unfortunately, the P wave is usually a low-amplitude wave and is therefore often difficult to detect. Conversely, the R wave is easy to detect and label with a fiducial point. The exact location of this marker is usually defined to be either the highest (or lowest) point, the QRS onset, or the center of mass of the QRS complex. Furthermore, the competing effects of the ANS branches lead to subtle changes in the features within the heartbeat. For instance, a sympathetic innervation of the SA node (from exercise, for example) will lead to an increased local heart rate, and an associated shortening of the PR interval [10], QT interval [21], QRS width [48], and T wave [18]. Since the magnitude of the beat-to-beat modulation of the PR interval is correlated with, and much less significant than that of the RR interval [10, 49], and the R peak is well defined and easy to locate, many researchers choose to analyze only the *RR tachogram* (of normal intervals). It is unclear to what extent the differences in fiducial point location affects measures of HRV, but the sensitivity of the spectral HRV metrics to sampling frequencies below 1 kHz indicates that even small differences may have a significant effect for such metrics under certain circumstances [50].

If we record a typical RR tachogram over at least 5 minutes, and calculate the power spectral density,[14] then two dominant peaks are sometimes observable; one in the low frequency (LF) range ($0.015 < f < 0.15$ Hz) and one in the high frequency (HF) region ($0.15 \leq f \leq 0.4$ Hz). In general, the activity in the HF band is thought to be due mainly to parasympathetic activity at the sinoatrial node. Since respiration is a parasympathetically mediated activity (through the vagal nerve), a peak corresponding to the rate of respiration can often be observed in this frequency band (i.e., RSA). However, not all the parasympathetic activity is due to respiration. Furthermore, the respiratory rate may drop below the (generally accepted) lower bound of the HF region and therefore confound measures in the LF region. The LF region is generally thought to reflect sympathetically mediated activity[15] such as

---

12. See Chapter 1 for more details.
13. The temporal sequence of events is therefore known as the NN tachogram, or more frequently the RR tachogram (to indicate that each point is between each normal R peak).
14. Care must be taken at this point, as the time series is unevenly sampled; see section 3.7.2.
15. Although there is some evidence to show that this distinction does not always hold [46].

blood pressure-related phenomena. Activity in bands lower than the LF region are less well understood but seem to be related to myogenic activity, physical activity, and circadian variations. Note also that these frequency bands are on some level quite ad hoc and should not be taken as the exact limits on different mechanisms within the ANS; there are many studies that have used variants of these limits with practical results.

Many metrics for evaluating HRV have been described in the literature, together with their varying successes for discerning particular clinical problems. In general, HRV metrics can be broken down into either statistical time-based metrics (e.g., variance), or frequency-based metrics that evaluate power, or ratios of power, in certain spectral bands. Furthermore, most metrics are calculated either on a short time scale (often about 5 minutes) or over extremely long periods of time (usually 24 hours). The following two subsections give a brief overview of many of the common metrics. A more detailed analysis of these techniques can be found in the references cited therein. A comprehensive survey of the field of HRV was conducted by Malik et al. [46, 51] in 1995, and although much of the material remains relevant, some recent notable recent developments are included below, which help clarify some of the problems noted in the book. In particular, the sensitivity (and lack of specificity) of HRV metrics in many experiments has been shown to be partly due to activity-related changes [52] and the widespread use of resampling [53]. These issues, together with some more recent metrics, will now be explored.

3.7.1 Time Domain and Distribution Statistics

Time domain statistics are generally calculated on RR intervals without resampling, and are therefore robust to aggressive data removal (of artifacts and ectopic beats; see Section 3.7.6). An excellent review of conventional time domain statistics can be found in [46, 51]. One recently revisited time domain metric is the $pNN50$; the percentage of adjacent NN intervals differing by more than 50 ms over an entire 24-hour ECG recording. Mietus et al. [54] studied the generalization of this technique; the $pNNx$ — the percentage of NN intervals in a 24-hour time series differing by more than x ms ($4 \leq x \leq 100$). They found that enhanced discrimination between a variety of normal and pathological conditions is possible by using a value of x as low as 20 ms or less, rather than the standard 50 ms threshold. This tool, and many of the standard HRV tools, are freely available from PhysioNet [2]. This work can be considered similar to recent work by Grogan et al. [55], who analyzed the predictive power of different bins in a smoothed RR interval histogram and termed the metric *cardiac volatility*. Histogram bins were isolated that were more predictive of deterioration in the ICU than conventional metrics, despite the fact that the data was averaged over many seconds. These results indicate that only certain frequencies of cardiac variability may be indicative of certain conditions, and that conventional techniques may be including confounding factors, or simply noise, into the metric and diminishing the metric's predictive power.

In Malik and Camm's collection of essays on HRV [51], metrics that involve a quantification of the probability distribution function of the NN intervals over a long period of time (such as the TINN, the "triangular index"), were referred to as *geometrical indices*. In essence, these metrics are simply an attempt at calculating robust approximations of the higher order statistics. However, the higher the moment, the more sensitive it is to outliers and artifacts, and therefore, such "geometrical" techniques have faded from the literature.

The fourth moment, kurtosis, measures how peaked or flat a distribution is, relative to a Gaussian (see Chapter 5), in a similar manner to the TINN. Approximations to kurtosis often involve entropy, a much more robust measure of non-Gaussianity. (A key result of information theory is that, for a set of independent sources, with the same variance, a Gaussian distribution has the highest entropy, of all the signals.) It is not surprising then, that entropy-based HRV measures are more frequently employed that kurtosis.

The third moment of a distribution, *skewness*, quantifies the asymmetry of a distribution and has therefore been applied to patients in which sudden accelerations in heart rate, followed by longer decelerations, are indicative of a clinical problem. In general, the RR interval sequence accelerates much more quickly than it decelerates.[16] Griffin and Moorman [56] have shown that a small difference in skewness (0.59 ± 0.10 for sepsis and 0.51 ± 0.012 for sepsis-like illness, compared with -0.10 ± 0.13 for controls) can be an early indicator (up to 6 hours) of an upcoming abrupt deterioration in newborn infants.

3.7.2 Frequency Domain HRV Analysis

Heart rate changes occur on a wide range of time scales. Millisecond sympathetic changes stimulated by exercise cause an immediate increase in HR resulting in a lower long-term baseline HR and increased HRV over a period of weeks and months. Similarly, a sudden increase in blood pressure (due to an embolism, for example) will lead to a sudden semipermanent increase in HR. However, over many months the baroreceptors will reset their operating range to cause a drop in baseline HR and blood pressure (BP). In order to better understand the contributing factors to HRV and the time scales over which they affect the heart, it is useful to consider the RR tachogram in the frequency domain.

3.7.3 Long-Term Components

In general, the spectral power in the RR tachogram is broken down into four bands [46]:

1. Ultra low frequency (ULF): 0.0001 Hz $\geq$ ULF < 0.003 Hz;
2. Very low frequency (VLF): 0.003 Hz $\geq$ VLF < 0.04 Hz;
3. Low frequency (LF): 0.04 Hz $\geq$ LF < 0.15 Hz;
4. High frequency (HF): 0.15 Hz $\geq$ HF < 0.4 Hz.

Other upper- and lower-frequency bands are sometimes used. Frequency domain HRV metrics are then formed by summing the power in these bands, taking ratios,

---

16. Parasympathetic withdrawal is rapid, but is damped out by either parasympathetic activation or a much slower sympathetic withdrawal.

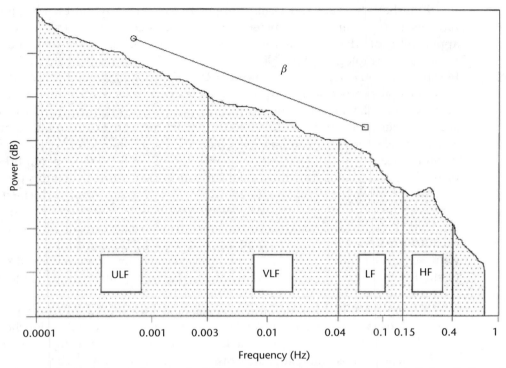

Figure 3.9   Typical periodogram of a 24-hour RR tachogram where power is plotted vertically and the frequency plotted horizontally on a log scale. Note that the gradient β of the $log - log$ plot is only meaningful for the longer scales. (*After:* [46].)

or calculating the slope,[17] β, of the $log - log$ power spectrum; see Figure 3.9. The motivation for splitting the spectrum into these frequency bands lies in the belief that the distinct biological regulatory mechanisms that contribute to HRV act at frequencies that are confined (approximately) within these bands. Fluctuations below 0.04 Hz in the VLF and ULF bands are thought to be due to long-term regulatory mechanisms such as the thermoregulatory system, the reninangiotensin system (related to blood pressure and other chemical regulatory factors), and other humoral factors [57]. In 1998 Taylor et al. [58] showed that the VLF fluctuations appear to depend primarily on the parasympathetic outflow. In 1999 Serrador et al. [59] demonstrated that the ULF band appears to be dominated by contributions from physical activity and that HRV in this band tends to increase during exercise. They therefore assert that any study that assesses HRV using data (even partially) from this frequency band should always include an indication of physical activity patterns. However, the effect of physical (and moreover, mental) activity on HRV is so significant that it has been suggested that controlling for activity for all metrics is extremely important [52].

Since spectral analysis was first introduced into HRV analysis in the late 1960s and early 1970s [60, 61], a large body of literature has arisen concerning this topic.

17. In the HRV literature, this slope is sometimes denoted by α.

In 1993, the U.S. Food and Drug Administration (FDA) withdrew its support of HRV as a useful clinical parameter due to a lack of consensus on the efficacy and applicability of HRV in the literature [62]. Although the Task Force of the European Society of Cardiology and the North American Society of Pacing Electrophysiology [46] provided an extensive overview of HRV estimation methods and the associated experimental protocols in 1996, the FDA has been reluctant to approve medical devices that calculate HRV unless the results are not explicitly used to make a specific medical diagnosis (e.g., see [63]). Furthermore, the clinical utility of HRV analysis (together with FDA approval) has only been demonstrated in very limited circumstances, where the patient undergoes specific tests (such as paced breathing or the Valsalva Maneuver) and the data are analyzed *off-line* by experts [64].

Almost all spectral analysis of the RR tachogram has been performed using some variant of autoregressive (AR) spectral estimation[18] or the FFT [46], which implicitly requires stationarity and regularly spaced samples. It should also be noted that most spectral estimation techniques such as the FFT require a windowing technique (e.g., the hamming window[19]), which leads to an implicit nonlinear distortion of the RR tachogram, since the value of the RR tachogram is explicitly joined to the time stamp.[20]

To mitigate for nonstationarities, linear and polynomial detrending is often employed, despite the lack of any real justification for this procedure. Furthermore, since the time stamps of each RR interval are related to the previous RR interval, the RR tachogram is inherently unevenly (or irregularly) sampled. Therefore, when using the FFT, the RR tachogram must either be represented in terms of power per cycle per beat (which varies based upon the local heart rate, and it is therefore extremely difficult, if not impossible, to compare one calculation with another) or a resampling method is required to make the time series evenly sampled.

Common resampling schemes involve either linear or cubic spline interpolative resampling. Resampling frequencies between 2 and 10 Hz have been used, but as long as the Nyquist criterion is satisfied, the resampling rate does not appear to have a serious effect on the FFT-based metrics [53]. However, experiments on both artificial and real data reveal that such processes overestimate the total power in the LF and HF bands [53] (although the increase is marginal for the cubic

---

18. Clayton et al. [65] have demonstrated that FFT and AR methods can provide a comparable measure of the low-frequency LF and high-frequency HF metrics on linearly resampled 5-minute RR tachograms across a patient population with a wide variety of ages and medical conditions (ranging from heart transplant patients who have the lowest known HRV to normals who often exhibit the highest overall HRV). AR models are particularly good at identifying line spectra and are therefore perhaps not an appropriate technique for analyzing HRV activity. Furthermore, since the optimal AR model order is likely to change based on the activity of the patient, AR spectral estimation techniques introduce an extra complication in frequency-based HRV metric estimation. AR modeling techniques will therefore not be considered in this chapter. As a final aside on AR analysis, it is interesting to note that measuring the width of a Poincaré plot is the same as treating the RR tachogram as an AR1 process and then estimating the process coefficient.

19. In the seminal 1978 paper on spectral windowing [66], Harris demonstrated that a hamming window (given by $W(t_j) = 0.54 - 0.46\cos(\omega t_j)$, $[j = 0, 1, 2, \ldots, N-1]$) provides an excellent performance for FFT analysis in terms of spectral leakage, side lobe amplitude, and width of the central peak (as well as a rapid computational time).

20. However, the window choice does not appear to affect the HRV spectral estimates significantly for RR interval variability.

spline resampling if the RR tachogram is smoothly varying and there are no missing or removed data points due to ectopy or artifact; see Section 3.7.6). The FFT over-estimates the $\frac{LF}{HF}$-ratio by about 50% with linear resampling and by approximately 10% with cubic spline resampling [53]. This error can be greater than the difference in the $\frac{LF}{HF}$-ratio between patient categories and is therefore extremely significant (see Section 3.7.7). One method for reducing (and almost entirely removing) this distortion is to use the Lomb-Scargle periodogram (LSP) [67–71], a method of spectral estimation which requires no explicit data replacement (nor assumes any underlying model) and calculates the PSD from only the known (observed) values in a time series.

3.7.4   The Lomb-Scargle Periodogram

Consider a physical variable X measured at a set of times t_j where the sampling is at equal times ($\Delta t = t_{j+1} - t_j = $ constant) from a stochastic process. The resulting time series data, $\{X(t_j)\}$ ($i = 1, 2, ..., N$), are assumed to be the sum of a signal X_s and random observational errors,[21] R;

$$X_j = X(t_j) = X_s(t_j) + R(t_j) \tag{3.2}$$

Furthermore, it is assumed that the signal is periodic, that the errors at different times are independent ($R(t_j) \neq f(R(t_k))$ for $j \neq k$) and that $R(t_j)$ is normally distributed with zero mean and constant variance, σ^2.

The N-point discrete Fourier transform (DFT) of this sequence is

$$FT_X(\omega) = \sum_{j=0}^{N-1} X(t_j)e^{-i\omega t_j} \tag{3.3}$$

($\omega_n = 2\pi f_n$, $n = 1, 2, ..., N$) and the power spectral density estimate is therefore given by the standard method for calculating a periodogram:

$$P_X(\omega) = \frac{1}{N} \sum_{j=0}^{N-1} \left| X(t_j)e^{-i\omega t_j} \right|^2 \tag{3.4}$$

Now consider arbitrary t_j's or uneven sampling ($\Delta t = t_{j+1} - t_j \neq$ constant) and a generalization of the N-point DFT [68]:

$$F : T_X(\omega) = \left(\frac{N}{2}\right)^{\frac{1}{2}} \sum_{j=0}^{N-1} X(t_j)[A\cos(\omega t_j) - iB\sin(\omega t_j)] \tag{3.5}$$

where $i = \sqrt{-1}$, j is the summation index, and A and B are as yet unspecified functions of the angular frequency ω. This angular frequency may depend on the

---

21. Due to the additive nature of the signal and the errors in measuring it, the errors are often referred to as noise.

vector of sample times, $\{t_j\}$, but not on the data, $\{X(t_j)\}$, nor on the summation index j. The corresponding (normalized) periodogram is then

$$P_X(\omega) = \frac{1}{N}|FT_X(\omega)|^2 = \frac{A^2}{2}\left[\sum_j X(t_j)\cos(\omega t_j)\right]^2$$

$$+ \frac{B^2}{2}\left[\sum_j X(t_j)\sin(\omega t_j)\right]^2 \tag{3.6}$$

If $A = B = \left(\frac{2}{N}\right)^{\frac{1}{2}}$, (3.5) and (3.6) reduce to the classical definitions [(3.3) and (3.4)] For even sampling ($\Delta t = $ constant) FT_X reduces to the DFT and in the limit $\Delta t \to 0$, $N \to \infty$, it is proportional to the Fourier transform. Scargle [68] shows how (3.6) is not unique and further conditions must be imposed in order to derive the corrected expression for the LSP:

$$P_N(\omega) \equiv \frac{1}{2\sigma^2}\left\{\frac{\left[\sum_j(x_j - \bar{x})\cos(\omega(t_j - \tau))\right]^2}{\sum_j\cos^2(\omega(t_j - \tau))}\right.$$

$$\left. + \frac{\left[\sum_j(x_j - \bar{x})\sin(\omega(t_j - \tau))\right]^2}{\sum_j\sin^2(\omega(t_j - \tau))}\right\} \tag{3.7}$$

where $\tau \equiv \tan^{-1}\left(\frac{\sum_j\sin(2\omega t_j)}{2\omega\sum_j\cos(2\omega t_j)}\right)$. τ is an offset that makes $P_N(\omega)$ completely independent of shifting all the t_j's by any constant. This choice of offset makes (3.7) exactly the solution that one would obtain if the harmonic content of a data set, at a given frequency ω, was estimated by linear least-squares fitting to the model $x(t) = A\cos(\omega t) + B\sin(\omega t)$. Thus, the LSP weights the data on a *per-point* basis instead of weighting the data on a *per-time interval* basis. Note that in the evenly sampled limit ($\Delta t = t_{j+1} - t_j = $ constant), (3.7) reduces to the classical periodogram definition [67]. See [67–72] for mathematical derivations and further details. C and Matlab code (*lomb.c* and *lomb.m*) for this routine are available from PhysioNet [2, 70] and the accompanying book Web site [73]. The well-known numerical computation library *Numerical Recipes in C* [74] also includes a rapid FFT-based method for computing the LSP, which claims not to use interpolation (rather *extirpolation*), but an implicit interpolation is still performed in the Fourier domain. Other methods for performing spectral estimation from irregularly sampled data do exist and include the min-max interpolation method [75] and the well-known geostatistical technique of *krigging*[22] [76]. The closely related fields of missing data *imputation* [77] and *latent variable discovery* [78] are also appropriate routes for dealing with missing data. However, the LSP appears to be sufficient for HRV analysis, even with a low SNR [53].

---

22. Instead of weighting nearby data points by some power of their inverted distance, krigging uses the spatial correlation structure of the data to determine the weighting values.

3.7.5 Information Limits and Background Noise

In order to choose a sensible window size, the requirement of stationarity must be balanced against the time required to resolve the information present. The European and North American Task Force on standards in HRV [46] suggests that the shortest time period over which HRV metrics should be assessed is 5 minutes. As a result, the lowest frequency that can be resolved is $\frac{1}{300} \approx 0.003$ Hz (just above the lower limit of the VLF region). Such short segments can therefore only be used to evaluate metrics involving the LF and HF bands. The upper frequency limit of the highest band for HRV analysis is 0.4 Hz [51]. Since the average time interval for N points over a time T is $\Delta t_{av} = \frac{T}{N}$, then the average Nyquist frequency [68] is then $f'_c = \frac{1}{2\Delta t_{av}} = \frac{N}{2T}$. Thus, a 5-minute window ($T = 300$) with the Nyquist constraint of $\frac{N}{2T} \geq 0.4$ for resolving the upper frequency band of the HF region, leads to a lower limit on N of 240 beats (an average heart rate of 48 bpm if all beats in a 5-minute segment are used). Utilization of the LSP, therefore, reveals a theoretical lower information threshold for accepting segments of an RR tachogram for spectral analysis in the upper HF region. If RR intervals of at least 1.25 seconds (corresponding to an instantaneous heart rate of $HR_i = \frac{60}{RR_i} = 48$ bpm) exist within an RR tachogram, then frequencies up to 0.4 Hz do exist. However, the accuracy of the estimates of the higher frequencies is a function of the number of RR intervals that exist with a value corresponding to this spectral region. Tachograms with no RR intervals smaller than 1.25s ($HR_i < 48$ bpm) can still be analyzed, but there is no power contribution at 0.4 Hz.

This line of thought leads to an interesting viewpoint on traditional short-term HRV spectral analysis; interpolation adds extra (erroneous) information into the time series and pads the FFT (in the time domain), tricking the user into assuming that there is a signal there, when really, there are simply not enough samples within a given range to allow the detection of a signal (in a statistically significant sense). Scargle [68] shows that at any particular frequency, f, and in the case of the null hypothesis, $P_X(\omega)$, has an exponential probability distribution with unit mean. Therefore, the probability that $P_X(\omega)$ will be between some positive value z and dz is $e^{-z} dz$, and hence, for a set of M independent frequencies, the probability that none give values larger than z is $(1 - e^{-z})^M$. The false alarm probability of the null hypothesis is therefore

$$P(> z) \equiv 1 - (1 - e^{-z})^M \tag{3.8}$$

Equation (3.8) gives the significance level for any peak in the LSP, $P_X(\omega)$ (a small value, say, $P < 0.05$ indicates a highly significant periodic signal at a given frequency). M can be determined by the number of frequencies sampled and the number of data points, N (see Press et al. [69]). It is therefore important to perform this test on each periodogram before calculating a frequency-based HRV metric, in order to check that there really are measurable frequencies that are not masked by noise or nonstationarity. There is one further caveat: Fourier analysis assumes that the signals at each frequency are independent. As we shall see in the next chapter on modeling, this assumption may be approximately true at best, and in some cases the coupling between different parts of the cardiovascular system may render Fourier-based spectral estimation inapplicable.

3.7.5.1   A Note on Spectral Leakage and Window Carpentry

The periodogram for unevenly spaced data allows two different forms of spectral adjustment: the application of time-domain (data) windows through weighting the signal at each point, and adjustment of the locations of the sampling times. The time points control the power in the window function, which leaks to the Nyquist frequency and beyond (the aliasing), while the weights control the side lobes. Since the axes of the RR tachogram are intricately linked (one is the first difference of the other), applying a windowing function to the amplitude of the data implicitly applies a nonlinear stretching function to the sample points in time. For an evenly sampled stationary signal, this distortion would affect all frequencies equally. Therefore, the reductions in LF and HF power cancel when calculating the $\frac{LF}{HF}$-ratio. For an irregularly sampled time series, the distortion will depend on the distribution of the sampling irregularity. A windowing function is therefore generally not applied to the irregularly sampled data. Distortion in the spectral estimate due to edge effects will not result as long as the start and end point means and first derivatives do not differ greatly [79].

3.7.6   The Effect of Ectopy and Artifact and How to Deal with It

To evaluate the effect of ectopy on HRV metrics, we can add artificial ectopic beats to an RR tachogram using a simple procedure. Kamath et al. [80] define ectopic beats (in terms of timing) as those which have intervals less than or equal to 80% of the previous sinus cycle length. Each datum in the RR tachogram represents an interval between two beats and the insertion of an ectopic beat therefore corresponds to the replacement of two data points as follows. The nth and $(n+1)$th beats (where n is chosen randomly) are replaced (respectively) by

$$RR'_n = \gamma RR_{n-1} \qquad (3.9)$$

$$RR'_{n+1} = RR_{n+1} + RR_n - RR'_n \qquad (3.10)$$

where the ectopic beat's timing is the fraction, γ, of the previous RR interval (initially 0.8). Note that the ectopic beat must be introduced at random within the central 50% of the 5-minute window to avoid windowing effects. Table 3.2 illustrates the effect of calculating the LF, HF, and $\frac{LF}{HF}$-ratio HRV metrics on an artificial RR tachogram with a known $\frac{LF}{HF}$-ratio (0.64) for varying levels of ectopy (adapted from [53]). Note that increasing levels of ectopy lead to an increase in HF power and a reduction in LF power, significantly distorting the $\frac{LF}{HF}$-ratio (even for just one beat).

It is therefore obvious that ectopic beats must be removed from the RR tachogram. In general, FFT-based techniques require the replacement of the removed beat with a *phantom* beat at a location where one would have expected the beat to have occurred if it was a sinus beat. Methods for performing phantom beat replacement range from linear and cubic spline interpolation,[23] AR model prediction, segment removal, and segment replacement.

---

23. Confusingly, phantom beat replacement is generally referred to as interpolation. In this chapter, it is referred
     to as phantom beat insertion, to distinguish it from the mathematical methods used to either place the
     phantom beat, or resample the unevenly sampled tachogram.

Table 3.2 LSP Derived Frequency Metrics for Different Magnitudes of Ectopy (γ)

Metric → Actual Value ↓	$\frac{LF}{HF}$	LF	HF	γ
0.64	0.64	0.39	0.61	†
0.64	0.60	0.37	0.62	0.8
0.64	0.34	0.26	0.74	0.7
0.64	0.32	0.25	0.76	0.6
0.64	0.47	0.32	0.68	0.8 ‡

† indicates no ectopy is present.
‡ indicates two ectopic beats are present.
Source: [52].

Although more robust and promising model-based techniques have been used [81], Lippman et al. [82] found that simply removing the signal around the ectopic beat performed as well as these more complicated methods. Furthermore, resampling the RR tachogram at a frequency (f_s) below the original ECG ($f_{ecg} > f_s$) from which it is derived effectively shifts the fiducial point by up to $\frac{1}{2}(\frac{1}{f_s} - \frac{1}{f_{ecg}})$s. The introduction of errors in HRV estimates due to low sampling rates is a well-known problem, but the additive effect from resampling is underappreciated. If a patient is suffering from low HRV (e.g., because they have recently undergone a heart transplant or are in a state of coma) then the sampling frequency of the ECG must be higher than normal. Merri et al. [83], and Abboud et al. [84] have shown that for such patients a sampling rate of at least 1,000 Hz is required. Work by Clifford et al. [85] and Ward et al. [50] demonstrate that a sampling frequency of 500 Hz or greater is generally recommended (see Figure 4.9 and Section 4.3.2).

The obvious choice for spectral estimation for HRV is therefore the LSP, which allows the removal of up to 20% of the data points in an RR tachogram without introducing a significant error in an HRV metric [53]. Therefore, if no morphological ECG is available, and only the RR intervals are available, it is appropriate to employ an aggressive beat removal scheme (removing any interval that changes by more than 12.5% on the previous interval [86]) to ensure that ectopic beats are not included in the calculation. Of course, since the ectopic beat causes a change in conduction, and momentarily disturbs the sinus rhythm, it is inappropriate to include the intervals associated with the beats that directly follow an ectopic beat (see Section 3.8.3.1) and therefore, all the affected beats should be removed at this nonstationarity. As long as there is no significant change in the phase of the sinus rhythm after the run of affected beats, then the LSP can be used without seriously affecting the estimate. Otherwise, the time series should be segmented at the nonstationarity.

3.7.7   Choosing an Experimental Protocol: Activity-Related Changes

It is well known that clinical investigations should be controlled for drugs, age, gender, and preexisting conditions. One further factor to consider is the activity of the patient population group, for this may turn out to be the single largest confounder of metrics, particularly in HRV studies. In fact, some HRV studies may be doing little more than identifying the difference in activity between two patient groups, something that can be more easily achieved by methods such as actigraphy, direct electrode noise analysis [87], or simply noting of the patient's activity using an empirical scale. Bernardi et al. [88] demonstrated that HRV in conscious patients (as measured by the $\frac{LF}{HF}$-ratio) changes markedly depending on a subject's activity. Their analysis involved measuring the ECG, respiration, and blood pressure of 12 healthy subjects, all aged around 29 years, for 5 minutes during a series of simple physical (verbal) and mental activities. Despite the similarity in subject physiology and physical activity (all remained in the supine position for at least 20 minutes prior to, and during the recording), the day-time $\frac{LF}{HF}$-ratio had a strong dependence on mental activity, ranging from 0.7 for controlled breathing to 3.6 for free talking. It may be argued that the changes in these values are simply an effect of changing breathing patterns (that modify the HF component). However, significant changes in both the LF component and blood pressure readings were also observed, indicating that the feedback loop to the central nervous system (CNS) was affected. The resultant change in HRV is therefore likely to be more than just a respiratory phenomenon.

Differences in mental as well as physical activity should therefore be minimized when comparing HRV metrics on an interpatient or intrapatient basis. Since it is probably impossible to be sure whether or not even a willing subject is controlling their thought processes for a few minutes (the shortest time window for traditional HRV metrics [46]), this would imply that HRV is best monitored while the subject is asleep, during which the level of mental activity can be more easily assessed.

Furthermore, artifact in the ECG is significantly reduced during sleep (because there is less physical movement by the subject) and the variation in $\frac{LF}{HF}$-ratio with respect to the mean value is reduced within a sleep state [52, 53, 72]. Sleep stages usually last more than 5 minutes [89], which is larger than the minimum required for spectral analysis of HRV [51]. Segmenting the RR time series according to sleep state basis should therefore provide data segments of sufficient length with minimal data corruption and departures from stationarity (which otherwise invalidate the use of Fourier techniques).

The standard objective scale for CNS activity during sleep was defined by Rechtschaffen and Kales [90], a set of heuristics known as the *R&K rules*. These rules are based partially on the frequency content of the EEG, assessed by expert observers over 30-second epochs. One of the five defined stages of sleep is termed dream, or rapid eye movement (REM), sleep. Stages 1–4 (light to deep) are non-REM (NREM) sleep, in which dreaming does not occur. NREM sleep can be further broken down into drowsy sleep (stage 1), light sleep, (stages 1 and 2), and deep sleep (stages 3 and 4), or slow wave sleep (SWS). Healthy humans cycle through these five sleep stages with a period of around 100 minutes, and each sleep stage can last up to 20 minutes during which time the cardiovascular system undergoes few changes, with the exception of brief arousals [89].

When loss of consciousness occurs, the parasympathetic nervous system begins to dominate with an associated rise in HF and decrease in $\frac{LF}{HF}$-ratio. This trend is more marked for deeper levels of sleep [91, 92]. PSDs calculated from 5 minutes of RR interval data during wakefulness and REM sleep reveal similar spectral components and $\frac{LF}{HF}$-ratios [92]. However, stage 2 sleep and SWS sleep exhibit a shift towards an increase in percentage contributions from the HF components

Table 3.3 $\frac{LF}{HF}$-Ratios During Wakefulness, NREM and REM Sleep

Activity → Condition ↓	Awake	REM Sleep	NREM Sleep
Normal [92]	N/A	2→2.5	0.5→1
Normal [46]	3.9	2.7	1.7
Normal [91]	4.0 ± 1.4	3.1 ± 0.7	1.2 ± 0.4
CNS Problem [93]	N/A	3.5→5.5	2→3.5
Post-MI [91]	2.4 ± 0.7	8.9 ± 1.6	5.1 ± 1.4

Note: N/A = not available; Post-MI = a few days after myocardial infarction; CNS = noncardiac related problem. Results quoted from [46, 91–93].

(above 0.15 Hz) with $\frac{LF}{HF}$-ratio values around 0.5 to 1 in NREM sleep and 2 to 2.5 in REM sleep [92]. In patients suffering from a simple CNS but noncardiac related problem, Lavie et al. [93] found slightly elevated NREM $\frac{LF}{HF}$-ratio values of between 2 and 3.5 and between 3.5 and 5.5 for REM sleep. Vanoli et al. [91] report that myocardial infarction (MI) generally results in a raised overall $\frac{LF}{HF}$-ratio during REM and NREM sleep with elevated LF and $\frac{LF}{HF}$-ratio (as high as 8.9) and lower HF. Values for all subjects during wakefulness in these studies (2.4 to 4.0) lie well within the range of values found during sleep (0.5 to 8.9) for the same patient population (see Table 3.3). This demonstrates that comparisons of HRV between subjects should be performed on a sleep-stage specific basis.

Recent studies [52, 53] have shown that the segmentation of the ECG into sleep states and the comparison of HRV metrics between patients on a per-sleep stage basis increases the sensitivity sufficiently to allow the separation of subtly different patient groups (normals and sleep apneics[24]), as long as a suitable spectral estimation technique (the LSP) is also employed. In particular, it was found that deep sleep or SWS gave the lowest variance in the $\frac{LF}{HF}$-ratio both in an intrapatient and interpatient basis, with the fewest artifacts, confirming that SWS is the most stable of all the sleep stages. However, since certain populations do not experience much SWS, it was found that REM sleep is an alternative (although slightly more noisy) state in which to compare HRV metrics. Further large-scale studies are required to prove that sleep-based segmentation will actually provide patient-specific assessments from HRV, although recent studies are promising.

3.8   Dealing with Nonstationarities

It should be noted at this point that all of the traditional HRV indices employ techniques that assume (weak) stationarity in the data. If part of the data in the window of analysis exhibits significant changes in the mean or variance over the length of the window, the HRV estimation technique can no longer be trusted. A cursory analysis of any real RR tachogram reveals that shifts in the mean or variance are a frequent occurrence [94]. For this reason it is common practice to *detrend* the signal by removing the linear or parabolic baseline trend from the window prior to calculating a metric.

---

24. Even when all data associated with the apneic episodes were excluded.

However, this detrending does not remove any changes in variance over a stationarity change, nor any changes in the spectral distribution of component frequencies. It is not only illogical to attempt to calculate a metric that assumes stationarity over the window of interest in such circumstances, it is unclear what the meaning of a metric taken over segments of differing autonomic tone could be. Moreover, changes in stationarity of RR tachograms are often joined by transient sections of heart rate overshoot and an accompanying increased probability of artifact on the ECG (and hence missing data) [86, 95].

In this section we will explore a selection of methods for dealing with nonstationarities, including multiscale techniques, detrending, segmentation (both statistically and from a clinical biological perspective), and the analysis of change points themselves.

3.8.1   Nonstationary HRV Metrics and Fractal Scaling

Empirical analyses employing detrending techniques can lead to metrics that appear to distinguish between certain patient populations. Such techniques include multiscale power analysis such as detrended fluctuation analysis (DFA) [96, 97]. Such techniques aid in the quantification of long-range correlations in a time series, and in particular, the *fractal scaling* of the RR tachogram. If a time series is self-similar over many scales, then the $log - log$ power-frequency spectrum will exhibit a $1/f^\beta$ scaling, where β is the slope of the spectrum. For a white noise process the spectrum is flat and $\beta = 0$. For pink noise processes, $\beta = 1$, and for Brownian processes, $\beta = 2$. Black noise has $\beta > 2$.

DFA is an alternative variance-based method for measuring the fractal scaling of a time series. Consider an N-sample time series x_k, which is integrated to give a time series y_k that is divided into boxes of equal length, m. In each box a least squares line fit is performed on the data (to estimate the trend in that box). The y coordinate of the straight line segments is denoted by $y_k^{(m)}$. Next, the integrated time series, y_k, is detrended by subtracting the local trend, $y_k^{(m)}$, in each box. The root-mean-square fluctuation of this integrated and detrended time series is calculated by

$$F(m) = \sqrt{\frac{1}{N}\left(\sum_{k=1}^{N}\left[y_k - y_k^{(m)}\right]^2\right)} \tag{3.11}$$

This computation is repeated over all time scales (box sizes) to characterize the relationship between $F(m)$, the average fluctuation, as a function of box size. Typically, $F(m)$ will increase with box size m. A linear relationship on a $log-log$ plot indicates the presence of power law (fractal) scaling. Under such conditions, the fluctuations can be characterized by a scaling exponent α, the slope of the line relating $\log F(m)$ to $\log m$, that is, $F(m) \sim m^\alpha$.

A direct link between DFA and conventional spectral analysis techniques and other fractal dimension estimation techniques exists [98–101]. These techniques include semivariograms (to estimate the Hausdorf dimension, H_a, [98]), the rescaled range (to estimate the Hurst exponent, H_u [98, 102]), wavelet transforms (to estimate the variance of the wavelets H_w [100, 103]), the Fano factor α_F [102, 104], and the Allan factor, α_A [102]. Their equivalences can be summarized as [105]

$$\beta = 2\alpha - 1$$
$$\beta = 2H_a + 1$$
$$\beta = 2H_u - 1 \qquad (3.12)$$
$$\beta = H_w$$
$$\beta = \alpha_F$$
$$\beta = \alpha_A$$

However, it is interesting to note that each of these fractal measures has limited ranges of applicability and suffer from differing problems [106]. In particular, the Fano factor is unsuitable for estimating $\beta > 1$, and the Allan factor (a ratio of the variance to the mean) is confined to $0 < \beta < 3$ [106]. Recently McSharry et al. [100] performed an analysis to determine the sensitivity of each of these metrics for determining fractal scaling in RR interval time series. They demonstrated that for a range of colored Gaussian and non-Gaussian processes ($-2 < \beta < 4$), H_w provided the best fractal scaling range ($-2 < \beta < 4$ for Gaussian and $-0.8 < \beta < 4$ for non-Gaussian processes).

3.8.1.1 Multiscale Entropy

Multiscale entropy (MSE) is a nonlinear variant of these multiscale metrics that uses an entropy-based metric known as the sample entropy.[25] For a time series of N points, $\{u(j) : 1 \leq j \leq N\}$ forms the $N - m + 1$ vectors $x_m(i)$ for $\{i | 1 \leq i \leq N - m + 1\}$, where $x_m(i) = u(i + k) : 0 \leq k \leq m - 1$ is the vector of m data points from $u(i)$ to $u(i + m - 1)$. If A_i is the number of vectors $x_{m+1}(j)$ within a given tolerance r of $x_{m+1}(i)$, B_i is the number of vectors $x_m(j)$ within r of $x_m(i)$ and $B(0) = N$, is the length of the input series, the sample entropy is given by

$$\text{SampEn}(k, r, N) = -\ln \frac{A(k)}{B(k-1)} \qquad (k = 0, 1, \ldots, m-1) \qquad (3.13)$$

Sample entropy is the negative natural logarithm of an estimate of the conditional probability that subseries (epochs) of length m that match point-wise within a tolerance r also match at the next point.

The algorithm for calculating sample entropy over many scales builds up runs of points matching within the tolerance r until there is not a match, and keeps track of template matches in counters $A(k)$ and $B(k)$ for all lengths k up to m. Once all the matches are counted, the sample entropy values are calculated by $\text{SampEn}(k, r, N) = -ln(\frac{A(k)}{B(k-1)})$ for $k = 0, 1, \ldots, m - 1$ with $B(0) = N$, the length of the input series.

---

25. Sample entropy has been shown to be a more accurate predictor of entropy in the RR tachogram than other traditional entropy estimation methods.

MSE does not change linearly with scale and therefore cannot be quantified by one exponent. In general, MSE increases (nonlinearly) with increasing N (or decreasing scale factor), reflecting the reduction in long-term coherence at longer and longer scales (shorter scale factors). This metric has been shown to be an independent descriptor of HRV to the fractal scaling exponent β [95]. An open-source implementation of this algorithm can be found on the PhysioNet Web site [107].

3.8.2   Activity-Related Changes

3.8.2.1   Segmentation of the Cardiac Time Series

Another possibility when dealing with nonstationarities is to simply segment the time series at an identifiable point of change and analyze the segments in isolation.[26] An early approach by Moody [110] involved a metric of nonstationarity that included mean heart rate and HRV. Later, Fukada et al. [111] used a modified t-test to identify shifts in the mean RR interval. If we assume that the RR tachogram is a series of approximately stationary states and measure the distribution of the frequency of length and size of the switching between states, we find that the distributions approximately fit specific power laws which vary depending on a subject's condition. Fukada et al. [111] achieved the segmentation of the time series by performing a t-test[27] to determine the most significant change in the mean RR interval. This process is repeated in a recursive manner on each bisection until the statistics of small numbers prevents any further divisions. One interesting result of the application of this method to the RR tachogram is the discovery that the scaling laws differ significantly depending on whether a subject is asleep or not. It is unclear if this is a reflection of the fact that differing parts of the human brain control these two major states, but the connections between the cardiovascular system and the mechanisms that control the interplay between sleep and arousals is rapidly becoming a research field of great interest [108, 109, 112, 113]. Models that reproduce this activity in a realistic manner are detailed in Chapter 4.

Unfortunately, empirical methods for segmenting the cardiac time series based purely on the RR tachogram have shown limited success and more detailed information is often needed. It has recently been shown [52] that by quantifying HRV only during sleep states, and comparing HRV between patients *only for* a particular sleep state, the sensitivity of a particular HRV metric is significantly increased. Furthermore, the deeper the sleep state, the more stationary the signal, the lower the noise, and the more sensitive is the HRV metric. Another method for segmenting the cardiac time series into active and inactive regions is based upon the work of Mietus et al. for quantifying sleep patterns from the ECG [87, 114].

---

26. Or some property derived from the frequency distribution of the means or lengths of the segments [108, 109].

27. The t-test is modified to account for the fact that each sample is not independent. This may not actually be necessary if each state is independent, although the success of modeling 24-hour fluctuations with hidden Markov models may indicate that there is some correlation between states, at least in the short term. However, the success of simple t-tests demonstrate that independence may be a reasonable approximation under certain circumstances [86].

3.8.2.2 Sleep Staging from the ECG

Respiratory rate may be derived from the body surface ECG by measuring the fluctuation of the mean cardiac electrical axis [115] or peak QRS amplitudes which accompany respiration. This phenomenon is known as ECG-derived respiration (EDR); see Chapter 8 for an in-depth analysis of this technique. The changes in the sequence of RR intervals during RSA are also heavily correlated with respiration through neurological modulation of the SA node. However, since the QRS morphology shifts due to respiration are mostly mechanically mediated, the phase difference between the two signals is not always constant. Recently Mietus et al. [114] demonstrated that by tracking changes in this coupling through cross-spectral analysis of the EDR and RSA time series, they were able to quantify the type and depth of sleep that humans experience into cyclic alternating pattern (CAP) and non-CAP sleep (rather than the traditional Rechtschaffen and Kales [90] scoring).

Following [114], frequency coupling can be measured using the cross-spectral density between RSA and EDR. There are two slightly different measures: coupling frequency with respect to magnitude of the sinusoidal oscillations $A(f)$ and the consistency in phase of the oscillations $\Theta(f)$. These are calculated separately such that

$$A(f) = \mathcal{E}\left[|P_{xy}^i(f)|^2\right] \tag{3.14}$$

and

$$\Theta(f) = \left|\mathcal{E}[P_{xy}^i(f)]\right|^2 \tag{3.15}$$

where $\mathcal{E}[.]$ denotes averaging across all the $i = 1, \ldots, N$ segments and $P_{xy}^i(f)$ is the cross-periodogram of the ith segment.

In general, $P_{xy}(f)$ is complex even if $X(t)$ and $Y(t)$ are real. Since $A(f)$ is calculated by taking the magnitude squared of $P_{xy}(f)$ in each block followed by averaging, it corresponds to the frequency coupling of the two signals due to the oscillations in amplitude only. Similarly, since $\Theta(f)$ is computed by first averaging the real and imaginary parts of $P_{xy}(f)$ across all blocks followed by magnitude squaring, it measures the consistency in phase of the oscillations across all blocks. $A(f)$ and $\Theta(f)$ are normalized and multiplied together to obtain the *cardiorespiratory coupling* (CRC), a measure of the strength of coupling between RSA and EDR as follows:

$$CRC(f) = \frac{A(f)}{\max[A(f)]} * \frac{\Theta(f)}{\max[\Theta(f)]} \tag{3.16}$$

CRC ranges between 0 and 1 with a low CRC indicating poor coupling and therefore increased activity. A high CRC (>0.4) indicates decreased activity that can be interpreted as sleep or sometimes sedation [87]. A value closer to 1 means strong coupling of RSA and EDR at a given frequency. It should be noted that this method,

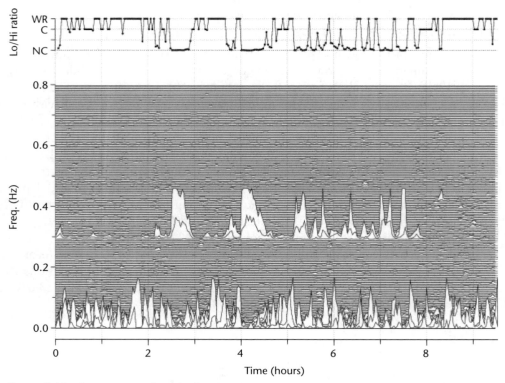

Figure 3.10 Spectrogram (lower) of EDR-RSA coherence, with associated sleep stability (upper) derived from thresholding a ratio of low frequency and high frequency (Lo/Hi) power for each segment. Note that this patient is on a ventilator so the respiratory frequency is sharp and fixed at 0.3 Hz. Stable non-CAP (NC) sleep is still observable despite the ventilation. (© 2005 J. Mietus. Reprinted with permission.)

is a slight modification of the one used in [114] (called cardiopulmonary coupling, or CPC), where the squaring of the phase is taken before the averaging.[28]

Figure 3.10 illustrates the application of this technique to a sedated and ventilated patient in an intensive care unit. The lower plot is a spectrogram; a time series of the cross spectral density between the EDR and RSA. The upper plot represents a stability of sleep from WR (wakefulness or REM sleep) to CAP sleep (C) to stable non-CAP (NC) sleep. This time series is derived by thresholding the ratio of the low (Lo) to high (Hi) frequency regions of the cross-spectral coherence. Note that despite the fact that this patient is ventilated (and hence the respiratory frequency is sharp and fixed at 0.3 Hz), stable (NC) sleep is still observable.

Coupling between RSA and EDR is more evident or easily obtainable when the subject is at rest (or in stable sleep, or perhaps, deep sleep) where there are fewer factors that may significantly influence changes in the respiratory rate or heart

---

28. These differences do not lead to significant differences in the metric as a predictor of stable (coupled high frequency) activity however. Furthermore, in CPC, the cross-power is thresholded at different frequencies to produce an output of wakefulness/REM sleep (WR), unstable/cyclic alternating pattern (CAP) sleep, or stable/non-CAP (NC) sleep. NC sleep is correlated with low sedation/agitation (Riker) levels [87, 116], and WR is correlated with medium to high agitation (Riker) scores.

rate. Therefore, this technique has also been employed to detect changes in activity or stationarity in patients [87]. Furthermore, the strongest coupling frequency is directly correlated with respiration, which is also a good index of activity, as well as an estimate of the prevailing respiratory rate. A sensitivity analysis of this technique also shows that the CPC metric is extremely robust to noise [87], since the presence of noise on the ECG is correlated with changes in activity [86].

It should be noted that the analysis of synchronization between the cardiac cycle and the respiratory frequency has been an area of interest for few years now [117], with promising results for determining the health of certain patient groups.

3.8.3 Perturbation Analysis

An alternative to detrending, or segmenting, the cardiac time series at nonstationary changes and analyzing the segments in isolation, is to perform an analysis of the ephemeral changes in the signal at the point of change. This type of *perturbation analysis* is a standard technique in clinical medicine and includes stress testing[29] and the Valsalva Maneuver.[30]

However, interventionist tests may not always be possible or appropriate, and a more passive analysis of change points is sometimes required. These include analyzing the periodicity of these changes, and the transient changes due to passive intrinsic shifts in cardiac activity, such as transitions between sleep states, changes due to arousals during sleep, or changes due to ectopy.

3.8.3.1 Heart Rate Turbulence

The changes in quasi-stationarity of the sinus rhythm due to the biphasic physiological change in SA node activity from PVCs is known as heart rate turbulence[31] (HRT) [118, 119]. In HRV analysis, this disturbance is removed from the RR tachogram, and an assumption is made that the phase of the RR tachogram is unchanged after the signal returns to the "undisturbed rhythm." In HRT, the changes in the "disturbed" section are analyzed to extract metrics to quantify the changes.

In general, HRT manifests as a short initial acceleration of the heart rate for a few beats, followed by a deceleration back to the basal value from before the PVC. HRT is usually quantified by two numerical parameters: turbulence onset (TO) and turbulence slope (TS). TO is defined as the percentage difference between the average value of the first two normal RR intervals following the PVC (RR^n, $n = 2, 3$) and of the last two normal intervals preceding the PVC (RR^{-n}, $n = 2, 1$) and is given by [119]:

$$TO = \frac{(RR^{+2} + RR^{+3}) - (RR^{-2} + RR^{-1})}{RR^{-2} + RR^{-1}} \times 100 \qquad (3.17)$$

---

29. A series of exercise tests that attempt to induce heart-related problems which manifest on the ECG at high heart rates or due to strong sympathetic innervation.
30. A pressure-inducing respiratory procedure which is thought to provide a rough guide to the integrity of the autonomic neural pathways involved in the response [51].
31. It should be noted that the term *turbulence* is a misnomer, since there is no strict evidence of actual turbulence in the neural modulation, electrophysical activity, or the resultant hemodynamic flow. A more appropriate term may be heart rate perturbation (HRP).

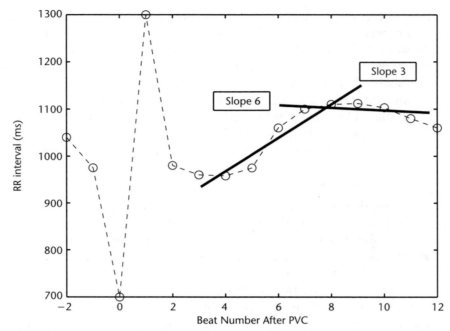

Figure 3.11   Example of HRT disturbance after PVC. Beat index denotes the RR interval associated with the beats surrounding the PVC (index zero). Note that the following beat after the PVC (RR^{+1}) has an associated elongated RR interval; the compensatory pause after the early (premature) preceding beat. Slopes are calculated for each following set of five consecutive beats (only slopes 3 and 6 are illustrated for clarity). (*After:* [120].)

where RR^{-2} and RR^{-1} are the first two normal intervals preceding the PVC and RR^{+2} and RR^{+3} the first two normal intervals following the PVC. (Note that there are two intervals associated with the PVC; the normal-PVC interval, RR^0, and the following PVC-normal interval RR^{+1}.) Therefore, positive TO values indicate deceleration and negative TO values indicate acceleration of the postectopic sinus rhythm. Although the TO can be determined for each individual PVC (and should be if performed online), TO has shown to be more (clinically) predictive if the average value of all individual measurements is calculated. For the calculation of the mean TO in the current version (1.11) of the freely available HRT-algorithm [121], at least 15 normal intervals after each single PVC are required.

TS is calculated by constructing an average ectopy-centered time series[32] and determining the steepest (linearly regressed) slope each possible sequence of five consecutive normal intervals in the post-PVC "disturbed" tachogram (usually taken to be up to RR^{+16}; the first 15 normal RR intervals). That is, all possible slopes from the set $\{RR^{+2,+3,...,+6}, \ldots, RR^{+17,+18,...,+16}\}$ are calculated, and the maximum of the 13 possible slopes is taken to be the TS. These values are usually averaged over all acceptable candidates, and can run into the tens of thousands for 24-hour Holter recordings. Figure 3.11 illustrates the calculation of TS after the disturbance

32. This averaging reduces the short-term noise from RSA and it is wise to use 20 or more ectopic examples to increase the statistical power of the technique. However, HRT estimation can be performed on as few as a single example.

in the RR tachogram due to a PVC. Note that the following beat after the PVC (RR^{+1}) has an associated elongated RR interval, the compensatory pause after the early (premature) preceding beat. Although slopes are calculated for each following set of five consecutive beats, only the third and sixth slopes are illustrated for clarity.

The criteria for excluding PVCs must be stringent, since HRT quantification can only deliver usable results if the triggering event was a true PVC (and not an artifact, T wave or similar non-PVC event). In addition, the sinus rhythm immediately preceding and following the PVC must be checked to ensure that it is free from arrhythmia, artifacts, and false beat classifications due to artifact. A useful set of exclusion criteria are:

- Remove all RR intervals < 300 ms or > 2, 000 ms;
- Remove all RR^n where $\| RR^{n-1} - RR^n \| > 200$ ms;
- Remove all RR intervals that change by more than > 20% with respect to the mean of the five last sinus intervals (the reference interval);
- Only use PVCs with a minimum prematurity of 20%;
- Exclude PVCs with a postextrasystole interval which is at least 20% longer than the normal interval.

TO values below 0 and TS values above 2.5 are considered normal, and abnormal otherwise (i.e., a healthy response to PVCs is a strong sinus acceleration followed by a rapid deceleration).

Although the exact mechanism that leads to HRT is unknown [120], it is thought to be an autonomous baroreflex whereby the PVC causes a brief disturbance of the arterial blood pressure [122]. Therefore, HRT can be measured around the point of atrial ectopy as well as ventricular ectopy. When the autonomic control system is healthy, this rapid change causes an instantaneous response in the following RR intervals. If the autonomic control system is impaired, the magnitude of this response is either diminished or possibly completely absent. From a clinical perspective, HRT metrics have been shown to be predictive of mortality and possibly cardiac arrest. Furthermore, HRT metrics have been shown to be particularly useful when the patients are taking beta-blockers. In one study [123], combined TO and TS was found to be the only independent predictor of mortality compared to otherwise predictive markers such as mean HR, previous myocardial infarction, and a low ejection fraction.

3.8.3.2   QT Turbulence and Other Measures

Many other studies indicate that this technique is useful [121], and in particular the application of HRT analysis to study of the QT interval variation after PVCs has shown that QT interval turbulence occurs in association with HR turbulence [124]. QT TO has been defined as the relative difference between the QT interval of the first sinus cycle after an induced PVC and the mean of the QT intervals of the two sinus cycles preceding the premature beat. Savelieva et al. [124] found that patients with ischemic VT and left ventricular dysfunction exhibited significantly lower QT TO values than those with nonischemic VT and normal ventricular function. Interestingly, neither induced APCs nor PVCs produced late QT dynamics equivalent to TS of HR turbulence, and the underlying mechanism of QT turbulence remains unclear. However, few studies in QT turbulence have been performed and difficulties in measuring and interpreting the QT interval may confound this type of analysis (see Section 3.4.1 and Chapter 11). It is therefore uncertain whether QT TS will prove to be a useful metric. Furthermore, many HRT-related metrics have been proposed with varying degrees of success, including:

- *Turbulence dynamics* [125]: The largest regressed slope between TS and heart rate in a particular individual over a sliding window of 10 bpm;
- *Turbulence timing* [126]: The beat number of the 5-RR interval sequence used in the TS calculation at which the largest slope occurs;
- *Correlation coefficient of TS* [127]: The correlation coefficient of the regression line fitted to the 5-RR intervals giving the maximum slope (i.e., where TS is defined);
- *Turbulence jump* [128]: The maximum difference between adjacent RR intervals;
- *Turbulence frequency decrease* [129]: A frequency-domain metric obtained by fitting a sine function to the postcompensatory pause.

Although many of these metrics have shown promise as independent disease predictors, further studies are required to determine whether any of these metrics provide significantly superior risk stratification to TO and TS. Furthermore, TO and TS are simpler to measure, and have been validated in large prospective studies. Further information is available from Schneider et al. [119, 121, 130].

3.9 Summary

Given the finite number of pages allowed in this book, all the possible metrics that researchers have chosen to quantify the EGG (and derived beat-to-beat timing sequences) cannot be detailed, nor all the possible applications of each metric be covered. Moreover, such a summary would be a transient document of only partial relevance in a few years from publication.

Rather, this chapter is intended to introduce the reader to the many different linear stationary and nonstationary qualities of the ECG, together with a selection of relevant metrics for evaluating these properties. This chapter is also intended to give an insight into possible approaches which are relevant to the different recording situations one may encounter (that vary based on activity, demographics and medical condition). It is important, although difficult, to differentiate between the concept of the nonstationary and the nonlinear nature of the ECG, since the application of a particular methodology or model will depend on prior beliefs concerning the relevance of these paradigms. In general, it is sufficient to apply linear techniques to quasi-stationary segments of ECG. However, to improve on such measures, it is important to understand the nonlinear nature of the ECG. Techniques for nonlinear analysis are therefore presented in Chapter 6. However, before reading the chapter on nonlinear analysis, it is advisable to read the following chapter, in which a selection of practically useful nonlinear and nonstationary models for both the ECG and the RR tachogram are presented.

References

[1] Welch, P. D., "The Use of Fast Fourier Transform for the Estimation of Power Spectra: A Method Based on Time Averaging over Short, Modified Periodograms," *IEEE Trans. Audio Electroacoust.*, Vol. AU-15, June 1967, pp. 70–73.

[2] Goldberger, A. L., R. G. Mark, and G. B. Moody, "PhysioNet: The Research Resource for Complex Physiologic Signals," http://www.physionet.org.

[3] Pettersson, J., O. Pahlm, and E. Carro, "Changes in High-Frequency QRS Components Are More Sensitive Than ST-Segment Deviation for Detecting Acute Coronary Artery Occlusion," *J. Am. Coll. Cardiol.*, Vol. 36, 2000, pp. 1827–1834.

[4] Schlegel, T. T., et al., "Real-Time 12-Lead High-Frequency QRS Electrocardiography for Enhanced Detection of Myocardial Ischemia and Coronary Artery Disease," *Mayo Clin Proc.*, Vol. 79, 2004, pp. 339–350.

[5] Spackman, T. N., M. D. Abel, and T. T. Schlegel, "Twelve-Lead High-Frequency QRS Electrocardiography During Anesthesia in Healthy Subjects," *Anesth. Analg.*, Vol. 100, No. 4, 2005, pp. 1043–1047.

[6] Hunt, A. C., "T Wave Alternans in High Arrhythmic Risk Patients: Analysis in Time and Frequency Domains: A Pilot Study," *BMC Cardiovasc. Disord.*, Vol. 2, No. 6, March 2002.

[7] Jarvis, M. R., and P. P. Mitra, "Apnea Patients Characterized by 0.02 Hz Peak in the Multitaper Spectrogram of Electrocardiogram Signals," *Computers in Cardiology*, Vol. 27, 2000, pp. 769–772.

[8] Zeng, W., and L. Glass, "Statistical Properties of Heartbeat Intervals During Atrial Fibrillation," *Phys. Rev. E*, 1996, pp. 1779–1784.

[9] Guyton, A. C., and J. E. Hall, *Textbook of Medical Physiology*, Philadelphia, PA: W. B. Saunders Company, 2001.

[10] Shouldice, R., et al., "Modulating Effect of Respiration on Atrioventricular Conduction Time Assessed Using PR Interval Variation," *Med. Biol. Eng. Comput.*, Vol. 40, No. 6, November 2002, pp. 609–617.

[11] Wagner, G. S., *Marriott's Practical Electrocardiography*, 9th ed., Baltimore, MD: Williams & Wilkins, 1994.

[12] Estes, N. A. M., et al., "ECG Findings in Active Patients; Differentiating the Benign from the Serious," *The Physician and Sportsmedicine*, Vol. 29, No. 3, 2001.

[13] Davey, P., "A New Physiological Method for Heart Rate Correction of the QT Interval," *Heart*, Vol. 82, 1999, pp. 183–186.

[14] Seed, W. A., et al., "Relation of Human Cardiac Action Potential Duration to the Interval Between Beats: Implications for the Validity of Rate Corrected QT Interval (QTc)," *British Heart Journal*, Vol. 57, 1987, pp. 32–37.

[15] Zabel, M., et al., "Assessment of QT Dispersion for Prediction of Mortality or Arrhythmic Events After Myocardial Infarction: Results of a Prospective, Long-Term Follow-Up Study," *Circulation*, No. 97, 1998, pp. 2543–2550.

[16] Coumel, P., P. Maison-Blanche, and F. Badilini, "Dispersion of Ventricular Repolarization: Reality? Illusion? Significance?" *Circulation*, No. 97, 1998, pp. 2491–2493.

[17] Rautaharju, P. M., "QT and Dispersion of Ventricular Repolarization: The Greatest Fallacy in Electrocardiography in the 1990s," *Circulation*, No. 99, 1999, pp. 2476–2479.

[18] di Bernardo, D., P. Langley, and A. Murray, "Effect of Changes in Heart Rate and in Action Potential Duration on the Electrocardiogram T Wave Shape," *Physiological Measurement*, Vol. 23, No. 2, 2002, pp. 355–364.

[19] Fletcher, G. F., et al., "Exercise Standards: A Statement for Healthcare Professionals from the American Heart Association," *Circulation*, Vol. 91, No. 2, 2001, pp. 580–615.

[20]   Malik, M., et al., "Relation Between QT and RR Intervals Is Highly Individual Among Healthy Subjects: Implications for Heart Rate Correction of the QT Interval," *Heart*, Vol. 87, No. 3, 2002, pp. 220–228.

[21]   Fossa, A. A., et al., "Dynamic Beat-to-Beat Modeling of the QT-RR Interval Relationship: Analysis of QT Prolongation During Alterations of Autonomic State Versus Human Ether A-Go-Go-Related Gene Inhibition," *J. Pharmacol. Exp. Ther.*, Vol. 312, No. 1, 2005, pp. 1–11.

[22]   Lehtinen, R., "ST/HR Hysteresis: Exercise and Recovery Phase ST Depression/Heart Rate Analysis of the Exercise ECG," *J. Electrocardiol.*, No. 32, 1999, pp. 198–204.

[23]   Lehtinen, R., "Diagnostic and Prognostic Value of ST/HR Hysteresis," *International Journal of Bioelectromagnetism*, Vol. 2, No. 1, 2000.

[24]   Shouldice, R., C. Heneghan, and P. Nolan, "Methods of Quantifying Respiratory Modulation in Human PR Electrocardiographic Intervals," *IEEE Engineering in Medicine and Biology Conference*, IEEE Engineering in Medicine and Biology Conference, Houston, TX, October 2002.

[25]   Moody, G. B., "PhysioNet: The Research Resource for Complex Physiologic Signals: Physiobank Annotations," http://www.physionet.org/physiobank/annotations.shtml.

[26]   Dingfei, G., N. Srinivasan, and S. M. Krishnan, "Cardiac Arrhythmia Classification Using Autoregressive Modeling," *Biomed. Eng. Online*, Vol. 1, No. 5, November 2002.

[27]   Owis, M. I., et al., "Study of Features Based on Nonlinear Dynamical Modeling in ECG Arrhythmia Detection and Classification," *IEEE Trans. Biomed. Eng.*, Vol. 49, No. 7, July 2002, pp. 733–736.

[28]   Moody, G. B., and R. G. Mark, "QRS Morphology Representation and Noise Estimation Using the Karhunen-Loève Transform," *Computers in Cardiology*, Vol. 16, 1989, pp. 269–272.

[29]   Mark, R. G., and G. B. Moody, "ECG Arrhythmia Analysis: Design and Evaluation Stratergies," Chapter 18, in I. Gath and G. F. Inbar, (eds.), *Advances in Processing and Pattern Analysis of Biological Signals*, New York: Plenum Press, 1996, pp. 251–272.

[30]   Coast, D. A., et al., "An Approach to Cardiac Arrhythmia Analysis Using Hidden Markov Models," *IEEE Trans. Biomed. Eng.*, No. 37, 1990, pp. 826–836.

[31]   Caswell, S. A., K. S. Kluge, and C. M. J. Chiang, "Pattern Recognition of Cardiac Arrhythmias Using Two Intracardiac Channels," *Computers in Cardiology*, Vol. 20, September 1993, pp. 181–184.

[32]   Zhou, S. H., P. M. Rautaharju, and H. P. Calhoun, "Selection of a Reduced Set of Parameters for Classification of Ventricular Conduction Defects by Cluster Analysis," *Computers in Cardiology*, Vol. 20, 1993, pp. 879–882.

[33]   Guvenir, H. A., et al., "Selection of a Reduced Set of Parameters for Classification of Ventricular Conduction Defects by Cluster Analysis," *Computers in Cardiology*, Vol. 24, 1997, pp. 433–436.

[34]   Maglaveras, N., et al., "ECG Pattern Recognition and Classification Using Non-Linear Transformations and Neural Networks: A Review," *International Journal of Medical Informatics*, Vol. 52, No. 1, October 1998, pp. 191–208.

[35]   Chazal, P., "Automatic Classification of the Frank Lead Electrocardiogram," Ph.D. dissertation, University of New South Wales, 1998.

[36]   Barro, S., et al., "Algorithmic Sequential Decision-Making in the Frequency Domain for Life Threatening Ventricular Arrhythmias and Imitative Artefacts: A Diagnostic System," *J. Biomed. Eng.*, No. 11, 1989, pp. 320–328.

[37]   Jekova, I., A. Cansell, and I. Dotsinsky, "Noise Sensitivity of Three Surface ECG Fibrillation Detection Algorithms," *Physiological Measurement*, Vol. 22, No. 2, 2001, pp. 287–297.

[38] Afonoso, V. X., and W. J. Tompkins, "Detecting Ventricular Fibrillation: Selecting the Appropriate Time-Frequency Analysis Tool for the Application," *IEEE Eng. Med. Biol. Mag.*, No. 14, 1995, pp. 152–159.

[39] Dokur, Z., T. Olmez, and E. Yazgan, "Comparison of Discrete Wavelet and Fourier Transforms for ECG Beat Classification," *Electronics Letters*, Vol. 35, No. 18, September 1999, pp. 1502–1504.

[40] deChazal, P., and R. B. Reilly, "A Comparison of the Use of Different Wavelet Coefficients for the Classification of the Electrocardiogram," *Proc. of the 14th International Conference on Pattern Recognition*, Barcelona, Spain, September 2000.

[41] Schulte-Frohlinde, V., et al., "Noise Effects on the Complex Patterns of Abnormal Heartbeats," *Phys. Rev. Lett.*, Vol. 87, No. 6, August 6, 2001, 068104.

[42] Schulte-Frohlinde, V., et al., "Complex Patterns of Abnormal Heartbeats," *Phys. Rev. E*, Vol. 66, No. 3, Pt. 1, September 2002, 031901.

[43] Schulte-Frohlinde, V., et al., "Heartprints: A Dynamical Portrait of Cardiac Arrhythmia," http://www.physionet.org/physiotools/heartprints/.

[44] deChazal, P., and R. B. Reilly, "Automatic Classification of ECG Beats Using Waveform Shape and Heart Beat Interval Features," *International Conference on Acoustics, Speech and Signal Processing (ICASSP'03)*, Hong Kong, Vol. 2, April 2003, pp. 269–272.

[45] Friesen, G. M., et al., "A Comparison of the Noise Sensitivity of Nine QRS Detection Algorithms," *IEEE Trans. Biomed. Eng.*, Vol. 37, No. 1, 1990, pp. 85–98.

[46] Malik, M., "Heart Rate Variability: Standards of Measurement, Physiological Interpretation, and Clinical Use," *Circulation*, Vol. 93, 1996, pp. 1043–1065.

[47] Kitney, R. I., and O. Rompelman, (eds.), *The Study of Heart Rate Variability*, London, U.K.: Oxford University Press, 1980.

[48] Yosefy, C., et al., "The Diagnostic Value of QRS Changes for Prediction of Coronary Artery Disease During Exercise Testing in Women: False-Positive Rates," *Coronary Artery Disease*, Vol. 15, No. 3, May 2004, pp. 147–154.

[49] Shouldice, R., C. Heneghan, and P. Nolan, "Methods of Quantifying Respiratory Modulation in Human pr Electrocardiographic Intervals," *Proc. 24th Annual IEEE International Conference on Engineering in Medicine and Biology (EMBS-BMES)*, October 2002.

[50] Ward, S., et al., "Electrocardiogram Sampling Frequency Errors in PR Interval Spectral Analysis," *Proc. IEEE PGBIOMED'04*, Southampton, U.K., August 2004.

[51] Malik, M., and A. J. Camm, *Heart Rate Variability*, Armonk, NY: Futura Publishing, 1995.

[52] Clifford, G. D., and L. Tarassenko, "Segmenting Cardiac-Related Data Using Sleep Stages Increases Separation Between Normal Subjects and Apnoeic Patients," *IOP Physiol. Meas.*, No. 25, 2004, pp. N27–N35.

[53] Clifford, G. D., and L. Tarassenko, "Quantifying Errors in Spectral Estimates of HRV Due to Beat Replacement and Resampling," *IEEE Trans. Biomed. Eng.*, Vol. 52, No. 4, April 2005.

[54] Mietus, J. E., et al., "The pNNx Files: Re-Examining a Widely Used Heart Rate Variability Measure," *Heart*, Vol. 88, No. 4, 2002, pp. 378–380.

[55] Grogan, E. L., et al., "Reduced Heart Rate Volatility: An Early Predictor of Death in Trauma Patients," *Annals of Surgery*, Vol. 240, No. 3, September 2004, pp. 547–556.

[56] Griffin, M. P., and J. R. Moorman, "Toward the Early Diagnosis of Neonatal Sepsis and Sepsis-Like Illness Using Novel Heart Rate Analysis," *Pediatrics*, Vol. 107, No. 1, 2001, pp. 97–104.

[57] Cerutti, S., A. M. Bianchi, and L. T. Mainardi, "Spectral Analysis of Heart Rate Variability Signal," in M. Malik and A. J. Camm, (eds.), *Heart Rate Variability*, Armonk, NY: Futura Publishing, 1995.

[58] Taylor, J. A., et al., "Mechanisms Underlying Very-Low-Frequency RR-Interval Oscillations in Humans," *Circulation*, Vol. 98, 1998, pp. 547–555.

[59] Serrador, J. M., H. C. Finlayson, and R. L. Hughson, "Physical Activity Is a Major Contributor to the Ultra Low Frequency Components of Heart Rate Variability," *Heart*, Vol. 82, No. e9, 1999, pp. 547–555.

[60] Galloway, D. G., and B. F. Womack, *An Application of Spectral Analysis and Digital Filtering to the Study of Respiratory Sinus Arrhythmia*, Technical Report 71, Bioengineering Research Lab, University of Texas, Electronics Research Center, Austin, TX, 1969.

[61] Sayers, B. McA., "Analysis of Heart Rate Variability," *Ergonomics*, Vol. 16, No. 1, 1969, pp. 17–32.

[62] Crawford, M. H., S. Bernstein, and P. Deedwania, "ACC/AHA Guidelines for Ambulatory ECG," *Circulation*, Vol. 100, 1999, pp. 886–893.

[63] Medical Predictive Science Corporation, 510(k) patent application no. K021230, FDA, 2003.

[64] Boston Medical Technologies, Inc., 510(k) patent application no. K010955, FDA, 2001, http://www.fda.gov/cdrh/pdf/k010955.pdf.

[65] Clayton, R. H., et al., "Comparison of Autoregressive and Fourier Transform Based Techniques for Estimating RR Interval Spectra," *Computers in Cardiology*, 1997, pp. 379–382.

[66] Harris, F. J., "On the Use of Windows for Harmonic Analysis with the Discrete Fourier Transform," *Proc. IEEE*, Vol. 66, No. 1, January 1978.

[67] Lomb, N. R., "Least-Squares Frequency Analysis of Unequally Spaced Data," *Astrophysical and Space Science*, Vol. 39, 1976, pp. 447–462.

[68] Scargle, J. D., "Studies in Astronomical Time Series Analysis. ii. Statistical Aspects of Spectral Analysis of Unevenly Spaced Data," *Astrophysical Journal*, Vol. 263, 1982, pp. 835–853.

[69] Press, W. H., et al., *Numerical Recipes in C*, 2nd ed., Cambridge, U.K.: Cambridge University Press, 1992.

[70] Moody, G. B., "Spectral Analysis of Heart Rate Without Resampling," *Computers in Cardiology*, No. 20, 1993, pp. 715–718.

[71] Laguna, P., G. B. Moody, and R. G. Mark, "Power Spectral Density of Unevenly Sampled Data by Least-Square Analysis: Performance and Application to Heart Rate Signals," *IEEE Trans. Biomed. Eng*, Vol. BME-45, 1998, pp. 698–715.

[72] Clifford, G. D., "Signal Processing Methods for Heart Rate Variability," Ph.D. dissertation, University of Oxford, 2002.

[73] Clifford, G. D., F. Azuaje, and P. E. McSharry, "Advanced Tools for ECG Analysis," http://www.ecgtools.org/.

[74] Press, W. H., et al., *Numerical Recipes in C: The Art of Scientific Computing*, 2nd ed., Cambridge, U.K.: Cambridge University Press, 1992.

[75] Fessler, J. A., and B. P. Sutton, "Nonuniform Fast Fourier Transforms Using Min-Max Interpolation," *IEEE Trans. Sig. Proc.*, Vol. 51, No. 2, 2003, pp. 560–574.

[76] den Hertog, D., J. P. C. Kleijnen, and A. Y. D. Siem, "The Correct Kriging Variance Estimated by Bootstrapping," Discussion Paper 46, Tilburg University, Center for Economic Research, 2004, available at http://ideas.repec.org/p/dgr/kubcen/200446.html.

[77] Brown, M. L., and J. F. Kros, "The Impact of Missing Data on Data Mining," in John Wang, (ed.), *Data Mining: Opportunities and Challenges*, Hershey, PA: IRM Press, 2003, pp. 174–198.

[78] Vermunt, J. K., "Causal Log-Linear Modeling with Latent Variables and Missing Data," in U. Engel and J. Reinecke, (eds.), *Analysis of Change: Advanced Techniques in Panel Data Analysis*, Berlin/New York: Walter de Gruyter, 1996, pp. 35–60.

[79] Schmitz, A., and T. Schreiber, "Testing for Nonlinearity in Unevenly Sampled Time Series," *Phys. Rev. E*, Vol. 59, 1999, p. 4044.

[80] Kamath, M. V., and F. L. Fallen, "Correction of the Heart Rate Variability Signal for Ectopics and Missing Beats," in M. Malik and A. J. Camm, (eds.), *Heart Rate Variability*, Armonk, NY: Futura Publishing, 1995, pp. 75–85.

[81] Mateo, J., and P. Laguna, "Improved Heart Rate Variability Signal Analysis from the Beat Occurrence Times According to the IPFM Model," *IEEE Trans. Biomed. Eng.*, Vol. 47, No. 8, 2000. pp. 985–996.

[82] Lippman, N., K. M. Stein, and B. B. Lerman, "Comparison of Methods for Removal of Ectopy in Measurement of Heart Rate Variability," *Am. J. Physiol., Heart Circ. Physiol. 36*, Vol. 267, No. 36, 1994, pp. H411–H418.

[83] Merri, M., et al., "Sampling Frequency of the Electrocardiogram for Spectral Analysis of the Heart Rate Variability," *IEEE Trans. Biomed. Eng.*, Vol. 37, No. 1, January 1990, pp. 99–106.

[84] Abboud, S., and O. Barnea, "Errors Due to Sampling Frequency of Electrocardiogram in Spectral Analysis of Heart Rate Signals with Low Variability," *Computers in Cardiology*, Vol. 22, 1995, pp. 113–116.

[85] Clifford, G. D., and P. E. McSharry, "Method to Filter ECGs and Evaluate Clinical Parameter Distortion Using Realistic ECG Model Parameter Fitting," *Computers in Cardiology*, Vol. 32, 2005.

[86] Clifford, G. D., P. E. McSharry, and L. Tarassenko, "Characterizing Abnormal Beats in the Normal Human 24-Hour RR Tachogram to Aid Identification and Artificial Replication of Circadian Variations in Human Beat to Beat Heart Rate," *Computers in Cardiology*, Vol. 29, 2002, pp. 129–132.

[87] Clifford, G. D., et al., "Segmentation of 24-Hour Cardiovascular Activity Using ECG-Based Sleep/Sedation and Noise Metrics," *Computers in Cardiology*, Vol. 32, 2005.

[88] Bernardi, L., et al., "Effects of Controlled Breathing, Mental Activity and Mental Stress with or without Verbalization on Heart Rate Variability," *Journal of the American College of Cardiology*, Vol. 35, No. 6, May 2000, pp. 1462–1469.

[89] Lavie, P., *The Enchanted World of Sleep*, New Haven, CT: Yale University Press, 1996.

[90] Rechtschaffen, A., and A. Kales, *A Manual of Standardized Terminology, Techniques and Scoring System for Sleep Stages of Human Subjects*, Public Health Service, Washington, D.C.: U.S. Government Printing Office, 1968.

[91] Vanoli, V., et al., "Heart Rate Variability During Specific Sleep Stages," *Circulation*, Vol. 91, 1995, pp. 1918–1922.

[92] Otzenberger, H., et al., "Dynamic Heart Rate Variability: A Tool for Exploring Sympathovagal Balance Continuously During Sleep in Men," *Am. J. Physiol.: Heart Circ. Physiol.*, Vol. 275, 1998, pp. H946–H950.

[93] Lavie, P., A. Shlitner, and R. Nave, "Cardiac Autonomic Function During Sleep in Psychogenic and Organic Erectile Dysfunction," *J. Sleep Res.*, Vol. 8, 1999, pp. 135–142.

[94] Clifford, G. D., and P. E. McSharry, "Generating 24-Hour ECG, BP and Respiratory Signals with Realistic Linear and Nonlinear Clinical Characteristics Using a Nonlinear Model," *Computers in Cardiology*, Vol. 31, 2004, pp. 709–712.

[95] McSharry, P. E., and G. D. Clifford, "A Statistical Model of the Sleep-Wake Dynamics of the Cardiac Rhythm," *Computers in Cardiology*, Vol. 32, 2005.

[96] Peng, C. -K., et al., "Quantification of Scaling Exponents and Crossover Phenomena in Nonstationary Heartbeat Time Series," *Chaos*, Vol. 5, 1995, pp. 82–87.

[97] Goldberger, A. L., et al., "Fractal Dynamics in Physiology: Alterations with Disease and Ageing" *Proc. Natl. Acad. Sci.*, Vol. 99, 2002, pp. 2466–2472.

[98] Schroeder, M. R., *Fractals, Chaos, Power Laws: Minutes from an Infinite Paradise*, New York: W. H. Freeman, 1991.

[99] Heneghan, C., and G. McDarby, "Establishing the Relation Between Detrended Fluctuation Analysis and Power Spectral Density Analysis for Stochastic Processes," *Phys. Rev. E*, Vol. 62, No. 5, 2000.

[100]   McSharry, P. E., and B. D. Malamud, "Quatifying Self-Similarity in Cardiac Inter-Beat Interval Time Series," *Computers in Cardiology*, Vol. 32, September 2005.

[101]   Willson, K., and D. P. Francis, "A Direct Analytical Demonstration of the Essential Equivalence of Detrended Fluctuation Analysis and Spectral Analysis of RR Interval Variability," *Physiological Measurement*, Vol. 24, No. 1, 2003, pp. N1–N7.

[102]   Teich, M. C., et al., *Heart Rate Variability: Measures and Models, Nonlinear Biomedical Signal Processing, Vol. II: Dynamic Analysis and Modeling*, Piscataway, NJ: IEEE Press, 2000.

[103]   Ivanov, P. C., et al., "Scaling Behaviour of Heartbeat Intervals Obtained by Wavelet-Based Time-Series Analysis," *Nature*, Vol. 383, September 1996, pp. 323–327.

[104]   Turcott, R. G., and M. C. Teich, "Fractal Character of the Electrocardiogram: Distinguishing Heart-Failure and Normal Patients," *Ann. Biomed. Eng.*, Vol. 2, No. 24, March–April 1996, pp. 269–293.

[105]   Malamud, B. D., and D. L. Turcotte, "Self-Affine Time Series: Measures of Weak and Strong Persistence," *Journal of Statistical Planning and Inference*, Vol. 80, No. 1–2, August 1999, pp. 173–196.

[106]   Lowen, S. B., et al., "Fractal Features of Dark, Maintained, and Driven Neural Discharges in the Cat Visual System," *AMethods*, Vol. 4, No. 24, August 2001, pp. 377–394.

[107]   Costa, M., A. L. Goldberger, and C. K. Peng, "Open Source Software for Multiscale Entropy Snalysis," http://www.physionet.org/physiotools/mse/.

[108]   Ivanov, P. C., et al., "Sleep Wake Differences in Scaling Behavior of the Human Heartbeat: Analysis of Terrestrial and Long-Term Space Flight Data," *Europhys. Lett.*, Vol. 48, No. 5, 1999, pp. 594–600.

[109]   Lo, C. C., et al., "Common Scale-Invariant Patterns of Sleep-Wake Transitions Across Mammalian Species," *PNAS*, Vol. 101, No. 50, 2004, pp. 17545–17548.

[110]   Moody, G. B., "ECG-Based Indices of Physical Activity," *Computers in Cardiology*, No. 19, 1992, pp. 403–406.

[111]   Fukada, K., H. E. Stanley, and L. A. N. Amaral, "Heuristic Segmentation of a Nonstationary Time Series," *Phys. Rev. E*, Vol. 69, 2004, pp. 021108.

[112]   Ferini-Strambi, L., et al., "The Impact of Cyclic Alternating Pattern on Heart Rate Variability During Sleep in Healthy Young Adults," *Clinical Neurophysiology*, Vol. 111, No. 1, January 2000, pp. 99–101.

[113]   Brown, E. N., et al., "A Statistical Model of the Human Core-Temperature Circadian Rhythm," *Am. J. Physiol. Endocrinol. Metab.*, Vol. 279, No. 3, 2000, pp. E669–683.

[114]   Thomas, R. J., et al., "An Electrocardiogram-Based Technique to Assess Cardiopulmonary Coupling During Sleep," *Sleep*, Vol. 28, No. 9, October 2005, pp. 1151–1161.

[115]   Moody, G. B., et al., "Derivation of Respiratory Signals from Multi-Lead ECGs," *Proc. Computers in Cardiology*, IEEE Computer Society Press, 1986, pp. 113–116.

[116]   Riker, R. R., J. T. Picard, and G. L. Fraser, "Prospective Evaluation of the Sedation-Agitation Scale for Adult Critically Ill Patients," *Crit. Care Med.*, Vol. 27, 1999, pp. 1325–1329.

[117]   Hoyer, D., et al., "Validating Phase Relations Between Cardiac and Breathing Cycles During Sleep," *IEEE Eng. Med. Biol.*, March/April 2001.

[118]   Schmidt, G., et al., "Chronotropy Following Ventricular Premature Beats Predicts Mortality After Acute Myocardial Infarction," *Circulation*, Vol. 98, No. 17, 1998, pp. 1–1016.

[119]   Schneider, R., P. Barthel, and G. Schmidt, "Methods for the Assessment of Heart Rate Turbulence in Holter-ECGs," *JACC*, Vol. 33, No. 2, 1999, p. 315A.

[120]   Watanabe, M. A., "Heart Rate Turbulence: A Review," *Indian Pacing Electrophysiol. J.*, Vol. 3, No. 1, 2003, p. 10.

[121]   Schmidt, G., et al., "Heart Rate Turbulence," http://www.h-r-t.org.

[122]   Watanabe, M. A., and G. Schmidt, "Heart Rate Turbulence: A 5-Year Review," *Heart Rhythm*, Vol. 1, No. 6, December 2004, pp. 732–738.

[123]   Schmidt, G., et al., "Heart Rate Turbulence in Post-MI Patients on and off β-Blockers," *PACE*, Vol. 23, No. II, 2000, p. 619.

[124]   Savelieva, I., D. Wichterle, and J. A. Camm, "QT-Interval Turbulence Induced by Atrial and Ventricular Extrastimuli in Patients with Ventricular Tachycardia," *Pacing and Clinical Electrophysiology*, Vol. 28, No. s1, 2005, pp. S187–S192.

[125]   Bauer, A., et al., "Turbulence Dynamics: An Independent Predictor of Late Mortality After Acute Myocardial Infarction," *International Journal of Cardiology*, No. 107, 2006, pp. 42–47.

[126]   Watanabe, M. A., et al., "Effects of Ventricular Premature Stimulus Coupling Interval on Blood Pressure and Heart Rate Turbulence," *Circulation*, Vol. 106, 2002, pp. 325–330.

[127]   Schneider, R., G. Schmidt, and P. Barthel, "Correlation Coefficient of the Heart Rate Turbulence Slope: New Risk Stratifier in Post-Infarction Patients," *European Heart Journal*, Vol. 22, 2001, p. 72.

[128]   Berkowitsch, A., et al., "Turbulence Jump: A New Descriptor of Heart-Rate Turbulence After Paced Premature Ventricular Beats, A Study in Dilated Cardiomyopathy Patients," *European Heart Journal*, Vol. 22, 2001, p. 547.

[129]   Schmidt, G., et al., "Heart-Rate Turbulence After Ventricular Premature Beats as a Predictor of Mortality After Acute Myocardial Infarction," *Lancet*, Vol. 353, No. 9162, 1999, pp. 1390–1396.

[130]   Schneider, R., et al., "Heart Rate Turbulence: Rate of Frequency Decrease Predicts Mortality in Chronic Heart Disease Patients," *PACE*, Vol. 22, No. 2, 1999, p. 879.

CHAPTER 4

Models for ECG and RR Interval Processes

Patrick E. McSharry and Gari D. Clifford

4.1 Introduction

The availability of open-source computational models and simulators can greatly facilitate the advancement of cardiovascular research by complementing clinical studies.[1] Such models provide the researcher with the means of formulating hypotheses that may be subsequently tested through investigations of both simulated biomedical signals and real-world signals obtained from clinical studies. There is a two-way relationship between the development of these models and the exploration of biomedical databases obtained from clinical studies. First, researchers can construct and evaluate their models using the biomedical signals. Access to these databases facilitates the estimation of important cardiovascular parameters and the comparison of different models. Second, the ability to simulate realistic signals using these models can be used to assess novel biomedical signal processing techniques. In addition, these models can be used to formulate new experimental hypotheses.

The ECG signal describes the electrical activity in the heart and each heartbeat traces the familiar morphology labeled by the P, Q, R, S, and T peaks and troughs. Since the R peak is typically associated with the largest deflection away from the baseline, this peak is generally taken as a marker for each heartbeat as it is the easiest to locate. As was pointed out in Chapter 3, the correct fiducial point for each heartbeat is the onset of the P wave. However, this point is both difficult to define and locate and the Q-R interval is often sufficiently short and of low variability that the R peak suffices to give an accurate fiducial marker of cardiac activity. The sequence of successive times, t_i ($i = 1, 2, \ldots, n$), produced by applying a QRS detector (see Chapter 7) to the ECG signal, are transformed into a sequence of RR intervals via

$$RR_i = t_i - t_{i-1} \tag{4.1}$$

This sequence of RR intervals forms the basis of the RR interval time series or *RR tachogram*. A corresponding sequence of instantaneous heart rates may also be defined by

$$f_i = \frac{1}{RR_i} \tag{4.2}$$

---

1. See http://www.physionet.org for a description of available databases and tools.

In the following sections, a number of useful models and related tools available for researchers within the field of biomedical signal processing are described. These models are grouped into two categories, the first relating to RR intervals and the second to ECG signals.

4.2 RR Interval Models

In the following sections, we review a variety of modeling approaches that are useful for understanding and investigating the processes underlying the RR tachogram. These models range from physiology-based to empirical data-based approaches and statistical descriptions that may be used for classification. Section 4.2.1 provides an overview of the cardiovascular system. Section 4.2.2 gives a summary of the DeBoer model. Section 4.2.3 discusses a freely available cardiovascular simulator available from PhysioNet. Section 4.2.4 describes the integral pulse frequency modulation model. Sections 4.2.5 and 4.2.6 present two data-driven modeling approaches using nonlinear deterministic models and a system of coupled oscillators. A more descriptive analysis from the point of scale invariance is given in Section 4.2.7. Finally, a selection of models that were entered in the 2002 PhysioNet Challenge are summarized in Section 4.2.8.

4.2.1 The Cardiovascular System

The cardiovascular system consists of a closed circuit of blood vessels. A continuous motion of blood from the left to the right heart provides the individual cells with sufficient nutrients. The flow in the vessels is controlled by the myogenic and neurogenic processes; the former refers to the contraction and relaxation of smooth muscle in the vessel wall whereas the latter is driven by the autonomic nervous system. Although the myogenic and neurogenic processes affect heart rate (and hence the ECG) over the long term, the dominant observable effects on the RR interval timing and ECG morphology are due to the regulation of the heart's pacemaker by the sympathetic and parasympathetic branches of the autonomic nervous system (see Chapters 1 and 3). In an oversimplistic sense, the sympathetic nervous system can be thought of as the body's *fight or flight* response, which acts quickly to increase heart rate, blood pressure, and respiration. Conversely, the parasympathetic system can be thought of as the *rest and digest* system, which acts to slow heart rate (HR) and respiration, as well as lowering blood pressure (BP) (e.g., when falling asleep).

Respiration, a mainly parasympathetically mediated process, is the most obvious observable phenomenon in the RR tachogram (and in the ECG; see Chapter 3 and Section 4.3.2). The normal variation in RR intervals (and R amplitudes) on a beat-to-beat basis, known as respiratory sinus arrhythmia [1, 2], is almost synchronous with the respiratory oscillations. The small phase differences between the two oscillations has been observed to be constant in some circumstances. However, this phase is known to change over even short periods of time, depending on the activity of the patient (see [3, 4] and Section 4.2.6). There is also a coupling between HR and BP and between BP and respiration (see [5] and Section 4.2.2). It should be noted at this point that BP measurements are a function of the location and time (in the cycle) at which they are measured. In this chapter, BP refers to the mean systemic arterial pressure (MAP), usually recorded from the brachial artery. Approximately two-thirds of the cardiac cycle is spent in diastole, and therefore MAP is often calculated as one-third of the difference between the maximum and minimum aortic pressure following ejection of blood from the left ventricle ($\frac{1}{3}$ systolic BP (SBP) $+\frac{2}{3}$ diastolic BP (DBP). Pulse pressure is simply the difference between the SBP and the DBP.

Since the effects of the myogenic and neurogenic processes on the RR interval time series are not well understood [6], the discussion of the biological processes in the context of the models presented in this chapter will be confined to short-term couplings of the cardiovascular system; HR (approximately $0.5 \rightarrow 5$ Hz), respiration (approximately $1/15 \rightarrow 0.5$ Hz), and BP (approximately $1/60 \rightarrow 1/5$ Hz). Longer term fluctuations are considered from an empirical standpoint in Sections 4.2.7 and 4.2.8 and in Chapter 3.

Any model that describes the changes in RR intervals over time, should allow for a description of heart rate variability (HRV) and its relationship to HR, BP, and respiration. There is no simple connection between HR, HRV, and BP. However, many measures of HR and HRV are often inversely correlated: Stimuli that increase HR often depress the variability of the HR in the short term. Conversely, activities that cause a drop in the average HR can lead to an increase in short-term HRV. Although the strength of this correlation can change over time and from individual to individual, it is useful to consider the cardiovascular system from a static perspective in order to investigate the relationship between the cardiovascular parameters.

The cardiovascular system may be viewed as a pressure controlled system, and therefore factors that influence changes in BP will also cause fluctuations in HR. In resting humans, beat-to-beat fluctuations in BP and HR are mainly due to respiratory influences and to the slower Mayer waves [5]. Sleight and Casadei [7] emphasize that there is much evidence to support the idea that beat-to-beat HR variations are a manifestation of a central nervous system oscillator which becomes entrained with respiration as a result of afferent input from bronchopulmonary receptors.

A variety of approaches have been employed to describe the short-term control of blood pressure. Ottesen et al. [8, 9] provide an excellent review of attempts at modeling the physiology of the cardiovascular system. Grodins [10] used algebraic equations for the steady controlled heart which can be rearranged to model mean arterial pressure by a sixth-order polynomial. Madwed et al. [11] provided a descriptive model using feedback control. Ursino et al. have produced a series of differential delay equation models to allow for changes in the venous capacity and cardiac pulsatility (see [12–14] and references therein). Seidel and Herzel [15] developed a hybrid model with continuous variables and an integrate and fire mechanism to generate a discrete heart rate. McSharry et al. [16] present a simple differential delay equation model of the cardiovascular system which is able to reproduce many of the empirical characteristics observed in biomedical signals such as heart rate, blood pressure, and respiration. The model also includes the effects of RSA, Mayer waves, and synchronization.

It is generally agreed [7], however, that coupling of HR, respiration, and the cardiac cycle (the flow of blood around the body with its consequent pressures) can be broadly explained as follows: inspiration lowers intrathoracic pressure and enhances filling of the right heart from extrathoracic veins. Right ventricular stroke volume, therefore, increases, and a consequent rise in the effective pressure of the rest of the circulation is observed. The rise in effective pressure in the pulmonary veins leads to an increased filling of the left heart and hence to an increased left ventricular stroke volume.

The resistance and hydraulic capacitances of the lesser circulation create a lag between inspiration and right ventricular output increase and between the rise of effective pulmonary venous pressure and left ventricular filling. A consequence of this is that stroke volume modulation will decrease with increasing respiratory rate (for a given respiratory depth). Furthermore, the phase lag of the stroke volume change with respect to the corresponding respiratory oscillation will increase for higher rates. In practice, at moderately rapid respiratory rates, the BP and stroke volume fall throughout most of the inspiration. Therefore, the fall in arterial pressure with inspiration is due to the preceding expiration. Furthermore, the strength of this relationship increases as the patient moves from a supine to upright position.

During expiration, the longer pulse or RR interval buffers any change in diastolic pressure caused by the resultant increase in stroke volume, so diastolic pressure changes may correlate poorly with reflex changes. This supports the notion that respiration drives BP changes, which in turn drive the RR and HR changes. Diastolic BP changes with respiration are quite small since the inspiratory tachycardia tends to reduce any inspiratory fall in diastolic pressure (as there is less time for the diastolic pressure to drop).

This observation was first explained by DeBoer in 1987 [5] and although there have been other mathematical models proposed since then (such as the Baselli model [17] and the Saul model [18]), most experimental evidence is thought to support DeBoer's model [7]. For a more detailed survey of the last 50 years of cardiovascular respiratory modeling, the reader is referred to Batzel et al. [19].

4.2.2 The DeBoer Model

The DeBoer model [5] is a beat-to-beat model of the cardiovascular system developed for investigating the spontaneous short-term variability in arterial BP and HR signals recorded from human subjects at rest. This model explains how the BP affects both RR interval length and peripheral (capillary) resistance through the actions of the baroreceptors and the central nervous system. Note that slow regulatory mechanisms (< 0.05 Hz) are not included in the model. Figure 4.1 shows how the cardiac output is governed by the current value of respiration and the previous RR interval. The new BP value is set by this value of cardiac output and the peripheral resistance. The new BP value then determines the new value for the RR interval. Therefore, the model assumes that respiration first affects BP, which in turn affects the RR interval. The low-frequency[2] peak in HR at 0.1 Hz observed in steady-state conditions for humans is explained as a resonance phenomenon due to the delay in the sympathetic control loop of the baroreflex: the reflex sympathetic neural outflow cannot follow beat-to-beat changes in the BP as sensed by the baroreceptors.

---

2.   See Chapter 3 for an exact definition of the low and high-frequency components.

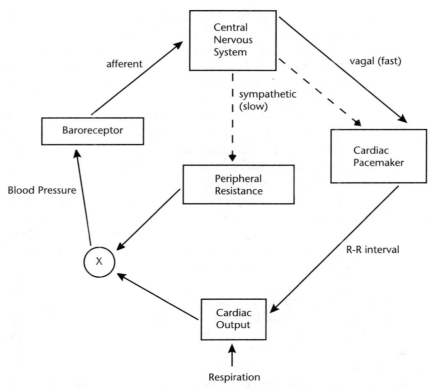

Figure 4.1 Schematic digram of the cardiovascular system following DeBoer [5]. Dashed lines indicate slow sympathetic control, and solid lines indicate faster parasympathetic control.

The respiratory signal that drives the high-frequency variations in the model is assumed to be unaffected by the other system parameters. DeBoer chose the respiratory signal to be a simple sinusoid, although other investigations have explored the use of more realistic signals [20]. DeBoer's model was the first to allow for the discrete (beat-to-beat) nature of the heart, whereas all previous models had used continuous differential equations to describe the cardiovascular system. The model consists of a set of difference equations involving systolic blood pressure (S), diastolic pressure (D), pulse pressure ($P = S - D$), peripheral resistance (R), RR interval (I), and an arterial time constant ($T = RC$), with C as the arterial compliance. The equations are then based upon four distinct mechanisms:

1. *Control of the HR and peripheral resistance by the baroreflex:* The current RR interval value, is a linear weighted combination of the last seven systolic BP values ($a_0 S_n...a_6 S_{n-6}$). The current systolic value, S_n, represents the vagal effect weighted by coefficient a_0 (fast with short delays), whereas $S_{n-2}...S_{n-6}$ represent sympathetic contributions (slower with longer delays). The previous systolic value, S_{n-1}, does not contribute ($a_1 = 0$) because its vagal effect has already died out and the sympathetic effect is not yet active.

2. *Windkessel properties of the systemic arterial tree:* This represents the sympathetic action of the baroreflex on the peripheral resistance. The Windkessel equation, $D_n = c_3 S_{n-1} \exp(-I_{n-1}/T_{n-1})$, describes the diastolic pressure

decay, governed by the ratio of the previous RR interval to the previous arterial time constant. The time constant of the decay, T_n, and thus (assuming a constant arterial compliance C) the current value of the peripheral resistance, R_n, depends on a weighted sum of the previous six values of S.

3. *Contractile properties of the myocardium:* The influence of the length of the previous interval on the strength of the ventricular contraction is given by $P_n = \gamma I_{n-1} + c_2$, where γ and c_2 are physiological constants. A longer pulse interval ($I_{n-1} > I_{n-2}$) therefore tends to increase the next pulse pressure (if $\gamma > 0$), P_n, a phenomenon motivated by the increased filling of the ventricles after a long interval, leading to a more forceful contraction (Starling's law) and by the restitution properties of the myocardium (which also leads to an increased strength of contraction after a longer interval).

4. *Mechanical effects of respiration on BP:* Respiration is simulated by disturbing P_n with a sinusoidal variation in I. Without this addition, the equations themselves do not imply any fluctuations in BP or HR but lead to stable values for the different variables.

Linearization of the equations of motion around operating points (normal human values for S, D, I, and T) was employed to facilitate an analysis of the model. Note that such a linearization is a good approximation when the subject is at rest. The addition of a simulated respiratory signal was shown to provide a good correspondence between the power spectra of real and simulated data. DeBoer also pointed out the need to perform cross-spectral analysis between the RR tachogram, the systolic BP, and respiration signals. Pitzalis et al. [21] performed such an analysis supporting DeBoer's model and showed that the respiratory rate modulates the interrelationship between the RR interval and S variabilities: the higher the rate of respiration, the smaller the gain and the smaller the phase difference between the two. Furthermore, the same response is found after administering a β-adrenoceptor blockade, suggesting that the sympathetic drive is not involved in this process. Sleight and Casadei [7] also present evidence to support the assumptions underlying the DeBoer model.

4.2.3   The Research Cardiovascular Simulator

The Research CardioVascular SIMulator (RCVSIM) [22–24] software[3] was developed in order to complement the experimental data sets provided by PhysioBank. The human cardiovascular model underlying RCVSIM is based upon an electrical circuit analog, with charge representing blood volume (Q, ml), current representing blood flow rate ($\dot{q}$, ml/s), voltage representing pressure (P, mmHg), capacitance representing arterial/vascular compliance (C), and resistance (R) representing frictional resistance to viscous blood flow. RCVSIM includes three major components.

The first component (illustrated in Figure 4.2) is a lumped parameter model of the pulsatile heart and circulation which itself consists of six compartments, the left ventricles, the right ventricles, the systemic arteries, the systemic veins, the

---

3.   Open-source code and further details are available from http://www.physionet.org/physiotools/rcvsim/.

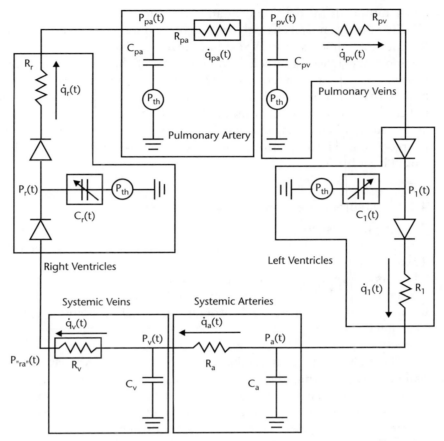

Figure 4.2 PhysioNet's RCVSIM lumped parameter model of the human heart-lung unit in terms of its electrical circuit analog. Charge is analogous to blood volume (Q, ml), current, to blood flow rate ($\dot{q}$, ml/s), and voltage, to pressure (P, mmHg). The model consists of six compartments which represent the left and right ventricles (l, r), systemic arteries and veins (a, v), and pulmonary arteries and veins (pa, pv). Each compartment consists of a conduit for viscous blood flow with resistance (R), a volume storage element with compliance (C) and unstressed volume (Q^0). The node labeled $P_{"ra"}(t)$ is the location of where the right atrium would be if it were explicitly included in the model. (*Adapted from:* [22] with permission. © 2006 R. Mukkamala.)

pulmonary arteries, and the pulmonary veins. Each compartment consists of a conduit for viscous blood flow with resistance (R), a volume storage element with compliance (C) and unstressed volume (Q^0). The second major component of the model is a short-term regulatory system based upon the DeBoer model and includes an arterial baroreflex system, a cardiopulmonary baroreflex system, and a direct neural coupling mechanism between respiration and heart rate. The third major component of RCVSIM is a model of resting physiologic perturbations which includes respiration, autoregulation of local vascular beds (exogenous disturbance to systemic arterial resistance), and higher brain center activity affecting the autonomic nervous system ($1/f$ exogenous disturbance to heart rate [25]).

The model is capable of generating realistically human pulsatile hemodynamic waveforms, cardiac function and venous return curves, and beat-to-beat hemodynamic variability. RCVSIM has been previously employed in cardiovascular research by its author for the development and evaluation of system identification methods aimed at the dynamical characterization of autonomic regulatory mechanisms [23]. Recent developments of RCVSIM have involved the development of a parallelized version and extensions for adaptation to space-flight data to describe the processes involved in orthostatic hypotension [26–28]. Simulink versions have been developed both with and without the baroreflex reflex mechanism, and an additional interstitial compartment to aid work fitting the model parameters to real data representing an instance of hemorrhagic shock [29]. These recent innovations are currently being redeveloped into a platform-independent version which will shortly be available from PhysioNet [22, 30].

4.2.4 Integral Pulse Frequency Modulation Model

The integral pulse frequency modulation (IPFM) model was developed for investigating the generation of a discrete series of events, such as a series of heartbeats [31]. This model assumes the existence of a continuous-time input modulation signal which possesses a particular physiological interpretation, such as describing the mechanisms underlying the autonomic nervous system [32]. The action of this modulation signal when integrated through the model generates a series of interbeat time intervals, which may be compared to RR intervals recorded from human subjects.

The IPFM model assumes that the autonomic activity, including both the sympathetic and parasympathetic influences, may be represented by a single modulating input signal $x(t)$. This input signal $x(t)$ is integrated until a threshold, R, is reached where a beat is generated. At this point, the integrator is reset to zero and the process is repeated [31, 33] (see Figure 4.3). The beat-to-beat time series may be expressed as a series of pulses,

$$p(t) = n = \int_0^{t_n} \frac{1 + x(t)}{T} dt, \qquad (4.3)$$

where n is an integer number representing the nth beat and t_n reflects its time stamp. The time T is the mean interbeat interval and $x(t)/T$ is the zero-mean modulating term. It is usual to assume that this modulation term is relatively small $(x(t) << 1)$

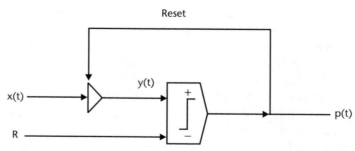

Figure 4.3 The integral pulse frequency modulation model. The input signal $x(t)$ is integrated yielding $y(t)$. When $y(t)$ reaches the fixed reference value R, a pulse is emitted and the integrator is reset to 0, whereupon the cycle starts again. Output of the model is the series of pulses $p(t)$. When used to model the cardiac pacemaker, the input is a signal proportional to the accelerating autonomic efferences on the pacemaker cells and the output is the RR interval time series.

in order to reflect that heart rate variability is usually smaller than the mean heart rate. The time-dependent value of $(1 + x(t))/T$ may be viewed as the instantaneous heart rate. For simplification, the first beat is assumed to occur at time $t_0 = 0$. Generally, $x(t)$ is assumed to be band-limited with negligible power for frequencies greater than 0.4 Hz.

In physiological terms, the output signal of the integrator can be viewed as the charging of the membrane potential of a sino-atrial pacemaker cell [34]. The potential increases until a certain threshold (R in Figure 4.3) is exceeded and then triggers an action potential which, when combined with the effect of many other action potentials, initiates another cardiac cycle.

Given that the assumptions underlying the IPFM are valid, the aim is to construct a method for obtaining information about the input signal $x(t)$ using the observed sequence of event times t_n. The various issues concerning a reasonable choice of time domain signal for representing the activity in the heart are discussed in [32].

The IPFM model has been extended to provide a time-varying threshold integral pulse frequency modulation (TVTIPFM) model [35]. This approach has been applied to RR intervals in order to discriminate between autonomic nervous modulation and the mechanical stretch induced effect caused by changes in the venous return and respiratory modulation.

4.2.5   Nonlinear Deterministic Models

A chaotic dynamic system may be capable of generating a wide range of irregular time series that would normally be associated with stochastic dynamics. The task of identifying whether a particular set of observations may have arisen from a chaotic system has given rise to a large body of research (see [36] and references therein). The method of surrogate data is particularly useful for constructing hypothesis tests for asking whether or not a given data set may have underlying nonlinear dynamics [37]. Nonlinear deterministic models come in a variety of forms ranging from local linear models [38–40] to radial basis functions and neural networks [41, 42].

The first step when constructing a model using nonlinear time series analysis techniques is to identify a suitable state space reconstruction. For a time series $s_n, (n = 1, 2, \ldots, N)$, a delay coordinate reconstruction is obtained using

$$x_n = \left[s_{n-(m-1)\tau}, \ldots, s_{n-2\tau}, s_n \right] \tag{4.4}$$

where m and τ are known as the reconstruction dimension and delay, respectively. The ability to accurately evaluate a particular reconstruction and compare various models requires an incorporation of the measurement uncertainty inherent in the data. McSharry and Smith give examples of how these techniques may be employed when analysing three different experimental datasets [43]. In particular, this investigation presents a consistency check that may be used to identify why and where a particular model is inadequate and suggests a means of resolving these problems.

Cao and Mees [44] developed a deterministic local linear model for analyzing nonlinear interactions between heart rate, respiration, and the oxygen saturation (SaO_2) wave in the cardiovascular system. This model was constructed using multichannel physiological signals from dataset B of the Santa Fe Time Series Competition [45]. They found that it was possible to construct a model that provides accurate forecasts of the next time step (next beat) in one signal using a combination of previous values selected from the other two signals. This demonstrates that heart rate, respiration, and oxygen saturation are three key interacting factors in the cardiorespiratory cycle since no other signal is required to provide accurate predictions. The investigation was repeated and it found similar results for different segments of the three signals. It should be emphasized, however, that this analysis was performed on only one subject who suffered from sleep apnea. In this case, a strong correlation between respiration and the cardiovascular effort is to be expected. For this reason, these results cannot be assumed to hold for normal subjects and the results may indeed be specific to only the Santa Fe Time Series. The question of whether parameters derived in specific situations are sufficiently distinct such that they can be used to identify improving or worsening conditions remains unanswered. A more detailed description of nonlinear techniques and their application to filtering ECG signals can be found in Chapter 6.

4.2.6   Coupled Oscillators and Phase Synchronization

Observations of the phase differences between oscillations in HR, BP, and respiration have shown that, although the phases drift in a highly nonstationary manner, at certain times, phase locking can occur [3, 46, 47]. These observations led Rosenblum et al. [48–51] to propose the idea of representing the cardiovascular system as a set of coupled oscillators, demonstrating that phase and frequency locking are not equivalent. In the presence of noise, the relative phase performs a biased random walk, resulting in no frequency locking, while retaining the presence of phase locking.

Bračič et al. [47, 52, 53] then extended this model, consisting of five linearly coupled oscillators,

$$\dot{x}_i = -x_i q_i - \omega_i y_i + g_{x_i}(\mathbf{x})$$

$$\dot{y}_i = -y_i q_i + \omega_i x_i + g_{y_i}(\mathbf{y}), \quad q_i = \alpha_i \left(\sqrt{x_i^2 + y_i^2} - a_i \right) \qquad (4.5)$$

where $\mathbf{x}$, $\mathbf{y}$ are state vectors, $g_{x_i}(\mathbf{x})$ and $g_{y_i}(\mathbf{y})$ are linear coupling vectors, and α_i, a_i, ω_i are constants governing the individual oscillators. For each oscillator i, the dynamics are described by the blood flow, x_i, and the blood flow rate, y_i.

Numerical simulation of this model generated signals which appeared similar to the observed signals recorded from human subjects. This model with linear couplings and added noise is capable of displaying similar forms of synchronization as that observed for real signals. In particular, short episodes of synchronization appear and disappear at random intervals as has been observed for human subjects.

One condition in which cardiorespiratory coupling is frequently observed is a type of sleep known as noncyclic alternating phase (NCAP) sleep (see Chapter 3). In fact, the changes in cardiovascular parameters over the sleep cycle and between wakefullness and sleep are an active current research field which is only just being explored (see [54–62]). In particular, Peng et al. [25, 57] have shown that the RR interval exhibits some interesting long-range (circadian) scaling characteristics over the 24-hour period (see Section 4.2.7). Since heart rate and HRV are known to be correlated with activity and sleep [56], Lo et al. [62] later followed up this work to show that the distribution of durations of wakefullness and sleep followed different distributions; sleep episode durations follow a scale-free power law independent of species, and sleep episode durations follow an exponential law with a characteristic time scale related to body mass and metabolic rate.

4.2.7 Scale Invariance

Many complex biological systems display scale-invariant properties and the absence of a characteristic scale (time and/or spatial domains) may suggest certain advantages in terms of the ability to easily adapt to changes caused by external sources. The traditional analysis of heart rate variability focuses on short time oscillations related to respiration (approximately between 0.15 and 0.4 Hz) and the influence of BP control mechanisms at approximately 0.1 Hz. The resting heartbeat of a healthy human tends to vary in an erratic manner and casts doubt on the homeostatic viewpoint of cardiovascular regulation in healthy humans. In fact, the analysis of a long time series of heartbeat interval time series (typically over 24 hours) gives rise to a $1/f$-like spectrum for frequencies less than 0.1 Hz, suggesting the possibility of scale-invariance in HRV [63].

The analysis of long records of RR intervals, with 24 hours giving approximately 10^5 data points, is possible using ambulatory (Holter) monitors. Peng et al. [25] found that in the case of healthy subjects, these RR intervals display scale-invariant, long-range anticorrelations up to 10^4 heartbeats. The histogram of increments of the RR intervals may be described by a Lévy stable distribution.[4] Furthermore, a group of subjects with severe heart disease had similar distributions but the long-range correlations vanished. This suggests that the different scaling behavior in health and disease must be related to the underlying dynamics of the cardiovascular system.

A log-log plot of the power spectra, $S(f)$, of the RR intervals displays a linear relationship, such that $S(f) \sim f^\beta$. The value of β can be used to distinguish between: (1) $\beta = 0$, an uncorrelated time series also known as "white noise"; (2) $-1 < \beta < 0$, correlated such that positive values are likely to be close in time to each other and the same is true for negative values; and (3) $0 < \beta < 1$, anticorrelated time series such that positive and negative values are more likely to alternate in time. The $1/f$ noise, $\beta = 1$, often called "pink noise," typically displayed by cardiac interbeat intervals is an intermediate compromise between the randomness of white noise, $\beta = 0$, and the much smoother Brownian motion, $\beta = 2$.

Although RR intervals from healthy subjects follow approximately $\beta \sim 1$, RR intervals from heart failure subjects have $\beta \sim 1.6$, which is closer to Brownian motion [65]. This variation in scaling suggests that the value of β may provide the basis of a useful medical diagnostic. While there are a number of techniques available

---

4. A heavy-tailed generalization of the normal distribution [64].

for quantifying self-similarity, detrended fluctuation analysis is often employed to measure the self-similarity of nonstationary biomedical signals [66]. DFA provides a scaling coefficient, α, which is related to β via $\beta = 2\alpha - 1$.

McSharry and Malamud [67] compared five different techniques for quantifying self-similarity in time series; these included power-spectral, wavelet variance, semivariograms, rescaled-range, and detrended fluctuation analysis. Each technique was applied to both normal and log-normal synthetic fractional noises and motions generated using a spectral method, where a normally distributed white noise was appropriately filtered such that its power-spectral density, S, varied with frequency, f, according to $S \sim f^{-\beta}$. The five techniques provide varying levels of accuracy depending on β and the degree of nonnormality of the time series being considered. For normally distributed time series, semivariograms provide accurate estimates for $1.2 < \beta < 2.5$, rescaled range for $0.0 < \beta < 0.8$, DFA for $-0.8 < \beta < 2.2$, and power spectra and wavelets for all values of β. All techniques demonstrate decreasing accuracy for log-normal fractional noises with increasing coefficient of variance, particularly for antipersistent time series. Wavelet analysis offers the best performance both in terms of providing accurate estimates for normally distributed time series over the entire range $-2 \leq \beta \leq 4$ and having the least decrease in accuracy for log-normal noises.

The existence of a power law spectrum provides a necessary condition for scale invariance in the process underlying heart rate variability. Ivanov et al. [68] demonstrated that the normal healthy human heartbeat, even under resting conditions, fluctuates in a complex manner and has a multifractal[5] temporal structure. Furthermore, there was evidence of a loss of multifractality (to monofractality) in cases of congestive heart failure. Scaling techniques adapted from statistical physics have revealed the presence of long-range, power-law correlations, as part of multifractal cascades operating over a wide range of time scales (see [65, 68] and references therein).

A number of different statistical models have been proposed to explain the mechanisms underlying the heart rate variability of healthy human subjects. Lin and Hughson [69] present a model motivated by an analogy with turbulence. This approach provides a cascade-type multifractal model for determining the deformation of the distribution of RR intervals. One feature of such a model is that of evolving from a Gaussian distribution at small scales to a stretched exponential at smaller scales. Kiyono et al. [70] argue that the healthy human heart rate is controlled to converge continually to a critical state and show that their model is capable of providing a better fit to the observed data than that of the random (multiplicative) cascade model reported in [69]. Kuusela et al. [71] present a model based on a simple one-dimensional Langevin-type stochastic difference equation, which can describe the fluctuations in the heart rate. This model is capable of explaining the multifractal behavior seen in real data and suggests how pathologic cases simplify the heart rate control system.

---

5. Monofractal signals are homogeneous in that only one scaling exponent is needed to describe all segments of the signal. In contrast, multifractal signals requires a range of different exponents to explain their scaling properties.

4.2.8   PhysioNet Challenge

The PhysioNet challenge of 2002[6] invited participants to design a numerical model for generating 24-hour records of RR intervals. A second part of the challenge asked participants to use their respective signal processing techniques to identify the real and artificial records from among a database of unmarked 24-hour RR tachograms. The wide range of models entered for the competition reflects the numerous approaches available for investigating heart rate variability. The following paragraphs summarize these approaches, which include a multiplicative cascade model, a Markovian model, and a heuristic multiscale approach based on empirical observations.

Lin and Hughson [69] explored the multifractal HRV displayed in healthy and other physiological conditions, including autonomic blockades and congestive heart failure, by using a multiplicative random cascade model. Their method used a bounded cascade model to generate artificial time series which was able to mimic some of the known phenomenology of HRV in healthy humans: (1) multifractal spectrum including $1/f$ power law, (2) the transition from stretch-exponential to Gaussian probability density function in the interbeat interval increment data and (3) the Poisson excursion law in small RR increments [72]. The cascade consisted of a discrete fragmentation process and assigned random weights to the cascade components of the fragmented time intervals. The artificial time series was finally constructed by multiplying the cascade components in each level.

Yang et al. [73] employed symbolic dynamics and probabilistic automaton to construct a Markovian model for characterizing the complex dynamics of healthy human heart rate signals. Their approach was to simplify the dynamics by mapping the output to binary sequences, where the increase and decrease of the interbeat interval were denoted by 1 and 0, respectively. In this way, it was also possible to define a m-bit symbolic sequence to characterize transitions of symbolic dynamics. For the simplest model consisting of 2-bit sequences, there are four possible symbolic sequences including 11, 10, 00, and 01. Moreover, each symbolic sequence has two possible transitions, for example, 1(0) can be transformed to (0)0, which results in decreasing RR intervals, or (0)1 and vice versa. In order to define the mechanism underlying these symbolic transitions, the authors utilized the concept of probabilistic automaton in which the transition from current symbolic sequence to next state takes place with a certain probability in a given range of RR intervals. The model used 8-bit sequences and a probability table obtained from the RR time series of healthy humans from Taipei Veterans General Hospital and PhysioNet. The resulting generator is comprised of the following major components: (1) the symbolic sequence as a state of RR dynamics, (2) the probability table defining transitions between two sequences, and (3) an absolute Gaussian noise process for governing increments of RR intervals.

McSharry et al. [74] used a heuristic empirical approach for modeling the fluctuations of the beat-to-beat RR intervals of a normal healthy human over 24 hours by considering the different time scales independently. Short range variability due to Mayer waves and RSA were incorporated into the algorithm using a

---

6.   See http://www.physionet.org/challenge/2002 for more details.

power spectrum with given spectral characteristics described by its low frequency and high frequency components, respectively [75]. Longer range fluctuations arising from transitions between physiological states were generated using switching distributions extracted from real data. The model generated realistic synthetic 24-hour RR tachograms by including both cardiovascular interactions and transitions between physiological states. The algorithm included the effects of various physiological states, including sleep states, using RR intervals with specific means and trends. An analysis of ectopic beat and artifact incidence in an accompanying paper [76] was used to provide a mechanism for generating realistic ectopy and artifact. Ectopic beats were added with an independent probability of one per hour. Artifacts were included with a probability proportional to mean heart rate within a state and increased for state transition periods. The algorithm provides RR tachograms that are similar to those in the MIT-BIH Normal Sinus Rhythm Database.

4.2.9   RR Interval Models for Abnormal Rhythms

Chapter 1 described some of the mechanisms that activate and mediate arrhythmias of the heart. Broadly speaking, modeling of arrhythmias can be broken down into two subgroups: ventricular arrhythmias and atrial arrhythmias. The models tend to describe either the underlying RR interval processes or the manifest waveform (ECG). Furthermore, the models are formulated either from the cellular conduction perspective (usually for RR interval models) or from an empirical standpoint. Since the connection between the underlying beat-to-beat interval process and the resultant waveform is complex, empirical models of the ECG waveform are common. These include simple time domain templates [77], Fourier and AR models [78], singular value decomposition-based techniques [79, 80], and more complex methods such as neural network classifiers [81–83], and finite element models [84]. Such models are usually applied on a beat-by-beat basis. Furthermore, due to the fact that the classifiers are trained using a cost function based upon a distance metric between waveforms, small deviations in the waveform morphology (such as that seen in atrial arrhythmias) are often poorly identified. In the case of atrial arrhythmias, unless a full three-dimensional model of the cardiac potentials is used (such as in Cherry et al. [85]), it is often more appropriate to analyze the RR interval process itself.

The following gives a chronological summary of the developments in modeling atrial fibrillation. In 1983, Cohen et al. [86] introduced a model for the ventricular response during AF that treated the atrio-ventricular junction as a lumped parameter structure with defined electrical properties such as the refactory period and period of autorhymicity, that is being continually bombarded by random AF impulses. Although this model could account for all the principal statistical properties of the RR interval distribution during AF, several important physiological properties of the heart were not included in the model (such as conduction delays within the AV junction and ventricle and the effect of ventricular pacing).

In 1988, Wittkampf et al. [87–89] explained the fact that short RR intervals during AF could be eliminated by ventricular pacing at relatively long cycle lengths through a model that modulates the AV node pacemaker rate and rhythm by AF impulses. However, this model failed to explain the relationship between most of the captured beats and the shortest RR interval length in a canine model.

In 1996, Meijler et al. [90] proposed an alternative model whereby the irregularity of RR intervals during AF are explained by modulation of the AV node through concealed AF impulses resulting in an inverse relationship between the atrial and ventricular rates. Unfortunately, recent clinical results do not support this prediction.

Around the same time Zeng and Glass [91] introduced an alternative model of AV node conduction which was able to correctly model much of the statistical distribution of the RR intervals during AF. This model was later extended by Tateno and Glass [92] and Jorgensen et al. [93] and includes a description of the AV delay time, τ^{AVD}, (which is known to be dependent on the AV junction recovery time) given by

$$\tau^{AVD} = \tau_{min}^{AVD} + \alpha e^{-T_R/c} \qquad (4.6)$$

where T_R is the AV junction recovery time, τ_{min}^{AVD} is the minimum AV delay when $T_R \to \infty$, α is the maximum extension of the AV delay when $T_R = 0$, and c is a time constant. Although this extension modeled many of the properties of AF, it failed to account for the dependence of the refactory period, τ^R, on the heart rate (the higher the heart rate, the shorter the refactory period) [86].

Lian et al. [94] recently proposed an extension of Cohen's model [86] which does model the refactory behavior of the AV junction as

$$\tau^{AVJ} = \tau_{min}^{AVJ} + \tau_{ext}^{AVJ}(1 - e^{-T_R/\tau_{ext}}) \qquad (4.7)$$

where τ_{min}^{AVJ} is the shortest AV junction refactory period corresponding to $T_R = 0$ and τ_{ext}^{AVJ} is the maximum extension of the refactory period when $T_R \to \infty$. The AV delay (4.6) is also included in this model together with a function which expresses the modulation of the AV junction refactory period by blocked impulses. If an impulse is blocked by the refactory AV junction, τ^{AVJ} is prolonged by the concealed impulse such that

$$\tau^{AVJ} \to \tau^{AVJ} + \tau_{min}^{AVJ}\left(\frac{t}{\tau^{AVJ}}\right)^{\theta}\left[\max\left(1, \frac{\Delta V}{(V_T - V_R)}\right)\right]^{\delta} \qquad (4.8)$$

where $\Delta V/(V_T - V_R)$ is the relative amplitude of the AF pulses and t ($0 < t < \tau^{AVJ}$) is the time when the impulse is blocked. θ and δ are independent parameters which modulate the timing and duration of the blocked impulse. With suitably chosen values for the above parameters, this model can account for all the statistical properties of observed RR intervals processes during AF (see Lian et al. [94] for further details and experimental results).

4.3 ECG Models

The following sections show two disparate approaches to modeling the ECG. While both paradigms can produce an ECG signal and are consistent with various aspects of the physiology, they attempt to replicate different observed phenomena on different temporal scales. Section 4.3.1 presents the first approach, based on computational physiology, which employs first principles to derive the fundamental equations and then integrates this information using a three-dimensional anatomical description of the heart. This approach, although complex and computationally intensive, often provides a model which furthers our understanding of the effects of small changes or defects in cardiac physiology. Section 4.3.2 describes the second approach which appeals to an empirical description of the ECG, whereby statistical quantities such as the temporal and spectral characteristics of both the ECG and associated heart rate are modeled. Given that these quantities are routinely used for clinical diagnosis, this latter approach is of interest in the field of biomedical signal processing.

4.3.1   Computational Physiology

While the ECG is routinely used to diagnose arrhythmias, it reflects an integrated signal and cannot provide information on the micro-spatial scales of cells and ionic channels. For this reason, the field of computational cardiac modeling and simulation has grown over the last decade. In the following, we consider a variety of approaches to whole heart modeling.

The fundamental approach to whole heart modeling is based on the finite element method, which partitions the entire heart and chest into numerous elements where each element represents a group of cells. The ECG may then be simulated by calculating the body surface potential of each cardiac element [95]. This approach, however, fails to relate the ECG waveform with the micro-scale cellular electrophysiology. The use of membrane equations is needed to incorporate the mechanisms at cell, channel, and molecular level [96]. In the following, we review some promising research in the area of whole heart modeling, such as cellular autonoma and multiscale modeling approaches.

Arrhythmias are often initiated by abnormal electrical activity at the cellular scale or the ionic channel level. Cellular automata provide an effective means of constructing whole heart models and of simulating such arrhythmias, which may display a spatio-temporal evolution within the heart [97]. Such models combine a differential description of electrical properties of cardiac cells using membrane equations. This approach relates the ECG waveform to the underlying cellular activity and is capable of describing a range of pathological conditions. Cluster computing is employed as a means of dealing with the necessary computationally intensive simulations.

A single autonoma cell may be viewed as a computing unit for the action potential and ECG simulation. The electrical activity of these cells is described by corresponding Hodgkin-Huxley action potential equations. Zhu et al. [97] constructed a three-dimensional heart model based on data from the axial images of the Visible Human Project digital male cadaver [98]. The anatomical model of the heart utilized a data file to describe the distribution of the cell array and the characteristics of each cell.

Understanding the complexity of the heart requires biological models of cells, tissues, organs, and organ systems. The present aim is to combine the bottom-up approach of investigating interactions at the lower spatial scales of proteins (receptors, transporters, enzymes, and so forth) with that of the top-down approach of modeling organs and organ systems [99]. Such a multiscale integrative approach relies on the computational solution of physical conservation laws and anatomically detailed geometric models [100].

Multiscale models are now possible because of three recent developments: (1) molecular and biophysical data on many proteins and genes is now available (e.g., ion transporters [101]); (2) models exist which can describe the complexity of biological processes [99]; and (3) continuing improvements in computing resources allow the simulation of complex cell models with hundreds of different protein functions on a single-processor computer whereas parallel computers can now deal with whole organ models [102].

The interplay between simulation and experimentation has given rise to models of sufficient accuracy for use in drug development. Numerous drugs have to be withdrawn during trials due to cardiac side effects that are usually associated with irregular heartbeats and abnormal ECG morphologies. Noble and Rudy [103] have constructed a model of the heart that is able to provide an accurate description at the cellular level. Simulations of this model have been of great value to improving the understanding of the complex interactions underlying the heart. Furthermore, such computer-based heart models, known as in silico screening, provide a means of simulating and understanding the effects of drugs on the cardiovascular system. In particular these models can now be used to investigate the regulation of drug therapy.

While the grand challenge of heart modeling is to simulate a full-scale coronary heart attack, this would require extensive computing power [99]. Another hindrance is the lack of transfer of both data and models between different research centers. In addition, there is no standard representation for these models, thereby limiting the communication of innovative ideas and decreasing the pace of research. Once these hurdles have been overcome, the eventual aim is the development of integrated models comprising cells, organs, and organ systems.

4.3.2   Synthetic Electrocardiogram Signals

When only a realistic ECG is required (such as in the testing of signal processing algorithms), we may use an alternative approach to modeling the heart. ECGSYN is a dynamical model for generating synthetic ECG signals with arbitrary morphologies (i.e., any lead configuration) where the user has the flexibility to choose the operating characteristics. The model was motivated by the need to evaluate and quantify the performance of the signal processing techniques on ECG signals with known characteristics. An early attempt to produce a synthetic ECG generator [104] (available from the PhysioNet Web site [30] along with ECGSYN) is not intended to be highly realistic, and includes no P wave, and no variations in timing or morphology and discontinuities. In contrast to this, ECGSYN is based upon time-varying differential equations and is continuous with convincing beat-to-beat variations in morphology and interbeat timing. ECGSYN may be employed to generate extremely realistic ECG signals with complete flexibility over the choice of parameters that govern the structure of these ECG signals in both the temporal and spectral domains. The model also allows the average morphology of the ECG

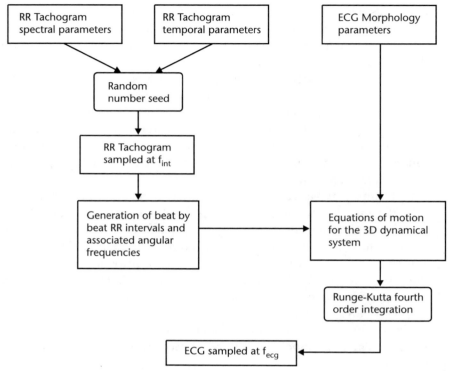

Figure 4.4   ECGSYN flow chart describing the procedure for specifying the temporal and spectral description of the RR tachogram and ECG morphology.

to be fully specified. In this way, it is possible to simulate ECG signals that show signs of various pathological conditions.

Open-source code in Matlab and C and further details of the model may be obtained from the PhysioNet Web site.[7] In addition a Java applet may be utilised in order to select model parameters from a graphical user interface, allowing the user to simulate and download an ECG signal with known characteristics. The underlying algorithm consists of two parts. The first stage involves the generation of an internal time series with internal sampling frequency f_{int} to incorporate a specific mean heart rate, standard deviation and spectral characteristics corresponding to a real RR tachogram. The second stage produces the average morphology of the ECG by specifying the locations and heights of the peaks that occur during each heartbeat. A flow chart of the various processes in ECGSYN for simulating the ECG is shown in Figure 4.4.

Spectral characteristics of the RR tachogram, including both RSA and Mayer waves, are replicated by describing a bimodal spectrum composed of the sum of

7.   See http://www.physionet.org/physiotools/ecgsyn/.

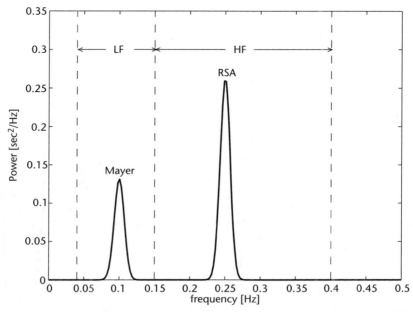

Figure 4.5 Spectral characteristics of (4.9), the RR interval generator for ECGSYN.

two Gaussian functions,

$$S(f) = \frac{\sigma_1^2}{\sqrt{2\pi c_1^2}} \exp\left(\frac{(f - f_1)^2}{2c_1^2}\right) + \frac{\sigma_2^2}{\sqrt{2\pi c_2^2}} \exp\left(\frac{(f - f_2)^2}{2c_2^2}\right) \qquad (4.9)$$

with means f_1, f_2 and standard deviations c_1, c_2. Power in the LF and HF bands is given by σ_1^2 and σ_2^2, respectively, whereas the variance equals the total area $\sigma^2 = \sigma_1^2 + \sigma_2^2$ and the LF/HF ratio is σ_1^2/σ_2^2 (see Figure 4.5).

A time series $T(t)$ with power spectrum $S(f)$ is generated by taking the inverse Fourier transform of a sequence of complex numbers with amplitudes $\sqrt{S(f)}$ and phases that are randomly distributed between 0 and 2π. By multiplying this time series by an appropriate scaling constant and adding an offset value, the resulting time series can be given any required mean and standard deviation. Different realizations of the random phases may be specified by varying the seed of the random number generator. In this way, many different time series $T(t)$ may be generated with the same temporal and spectral properties. Alternatively a real RR interval time series could be used instead. This has the advantage of increased realism, but the disadvantage of unknown spectral properties of the RR tachogram. However, if all the beat intervals are from sinus beats, the Lomb periodogram can produce an accurate estimate of the spectral characteristics of the time series [105, 106].

During each heartbeat, the ECG traces a quasi-periodic waveform where the morphology of each cycle is labeled by its peaks and troughs, P, Q, R, S, and T, as shown in Figure 4.6. This quasi-periodicity can be reproduced by constructing a dynamical model containing an attracting limit cycle; each heartbeat corresponds to one revolution around this limit cycle, which lies in the (x, y)-plane as shown in Figure 4.7. The morphology of the ECG is specified by using a series of exponentials

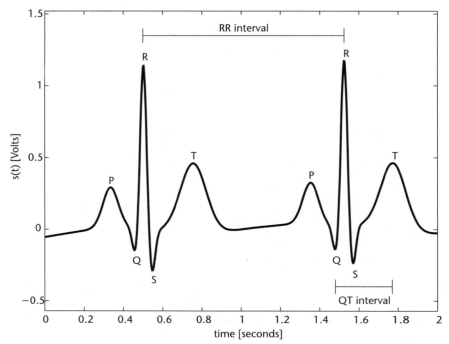

Figure 4.6 Two seconds of synthetic ECG reflecting the electrical activity in the heart during two beats. Morphology is shown by five extrema P, Q, R, S, and T. Time intervals corresponding to the RR interval and the surrogate QT interval are also indicated.

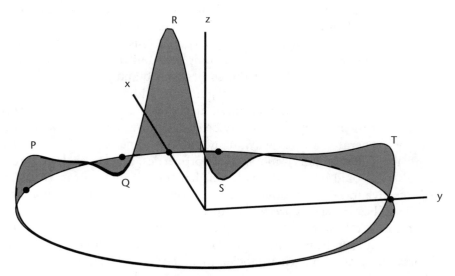

Figure 4.7 Three-dimensional state space of the dynamical system given by integrating (4.10) showing motion around the limit cycle in the horizontal (x, y)-plane. The vertical z-component provides the synthetic ECG signal with a morphology that is defined by the five extrema P, Q, R, S, and T.

to force the trajectory to trace out the PQRST-waveform in the z-direction. A series of five angles, $(\theta_P, \theta_Q, \theta_R, \theta_S, \theta_T)$, describes the extrema of the peaks (P, Q, R, S, T), respectively.

The dynamical equations of motion are given by three ordinary differential equations [107],

$$
\begin{aligned}
\dot{x} &= \alpha x - \omega y \\
\dot{y} &= \alpha y + \omega x \\
\dot{z} &= - \sum_{i \in \{P, Q, R, S, T^-, T^+\}} a_i \Delta\theta_i \exp(-\Delta\theta_i^2 / 2b_i^2) - (z - z_0)
\end{aligned}
\tag{4.10}
$$

where $\alpha = 1 - \sqrt{x^2 + y^2}$, $\Delta\theta_i = (\theta - \theta_i) \bmod 2\pi$, $\theta = \mathrm{atan2}(y, x)$ and ω is the angular velocity of the trajectory as it moves around the limit cycle. The coefficients a_i govern the magnitude of the peaks whereas the b_i define the width (time duration) of each peak. Note that the T wave is often asymmetrical and therefore requires two Gaussians, T^- and T^+ (rather than one), to correctly model this asymmetry (see [108]). Baseline wander may be introduced by coupling the baseline value z_0 in (4.10) to the respiratory frequency f_2 in (4.9) using $z_0(t) = A \sin(2\pi f_2 t)$. The output synthetic ECG signal, $s(t)$, is the vertical component of the three-dimensional dynamical system in (4.10): $s(t) = z(t)$.

Having calculated the internal RR tachogram expressed by the time series $T(t)$ with power spectrum $S(f)$ given by (4.9), this can then be used to drive the dynamical model (4.10) so that the resulting RR intervals will have the same power spectrum as that given by $S(f)$. Starting from the auxiliary[8] time t_n, with angle $\theta = \theta_R$, the time interval $T(t_n)$ is used to calculate an angular frequency $\Omega_n = \frac{2\pi}{T(t_n)}$. This particular angular frequency, Ω_n, is used to specify the dynamics until the angle θ reaches θ_R again, whereby a complete revolution (one heartbeat) has taken place. For the next revolution, the time is updated, $t_{n+1} = t_n + T(t_n)$, and the next angular frequency, $\Omega_{n+1} = \frac{2\pi}{T(t_{n+1})}$, is used to drive the trajectory around the limit cycle. In this way, the internally generated beat-to-beat time series, $T(t)$, can be used to generate an ECG signal with associated RR intervals that have the same spectral characteristics. The angular frequency $\omega(t)$ in (4.10) is specified using the beat-to-beat values Ω_n obtained from the internally generated RR tachogram:

$$
\omega(t) = \Omega_n, \qquad t_n \le t < t_{n+1}
\tag{4.11}
$$

A fourth-order Runge-Kutta method [109] is used to integrate the equations of motion in (4.10) using the beat-to-beat values of the angular frequency Ω. The time series $T(t)$ used for defining the values of Ω_n has a high sampling frequency of f_{int}, which is effectively the step size of the integration. The final output ECG signal is then downsampled to f_{ecg} if $f_{\mathrm{int}} > f_{\mathrm{ecg}}$ by a factor of $\frac{f_{\mathrm{int}}}{f_{\mathrm{ecg}}}$ in order to generate an ECG signal at the requested sampling frequency. In practice f_{int} is taken as an integer multiple of f_{ecg} for simplicity.

---

8. This auxiliary time axis is used to calculate the values of Ω_n for consecutive RR intervals, whereas the time axis for the ECG signal is sampled around the limit cycle in the (x, y)-plane.

Table 4.1 Morphological Parameters of the ECG Model with Modulation Factor $\alpha = \sqrt{h_{mean}/60}$

Index (i)	P	Q	R	S	T^-	T^+
Time (seconds)	$-0.2\sqrt{\alpha}$	-0.05α	0	0.05α	$0.277\sqrt{\alpha}$	$0.286\sqrt{\alpha}$
θ_i (radians)	$-\frac{\pi\sqrt{\alpha}}{3}$	$-\frac{\pi\alpha}{12}$	0	$\frac{\pi\alpha}{12}$	$\frac{5\pi\sqrt{\alpha}}{9} - \frac{\pi\sqrt{\alpha}}{60}$	$\frac{5\pi\sqrt{\alpha}}{9}$
a_i	0.8	-5.0	30.0	-7.5	$0.5\alpha^{2.5}$	$0.75\alpha^{2.5}$
b_i	0.2α	0.1α	0.1α	0.1α	$0.4\alpha^{-1}$	0.2α

The size of the mean heart rate affects the shape of the ECG morphology. An analysis of real ECG signals from healthy human subjects for different heart rates shows that the intervals between the extrema vary by different amounts; in particular, the QRS width decreases with increasing heart rate. This is as one would expect; when sympathetic tone increases, the conduction velocity across the ventricles increases together with an augmented heart rate. The time for ventricular depolarization (represented by the QRS complex of the ECG) is therefore shorter. These changes are replicated by modifying the width of the exponentials in (4.10) and also the positions of the angles θ. This is achieved by using a heart rate dependent factor $\alpha = \sqrt{h_{mean}/60}$ where h_{mean} is the mean heart rate expressed in units of bpm (see Table 4.1). The well-documented [110] asymmetry of the T wave and heart rate related changes in the T wave [111] are emulated by adding an extra Gaussian to the T wave section (denoted T^- and T^+ because they are placed just before and just after the peak of the T wave in the original model). To replicate the increasing T wave symmetry and amplitude observed with increasing heart rate [111], the Gaussian heights associated with the T wave are increased by an empirically derived factor $\alpha^{2.5}$. The increasing symmetry for increasing heart rates is emulated by shrinking a^{T+} by a factor α^{-1}. Perfect T wave symmetry would therefore be achieved at about 134 bpm if $a^{T+} = a^{T-}$ ($0.4\alpha^{-1} = 0.2\alpha$). In practice, this symmetry is asymptotic as $a^{T+} \neq a^{T-}$. In order to employ ECGSYN to simulate an ECG signal, the user must select from the list of parameters given in Tables 4.1 and 4.2, which specify the model's behavior in terms of its spectral characteristics given by (4.9) and time domain dynamics given by (4.10).

As illustrated in Figure 4.8, ECGSYN is capable of generating realistic ECG signals for a range of heart rates. The temporal modulating factors provided in

Table 4.2 Temporal and Spectral Parameters of the ECG Model

Description	Notation	Defaults
Approximate number of heartbeats	N	256
ECG sampling frequency	f_{ecg}	256 Hz
Internal sampling frequency	f_{int}	512 Hz
Amplitude of additive uniform noise	A	0.1 mV
Heart rate mean	h_{mean}	60 bpm
Heart rate standard deviation	h_{std}	1 bpm
Low frequency	f_1	0.1 Hz
High frequency	f_2	0.25 Hz
Low-frequency standard deviation	c_1	0.1 Hz
High-frequency standard deviation	c_2	0.1 Hz
LF/HF ratio	γ	0.5

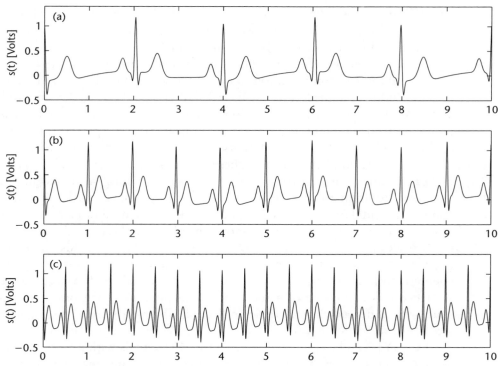

Figure 4.8 Synthetic ECG signals for different mean heart rates: (a) 30 bpm, (b) 60 bpm, and (c) 120 bpm.

Table 4.1 ensure that the various intervals, such as the PR, QT, and QRS, decrease with increasing heart rate. A nonlinear relationship between the morphology modulation factor α and the mean heart rate h_{mean} decreases the temporal contraction of the overall PQRST morphology with respect to the refractory period (the minimum amount of time in which depolarization and repolarization of the cardiac muscle can occur). This is consistent with the changes in parasympathetic stimulation connected to changes in heart rate; a higher heart rate due to sympathetic stimulation leads to an increase in conduction velocity across the ventricles and an associated reduction in QRS width. Note that the changes in angular frequency, ω, around the limit cycle, resulting from the period changes in each RR interval, do not lead to temporal changes, but to amplitude changes. For example, decreases in RR interval (higher heart rates) will not only lead to less broad QRS complexes, but also to lower amplitude R peaks, since the limit cycle will have less time to reach the maximum value of the Gaussian contribution given by a_R, b_R, and θ_R. This realistic (parasympathetically mediated) amplitude variation [112, 113], which is due to respiration-induced mechanical changes in the heart position with respect to the electrode positions in real recordings, is dominated by the high-frequency component in (4.9), which reflects parasympathetic activity in our model. This phenomenon is independent of the respiratory-coupled baseline wander in this model which is coupled to the peak HF frequency in a rather ad hoc manner. Of course, this part of the model could be made more realistic by coupling the baseline wander to a phase-lagged signal derived from highpass filtering ($f_c = 0.15$ Hz) the RR interval time series. The phase lag is important, since RSA and mechanical effects on the ECG and RR time series are not in phase (and often drift based on a subject's activity [3]). The beat-to-beat changes in RR intervals in this model faithfully reproduce RSA effects (decreases in RR interval with inspiration and increases with expiration) for lead configurations taken in the sense of lead I. Therefore, although the morphologies in the figures are modeled after lead II or V5, the amplitude modulation of the R peaks acts in the opposite sense to that which is seen on real lead II or V5 electrode configurations. That is, on inspiration (expiration) the amplitude of the model-derived R peaks decrease (increase) rather than increase (decrease). This is a reflection of the fact that these changes are a mechanical artifact on real ECG recordings, rather than a direct result of the neural mediated mechanisms. (A recent addition to the model, proposed by Amann et al. [114], includes an amplitude modulation term in $\dot{z}$ in (4.10) and may be used to provide the required modulation in such cases.) Furthermore, the phase lag between the RSA effect and the R peak modulation effect is fixed, reflecting the fact that this model is assuming a stationary state for each instance of generation. Extensions to this model, to couple it to a 24-hour RR time series, were presented in [115], where the entire sequence was composed of a series of RR tachograms, each having a stationary state with different characteristics reflecting observed normal circadian changes (see [74] and Section 4.2.8).

ECGSYN can be employed to generate ECG signals with known spectral characteristics and can be used to test the effect of varying the ECG sampling frequency f_{ecg} on the estimation of HRV metrics. In the following analysis, estimates of the LF/HF ratio were calculated for a range of sampling frequencies (Figure 4.9). ECGSYN was operated using a mean heart rate of 60 bpm, a standard deviation of 3 bpm, and a LF/HF ratio of 0.5. Error bars representing one standard deviation on either side of the means (dots) using a total of 100 Monte Carlo runs are also shown.

The LF/HF ratio was estimated using the Lomb periodogram. As this technique introduces negligible variance into the estimate [105, 106, 116], it may be concluded that the underestimation of the LF/HF ratio is due to the sampling frequency being too small. The analysis indicates that the LF/HF ratio is considerably underestimated for sampling frequencies below 512 Hz. This result is consistent with previous investigations performed on real ECG signals [61, 106, 117]. In addition, it provides a guide for clinicians when selecting the sampling frequency of the ECG based on the required accuracy of the HRV metrics.

The key features of ECGSYN which make this type of model such a useful tool for testing signal processing algorithms are as follows:

1. A user can rapidly generate many possible morphologies at a range of heart rates and HRVs (determined separately by the standard deviation and the LF/HF ratio). An algorithm can therefore be tested on a vast range of ECGs (some of which can be extremely rare and therefore underrepresented in databases).
2. The sampling frequency can be varied and the response of an algorithm can be evaluated.

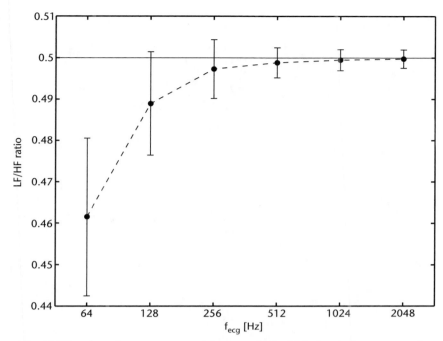

Figure 4.9 LF/HF ratio estimates computed from synthetic ECG signals for a range of sampling frequencies using an input LF/HF ratio of 0.5 (horizontal line). The distribution of estimates is shown by the mean (dot) and plus/minus one standard deviation error bars. The simulations used 100 realizations of noise-free synthetic ECG signals with a mean heart rate of 60 bpm and standard deviation of 3 bpm.

3. The signal is noise free, so noise may be incrementally added and a filter response at different frequencies and noise levels can be evaluated for differing physiological events.

4. Abnormal events (such as arrhythmias or ST-elevation) may be incorporated into the algorithm, and detectors of these events can be evaluated under varying noise conditions and for a variety of morphologies.

Although the model is designed to provide a realistic emulation of a sinus rhythm ECG, the fact that the RR interval process can be decoupled from the waveform generator, it is possible to reproduce the waveforms of particular arrhythmias by selecting a suitable RR interval process generator and altering the morphological parameters (θ_i, a_i, and b_i) together with the number of events, i, on the limit cycle. Healey et al. [118] have used ECGSYN to simulate AF by extending the AF RR interval model of Zeng and Glass [91] and coupling the conducted and nonconducted RR intervals to two different ECGSYN models (one with no P wave and one with only a P wave). Moreover, the concept behind ECGSYN could be used to simulate any quasi-periodic signal. In [119] the model was extended to produce BP and respiration waveforms, with realistic coupling to the ECG. The model has also been use to generate a 12-lead simulator for training in coronary artery disease identification as part of American Board of Family Practice Maintenance of

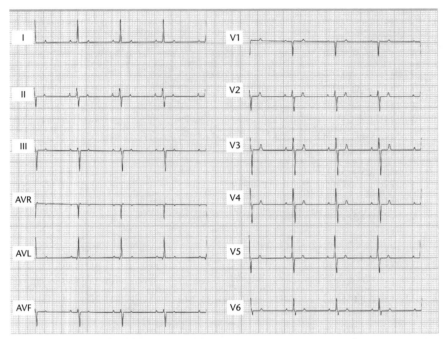

Figure 4.10 Example of a 12-lead version of ECGSYN, produced for [120] by Dr. Guy Roussel of the American Board of Family Practice. Standard lead labels and graph paper has been used. One small square = 1 mm, = 0.1 mV amplitude vertically (one large square = 0.5 mV) and 5 large boxes horizontally represent 1 second; paper moves at 25 mm/s. (*From:* [120]. © 2006 Guy Roussel. Reproduced with permission.)

Certification [120]. An example of a 12-lead output from the model can be found in Figure 4.10. The model has also been used to generate realistic ST-depressions on leads V5 and V6.

Other recent developments have included the automatic derivation of model parameters for a specific patient [108], and the transposition of the differential equations into polar coordinates [114, 121]. Further developments to improve the model should include the variation of ω within the limit cycle (to reflect changes in conduction velocity) and the generalization to a three-dimensional dipole model. These are current active areas of research (see [122]). Chapter 6 illustrates the application of the ECG model to filtering, compression and parameter extraction through a gradient descent, including a Kalman filter formulation to track the changes in the model parameters over time.

4.4 Conclusion

The models presented in this chapter are intended to provide the reader with an overview of the variety of cardiovascular models available to the researcher. Models for describing RR interval dynamics and ECG signals range from physiological-based to data-based approaches. The motivation behind these models often varies with the intended application: whether to improve understanding of the underlying control mechanisms or to attempt to obtain a better fit to the observed biomedical signals.

Applications of these models have included model fitting [29, 108], compression and filtering [119, 123], and classification [124]. However, the required complexity for realistic models (particularly for ECG generation) has limited the development of using model parameters for classifying hemodynamic and cardiac states. The assumed increase in computing power and utilization of parallel processing is likely to stimulate research in these fields in the near future. Simplified (and tractable) models such as ECGSYN provide a realistic current alternative. Chapter 6 describes a model fitting procedure that can run on a beat-by-beat basis in real time on a modern desktop computer.

Computational physiology is now at the stage where it is possible to integrate models from the level of the cell to that of the organ. By taking a multidisciplinary approach to systems biology, the ability to construct in silico models that reflect the underlying physiology and match the observed signals has the potential to deliver considerable advances in the field of biomedical science.

References

[1] Hales, S., *Statical Essays II, Haemastaticks*, London, U.K.: Innings and Manby, 1733.

[2] Ludwig, C., "Beiträge zur Kenntnis des Einflusses der Respirationsbewegung auf den Blutlauf im Aortensystem," *Arch. Anat. Physiol.*, Vol. 13, 1847, pp. 242–302.

[3] Hoyer, D., et al., "Validating Phase Relations Between Cardiac and Breathing Cycles During Sleep," *IEEE Eng. Med. Biol.*, March/April 2001.

[4] Thomas, R. J., et al., "An Electrocardiogram-Based Technique to Assess Cardiopulmonary Coupling During Sleep," *Sleep*, Vol. 28, No. 9, October 2005, pp. 1151–1161.

[5] DeBoer, R. W., J. M. Karemaker, and J. Strackee, "Hemodynamic Fluctuations and Baroreflex Sensitivity in Humans: A Beat-to-Beat Model," *Am. J. Physiol.*, Vol. 253, 1987, pp. 680–689.

[6] Malik, M., "Heart Rate Variability: Standards of Measurement, Physiological Interpretation, and Clinical Use," *Circulation*, Vol. 93, 1996, pp. 1043–1065.

[7] Sleight, P., and B. Casadei, "Relationships Between Heart Rate, Respiration and Blood Pressure Variabilities," in M. Malik and A. J. Camm, (eds.), *Heart Rate Variability*, Armonk, NY: Futura Publishing, 1995, pp. 311–327.

[8] Ottesen, J. T., "Modeling of the Baroreflex-Feedback Mechanism with Time-Delay," *J. Math. Biol.*, Vol. 36, 1997, pp. 41–63.

[9] Ottesen, J. T., M. S. Olufsen, and J. K. Larsen, *Applied Mathematical Models in Human Physiology*, Philadelphia, PA: SIAM Monographs on Mathematical Modeling and Computation, 2004.

[10] Grodins, F. S., "Integrative Cardiovascular Physiology: A Mathematical Synthesis of Cardiac and Blood Pressure Vessel Hemodynamics," *Q. Rev. Biol.*, Vol. 34, 1959, pp. 93–116.

[11] Madwed, J. B., et al., "Low Frequency Oscillations in Arterial Pressure and Heart Rate: A Simple Computer Model," *Am. J. Physiol.*, Vol. 256, 1989, pp. H1573–H1579.

[12] Ursino, M., M. Antonucci, and E. Belardinelli, "Role of Active Changes in Venous Capacity by the Carotid Beroreflex: Analysis with a Mathematical Model," *Am. J. Physiol.*, Vol. 267, 1994, pp. H2531–H2546.

[13]   Ursino, M., A. Fiorenzi, and E. Belardinelli, "The Role of Pressure Pulsatility in the Carotid Baroreflex Control: A Computer Simulation Study," *Comput. Bio. Med.*, Vol. 26, No. 4, 1996, pp. 297–314.

[14]   Ursino, M., "Interaction Between Carotid Baroregulation and the Pulsating Heart: A Mathematical Moodel," *Am. J. Physiol.*, Vol. 275, 1998, pp. H1733–H1747.

[15]   Seidel, H., and H. Herzel, "Bifurcations in a Nonlinear Model of the Baroreceptor Cardiac Reflex," *Physica D*, Vol. 115, 1998, pp. 145–160.

[16]   McSharry, P. E., M. J. McGuinness, and A. C. Fowler, "Comparing a Cardiovascular System Model with Heart Rate and Blood Pressure Data," *Computers in Cardiology*, Vol. 32, September 2005, pp. 587–590.

[17]   Baselli, G., S. Cerutti, and S. Civardi, "Cardiovascular Variability Signals: Toward the Identification of a Closed-Loop Model of the Neural Control Mechanisms," *IEEE Trans. Biomed. Eng.*, Vol. 35, 1988, pp. 1033–1046.

[18]   Saul, J. P., R. D. Berger, and P. Albrecht, "Transfer Function Analysis of the Circulation: Unique Insights into Cardiovascular Regulation," *Am. J. Physiol. (Heart Circ. Physiol.)*, Vol. 261, No. 4, 1991, pp. H1231–H1245.

[19]   Batzel, J., and F. Kappel, "Survey of Research in Modeling the Human Respiratory and Cardiovascular Systems," in R. C. Smith and M. A. Demetriou, (eds.), *Research Directions in Distributed Parameter Systems*, SIAM Series: Frontiers in Applied Mathematics, Philadelphia, PA: SIAM, 2003.

[20]   Whittam, A. M., et al., "Computer Modeling of Heart Rate and Blood Pressure," *Computers in Cardiology*, Vol. 25, 1998, pp. 149–152.

[21]   Pitzalis, M. V., et al., "Effect of Respiratory Rate on the Relationship Between π Interval and Systolic Blood Pressure Fluctuations: A Frequency-Dependent Phenomenon," *Cardiovascular Research*, Vol. 38, 1998, pp. 332–339.

[22]   Mukkamala, R., and R. J. Cohen, "A Cardiovascular Simulator for Research," http://www.physionet.org/physiotools/rcvsim/.

[23]   Mukkamala, R., and R. J. Cohen, "A Forward Model-Based Validation of Cardiovascular System Identification," *Am. J. Physiol.: Heart Circ. Physiol.*, Vol. 281, No. 6, 2001, pp. H2714–H2730.

[24]   Mukkamala, R., K. Toska, and R. J. Cohen, "Noninvasive Identification of the Total Peripheral Resistance Baroreflex," *Am. J. Physiol.*, Vol. 284, No. 3, 2003, pp. H947–H959.

[25]   Peng, C. K., et al., "Long-Range Anticorrelations and Non-Gaussian Behavior of the Heartbeat," *Physical Review Letters*, Vol. 70, No. 9, 1993, pp. 1343–1346.

[26]   Heldt, E. B., et al., "Computational Modeling of Cardiovascular Responses to Orthostatic Stress," *Journal of Applied Physiology*, Vol. 92, 2002, pp. 1239–1254, http://mimic.mit.edu/Archive/Papers/heldtpaper2.pdf.

[27]   Heldt, T., and R. G. Mark, "Scaling Cardiovascular Parameters for Population Simulation," *Computers in Cardiology*, IEEE Computer Society Press, Vol. 31, September 2004, pp. 133–136, http://mimic.mit.edu/Archive/Papers/heldtpaper2.pdf.

[28]   Heldt, T., "Orthostatic Hypotension," Ph.D. dissertation, Massachusetts Institute of Technology, 2005.

[29]   Samar, Z., "Parameter Fitting of a Cardiovascular Model," M.S. thesis, Massachusetts Institute of Technology, 2005.

[30]   Goldberger, A. L., et al., "Physiobank, Physiotoolkit, and Physionet: Components of a New Research Resource for Complex Physiologic Signals," *Circulation*, Vol. 101, No. 23, 2000, pp. e215–e220.

[31]   Rompelman, O., A. J. R. M. Coenen, and R. I. Kitney, "Measurement of Heart-Rate Variability—Part 1: Comparative Study of Heart-Rate Variability Analysis Methods," *Med. Biol. Eng. & Comput.*, Vol. 15, 1977, pp. 239–252.

[32] Mateo, J., and P. Laguna, "Improved Heart Rate Variability Signal Analysis from the Beat Occurrence Times According to the IPFM Model," *IEEE Trans. Biomed. Eng.*, Vol. 47, No. 8, 2000, pp. 985–996.

[33] Rompelman, O., J. D. Snijders, and C. van Spronsen, "The Measurement of Heart Rate Variability Spectra with the Help of a Personal Computer," *IEEE Trans. Biomed. Eng.*, Vol. 29, 1982, pp. 503–510.

[34] Hyndman, B. W., and R. K. Mohn, "A Model of the Cardiac Pacemaker and Its Use in Decoding the Information Content of Cardiac Intervals," *Automedia*, Vol. 1, 1975, pp. 239–252.

[35] Seydnejad, S. R., and R. I. Kitney, "Time-Varying Threshold Integral Pulse Frequency Modulation," *IEEE Trans. Biomed. Eng.*, Vol. 48, No. 9, 2001, pp. 949–962.

[36] Kantz, H., and T. Schreiber, *Nonlinear Time Series Analysis*, Cambridge, U.K.: Cambridge University Press, 1997.

[37] Theiler, J., et al., "Testing for Nonlinearity in Time Series: The Method of Surrogate Data," *Physica D*, Vol. 58, 1992, pp. 77–94.

[38] Farmer, J. D., and J. J. Sidorowich, "Predicting Chaotic Time Series," *Phys. Rev. Lett.*, Vol. 59, No. 8, 1987, pp. 845–848.

[39] Casdagli, M., "Nonlinear Prediction of Chaotic Time Series," *Physica D*, Vol. 35, 1989, pp. 335–356.

[40] Smith, L. A., "Identification and Prediction of Low-Dimensional Dynamics," *Physica D*, Vol. 58, 1992, pp. 50–76.

[41] Broomhead, D. S., and D. Lowe, "Multivariable Functional Interpolation and Adaptive Networks," *J. Complex Systems*, Vol. 2, 1988, pp. 321–355.

[42] Bishop, C., *Neural Networks for Pattern Recognition*, New York: Oxford University Press, 1995.

[43] McSharry, P. E., and L. A. Smith, "Consistent Nonlinear Dynamics: Identifying Model Inadequacy," *Physica D*, Vol. 192, 2004, pp. 1–22.

[44] Cao, L., and A. Mees, "Deterministic Structure in Multichannel Physiological Data," *International Journal of Bifurcation and Chaos*, Vol. 10, No. 12, 2000, pp. 2767–2780.

[45] Weigend, A. S., and N. A. Gershenfeld, *Time Series Prediction: Forecasting the Future and Understanding the Past*, Volume 15, SFI Studies in Complexity, Reading, MA: Addison-Wesley, 1993.

[46] Petrillo, G. A., L. Glass, and T. Trippenbach, "Phase Locking of the Respiratory Rhythm in Cats to a Mechanical Ventilator," *Canadian Journal of Physiology and Pharmacology*, Vol. 61, 1983, pp. 599–607.

[47] Bračič Lotrič, A., and M. Stefanovska, "Synchronization and Modulation in the Human Cardiorespiratory System," *Physica A*, Vol. 283, 2000, p. 451.

[48] Rosenblum, M. G., et al., "Synchronization in Noisy Systems and Cardiorespiratory Interaction," *IEEE Eng. Med. Biol. Mag.*, Vol. 17, No. 6, November–December 1998, pp. 46–53.

[49] Schäfer, C., et al., "Heartbeat Synchronization with Ventilation," *Nature*, Vol. 392, March 1998, pp. 239–240.

[50] Toledo, E., et al., "Quantification of Cardiorespiratory Synchronization in Normal and Heart Transplant Subject," *Proc. of Int. Symposium on Nonlinear Theory an Applications (NOLTA)*, Vol. 1, Presses Polytechnique et Universitaires Romandes, September 1998, pp. 171–174.

[51] Toledo, E., et al., "Cardiorespiratory Synchronization: Is It a Real Phenomenon?" in A. Murray and S. Swiryn, (eds.), *Computers in Cardiology*, Hannover, Germany: IEEE Computer Society, Vol. 26, 1999, pp. 237–240.

[52]   Stefanovska, A., et al., "The Cardiovascular System as Coupled Oscillators?" *Physiol. Meas.*, Vol. 22, 2001, pp. 535–550.

[53]   Stefanovska, A., D. G. Luchinsky, and V. E. McClintock, "Modeling Couplings Among the Oscillators of the Cardiovascular System," *Physiol. Meas.*, Vol. 22, 2001, pp. 551–564.

[54]   Ichimaru, Y., et al., "Effect of Sleep Stage on the Relationship Between Respiration and Heart Rate Variability," *Computers in Cordiology*, Vol. 17, 1990, pp. 657–660.

[55]   Lavie, P., A. Schlitner, and R. Nave, "Cardiac Automatic Function During Sleep in Psychogenic and Organic Erectile Dysfunction," *J. Sleep Res.*, Vol. 8, 1999, pp. 135–142.

[56]   Otzenberger, H., et al., "Dynamic Heart Rate Variability: A Tool for Exploring Sympathovagal Balance Continuously During Sleep in Men," *Am. J. Physiol.: Heart Circ. Physiol.*, Vol. 275, 1998, pp. H946–H950.

[57]   Ivanov, P. C., et al., "Sleep Wake Differences in Scaling Behavior of the Human Heartbeat: Analysis of Terrestrial and Long-Term Space Flight Data," *Europhys. Lett.*, Vol. 48, No. 5, 1999, pp. 594–600.

[58]   Bunde, A., et al., "Correlated and Uncorrelated Regions in Heart-Rate Fluctuations During Sleep," *Phy. Rev. Lett.*, Vol. 85, No. 17, October 2000.

[59]   Ferini-Strambi, L., et al., "The Impact of Cyclic Alternating Pattern on Heart-Rate Variability During Sleep in Healthy Young Adults," *Clinical Neurophysiology*, Vol. 111, No. 1, January 2000, pp. 99–101.

[60]   Ferri, R., et al., "Cyclic Alternating Pattern and Spectral Analysis of Heart Rate Variability During Normal Sleep," *J. Sleep Res.*, Vol. 9, 2000, pp. 13–18.

[61]   Clifford, G. D., and L. Tarassenko, "Segmenting Cardiac-Related Data Using Sleep Stages Increases Separation Between Normal Subjects and Apnoeic Patients," *IOP Physiol. Means.*, 2004.

[62]   Lo, C. -C., et al., "Common Scale-Invariant Patterns of Sleep-Wake Transitions Across Mammalian Species," *PNAS*, Vol. 101, No. 50, 2004, pp. 17545–17548.

[63]   Kobayashi, M., and T. Musha, "1/f Fluctuation of Heartbeat Period," *IEEE Trans. Biomed. Eng.*, Vol. 29, 1982, p. 456.

[64]   *Théorie de l'Addition des Variables Aléatoires*, Paris, France: Gauthier Villars, 1937.

[65]   Goldberger, A. L., et al., "Fractal Dynamics in Physiology: Alterations with Disease and Ageing," *Proc. Natl. Acad. Sci.*, Vol. 99, 2002, pp. 2466–2472.

[66]   Peng, C. -K., et al., "Quantification of Scaling Exponents and Crossover Phenomena in Nonstationary Heartbeat Time Series," *Chaos*, Vol. 5, 1995, pp. 82–87.

[67]   McSharry, P. E., and B. D. Malamud, "Quantifying Self-Similarity in Cardiac Inter-Beat Interval Time Series," *Computers in Cardiology*, Vol. 32, September 2005, pp. 462–495.

[68]   Ivanov, P. C., et al., "Multifractality in Human Heartbeat Dynamics," *Nature*, Vol. 399, 1999, pp. 461–465.

[69]   Lin, D. C., and R. L. Hughson, "Modeling Heart Rate Variability in Healthy Humans: A Turbulence Analogy," *Phys. Rev. Lett.*, Vol. 86, No. 8, 2001, pp. 1650–1653.

[70]   Kiyono, K., et al., "Critical Scale Invariance in a Healthy Human Heart Rate," *Phys. Rev. Lett.*, Vol. 93, No. 17, 2004, pp. 178103–17.

[71]   Kuusela, T., "Stochastic Heart-Rate Model Can Reveal Pathologic Cardiac Dynamics," *Phys. Rev. E*, Vol. 69, 2004, p. 031916.

[72]   Lin, D. C., and J. Thevaril, "Simulate Heart Rate Variability in Different Physiological Conditions," *Computers in Cardiology*, Vol. 29, 2002, pp. 149–152.

[73]   Yang, C. C., et al., "Simulating Healthy Humans Heart Rate: A Model Using Symbolic Dynamics and Probabilistic Automaton," *Computers in Cardiology*, Vol. 29, 2002, pp. 229–232.

[74]   McSharry, P. E., et al., "Method for Generating an Artificial RR Tachogram of a Typical Healthy Human over 24-Hours," *Computers in Cardiology*, Vol. 29, September 2002, pp. 225–228.

[75]   McSharry, P. E., et al., "A Dynamical Model for Generating Synthetic Electrocardiogram Signals," *IEEE Trans. Biomed. Eng.*, Vol. 50, No. 3, 2003, pp. 289–294.

[76]   Clifford, G., P. E. McSharry, and L. Tarassenko, "Characterizing Artifact in the Normal Human 24-Hour RR Time Series to Aid Identification and Artificial Replication of Circadian Variations in Human Beat to Beat Heart Rate Using a Simple Threshold," *Computers in Cardiology*, Vol. 29, September 2002, pp. 129–132.

[77]   *Medilog Manual*, Old Woking: Oxford Medical Instruments.

[78]   Dingfei, G., N. Srinivasan, and S. Krishnan, "Cardiac Arrhythmia Classification Using Autoregressive Modeling," *BioMedical Engineering OnLine*, Vol. 1, No. 1, 2002, p. 5.

[79]   Moody, G. B., and R. G. Mark, "QRS Morphology Representation and Noise Estimation Using the Karhunen-Loève Transform," *Computers in Cardiology*, Vol. 16, 1989, pp. 269–272.

[80]   Mark, R. G., and G. B. Moody, "ECG Arrhythmia Analysis: Design and Evaluation Strategies," Chapter 18, in I. Gath and G. F. Inbar, (eds.), *Advances in Processing and Pattern Analysis of Biological Signals*, New York: Plenum Press, 1996, pp. 251–272.

[81]   Clifford, G. D., L. Tarassenko, and N. Townsend, "Fusing Conventional ECG QRS Detection Algorithms with an Auto-Associative Neural Network for the Detection of Ectopic Beats," *5th International Conference on Signal Processing*, Beijing, China, August 2000, IFIP, World Computer Congress, pp. 1623–1628.

[82]   Tarassenko, L., G. D. Clifford, and N. Townsend, "Detection of Ectopic Beats in the Electrocardiogram Using an Auto-Associative Neural Network," *Neural Processing Letters*, Vol. 14, No. 1, 2001, pp. 15–25.

[83]   Clifford, G. D., and L. Tarassenko, "One-Pass Training of Optimal Architecture Auto-Associative Neural Network for Detecting Ectopic Beats," *IEE Electronic Letters*, Vol. 37, No. 18, August 2001, pp. 1126–1127.

[84]   Hastings, H., et al., "Alternans and the Onset of Ventricular Fibrillation," *Physical Review E*, 2000, pp. 4043–4048.

[85]   Cherry, E. M., et al., "The Role of Decreased Conduction Velocity in the Initiation and Maintenance of Atrial Fibrillation in a Computer Model of Human Atria," *Pacing and Clinical Electrophysiology*, Part II, 2002, p. 538.

[86]   Cohen, R. J., R. D. Berger, and T. E. Dushane, "A Quantative Model for the Ventricular Escape Response During Atrial Fibrillation," *IEEE Trans. Biomed. Eng.*, 1983, pp. 769–781.

[87]   Wittkampf, F. H., et al., "Effect of Right Ventricular Pacing on Ventricular Rhythm During a Atrial Fibrillation," *J. Am. Coll. Cardiol.*, 1988, pp. 539–545.

[88]   Wittkampf, F. H., M. J. L. DeJongste, and F. L. Meijler, "Atrioventricular Nodal Response to Retrograde Action in Atrial Fibrillation," *J. Cardiovascular Electro-Physiology*, 1990, pp. 437–447.

[89]   Wittkampf, F. H., M. J. L. DeJongste, and F. L. Meijler, "Competitive Antegrade and Retrograde Atrioventricular Junctional Activation in Atrial Fibrillation," *J. Cardiovascular Electrophysiology*, 1990, pp. 448–456.

[90]   Meijler, F. L., et al., "AV Nodal Function During Atrial Fibrillation: The Role of Electronic Modulation of Propagation," *J. Cardiovascular Electrophysiology*, 1996, pp. 843–861.

[91]   Zeng, W., and L. Glass, "Statistical Properties of Heartbeat Intervals During Atrial Fibrillation," *Phys. Rev. E*, 1996, pp. 1779–1784.

[92]   Glass, L., and K. Tateno, "Automatic Detection of Atrial Fibrillation Using the Coefficient of Variation and Density Histograms of RR and DRR Intervals," *Medical and Biological Engineering and Computing*, 2001, pp. 664–671.

[93]   Jorgensen, P., et al., "A Mathematical Model of Human Atrioventricular Nodal Function Incorporating Concealed Conduction," *Bulletin of Mathematical Biology*, 2002, pp. 1083–1099.

[94]   Lian, J., D. Müssig, and V. Lang, "Computer Modeling of Ventricular Rhythm During Atrial Fibrillation and Ventricular Pacing," *IEEE Trans. Biomed. Eng.*, Vol. 53, No. 8, 2006, pp. 1512–1520.

[95]   Shahidi, A. V., and P. Savard, "Forward Problem of Electrocardiography: Construction of Human Torso Models and Field Calculations Using Finite Element Method," *Med. Biol. Eng. Comput.*, Vol. 32, 1994, pp. S25–S33.

[96]   Thakor, N. V., et al., "Electrophysiologic Models of Heart Cells and Cell Networks," *IEEE Engineering in Medicine and Biology*, Vol. 17, No. 5, 1998, pp. 73–83.

[97]   Zhu, H., et al., "Facilitating Arrhythmia Simulation: The Method of Quantitative Cellular Automata Modeling and Parallel Running," *BioMedical Engineering OnLine*, Vol. 3, 2004, p. 29.

[98]   Ackerman, M. J., "The Visible Human Project: A Resource for Anatomical Visualization," *Medinfo*, Vol. 9, 1998, pp. 1030–1032.

[99]   Noble, D., "Modeling the Heart: From Genes to Cells to the Whole Organ," *Science*, Vol. 295, 2002, pp. 1678–1682.

[100]   Crampin, E. J., et al., "Computational Physiology and the Physiome Project," *Experimental Physiology*, Vol. 89, No. 1, 2004, pp. 1–26.

[101]   Ashcroft, F. M., *Ion Channels and Disease*, San Diego, CA: Academic Press, 2000.

[102]   Kohl, P., et al., "Computational Modeling of Biological Systems: Tools and Visions," *Phil. Trans. Roy. Soc. A*, Vol. 358, 2000, pp. 579–610.

[103]   Noble, D., and Y. Rudy, "Models of Cardiac Ventricular Action Potentials: Iterative Interaction Between Experiment and Simulation," *Phil. Trans. R. Soc. A*, Vol. 359, 2001, pp. 1127–1142.

[104]   Ruha, A., and S. Nissila, "A Real-Time Microprocessor QRS Detector System with a 1-ms Timing Accuracy for the Measurement of Ambulatory HRV," *IEEE Trans. Biomed. Eng.*, Vol. 44, No. 3, 1997, pp. 159–167.

[105]   Laguna, P., G. B. Moody, and R. G. Mark, "Power Spectral Density of Unevenly Sampled Data by Least-Square Analysis: Performance and Application to Heart Rate Signals," *IEEE Trans. Biomed. Eng*, Vol. BME-45, 1998, pp. 698–715.

[106]   Clifford, G. D., and L. Tarassenko, "Quantifying Errors in Spectral Estimates of HRV Due to Beat Replacement and Resampling," *IEEE Trans. Biomed. Eng.*, Vol. 52, No. 4, April 2005.

[107]   McSharry, P. E., et al., "A Dynamical Model for Generating Synthetic Electrocardiogram Signals," *IEEE Trans. Biomed. Eng.*, Vol. 50, No. 3, 2003, pp. 289–294.

[108]   Clifford, G. D., et al., "Model-Based Filtering, Compression and Classification of the ECG," *Joint Meeting of 5th International Conference on Bioelectromagnetism and 5th International Symposium on Noninvasive Functional Source Imaging within the Human Brain and Heart (BEM & NFSI)*, Minnesota, May 2005, invited paper.

[109]   Press, W. H., et al., *Numerical Recipes in C*, 2nd ed., Cambridge, U.K.: Cambridge University Press, 1992.

[110]   Zareba, W., and A. J. Moss, "Dispersion of Repolarization; Relation to Heart Rate and Repolarization Duration," *J. Electrocardiol.*, No. 28, 1995, pp. 202–206.

[111]   di Bernardo, D., P. Langley, and A. Murray, "Effect of Changes in Heart Rate and in Action Potential Duration on the Electrocardiogram T Wave Shape," *Physiological Measurement*, Vol. 23, No. 2, 2002, pp. 355–364.

[112]   Moody, G. B., et al., "Derivation of Respiratory Signals from Multi-Lead ECGs," *Computers in Cardiology*, Vol. 12, 1985, pp. 113–116.

[113]   Moody, G. B., et al., "Clinical Validation of the ECG-Derived Respiration (EDR) Technique," *Computers in Cardiology*, Vol. 13, 1986, pp. 507–510.

[114]   Amann, A., and K. Klotz, "Improved Models for Generating Synthetic Electrocardiogram Signals," *IEEE Trans. Biomed. Eng.*, 2005, in submission.

[115]   Clifford, G. D., and P. E. McSharry, "Generating 24-Hour ECG, BP and Respiratory Signals with Realistic Linear and Nonlinear Clinical Characteristics Using a Nonlinear Model," *Computers in Cardiology*, Vol. 31, 2004, pp. 709–712.

[116]   Clifford, G. D., "Signal Processing Methods for Heart Rate Variability," Ph.D. dissertation, University of Oxford, 2002.

[117]   Abboud, S., and O. Barnea, "Errors Due to Sampling Frequency of Electrocardiogram in Spectral Analysis of Heart Rate Signals with Low Variability," *Computers in Cardiology*, Vol. 22, September 1995, pp. 461–463.

[118]   Healey, J., et al., "An Open-Source Method for Simulating Atrial Fibrillation Using ECGSYN," *Computers in Cardiology*, Vol. 31, No. 19–22, September 2004, pp. 425–428.

[119]   Clifford, G. D., and P. E. McSharry, "A Realistic Coupled Nonlinear Artificial ECG, BP, and Respiratory Signal Generator for Assessing Noise Performance of Biomedical Signal Processing Algorithms," *Proc of SPIE International Symposium on Fluctuations and Noise*, Vol. 5467, No. 34, 2004, pp. 290–301.

[120]   Roussel, G., "Coronary Artery Disease Simulation," American Board of Family Medicine Maintenance of Certification for Family Physicians, 2006, https://www.theabfm.org/moc/.

[121]   Sameni, R., M. B. Shamsollahi, and C. Jutten, "Filtering Noisy Signals Using the Extended Kalman Filter Based on a Modified Dynamic ECG Model," *Computers in Cardiology*, Vol. 32, September 2005, pp. 5639–5642.

[122]   Sameni, R., et al., "A Nonlinear Bayesian Filtering Framework for ECG Denoising," submitted to *IEEE Trans. Biomed. Eng.*, 2005.

[123]   McSharry, P. E., and G. D. Clifford, "A Comparison of Nonlinear Noise Reduction and Independent Component Analysis Using a Realistic Dynamical Model of the Electrocardiogram," *Proc. of SPIE International Symposium on Fluctuations and Noise*, Vol. 5467, No. 9, 2004, pp. 78–88.

[124]   Heldt, T., et al., "Computational Model of Cardiovascular Function During Orthostatic Stress," *Computers in Cardiology*, Vol. 27, 2000, pp. 777–780.

CHAPTER 5
Linear Filtering Methods

Gari D. Clifford

5.1 Introduction

In this chapter a basic knowledge of the ECG and signal processing is assumed, including time-domain infinite impulse response (IIR) filters, finite impulse response (FIR) filters, and basic Fourier theory. As background references, the reader is encouraged to read Chapter 7 in [1] and Chapter 3 in [2]. From this base, we will explore a range of modern filtering techniques including wavelets, principal component analysis, and independent component analysis. Furthermore, the selection of the appropriate filtering technique for a particular situation is not always obvious, and sometimes it is appropriate to cascade a series of filters. Methods and metrics for evaluating filters are therefore described both in this chapter and in the following chapter on nonlinear filtering techniques.

The simplest filtering of a time series involves the transformation of a discrete one-dimensional ($M = 1$) time series $\mathbf{x}[n]$, consisting of N points such that $\mathbf{x}[n] = (x_1, x_2, x_3 ... x_N)^T$, into a new representation, $\mathbf{y}[n] = (y_1, y_2, y_3 ... y_N)^T$. If $\mathbf{x}[n]$ ($t = 1, 2, ..., N$) is a column vector that represents a channel of ECG, then we can generalize this representation so that M channels of ECG, $\mathbf{X}$, and their transformed representation $\mathbf{Y}$ are given by

$$\mathbf{X} = \begin{bmatrix} x_{11} & x_{12} & \cdots & x_{1M} \\ x_{21} & x_{22} & \cdots & x_{2M} \\ \vdots & \vdots & & \vdots \\ x_{N1} & x_{N2} & \cdots & x_{NM} \end{bmatrix}, \quad \mathbf{Y} = \begin{bmatrix} y_{11} & y_{12} & \cdots & y_{1M} \\ y_{21} & y_{22} & \cdots & y_{2M} \\ \vdots & \vdots & & \vdots \\ y_{N1} & y_{N2} & \cdots & y_{NM} \end{bmatrix} \tag{5.1}$$

An ($M \times M$) transformation matrix $\mathbf{W}$ can then be applied to $\mathbf{X}$ to create the transformed matrix $\mathbf{Y}$ such that

$$\mathbf{Y}^T = \mathbf{W}\mathbf{X}^T \tag{5.2}$$

The purpose of a transformation is to map (or *project*) data into another space which serves to highlight patterns in data and identify interesting projections. To filter data we discard the noise, or uninteresting parts of the signal, which are masking the interesting information. This amounts to a dimensionality reduction, as we are discarding the dimensions (or subspace) that correspond to the noise.

In general, transforms can be categorized as *orthogonal* or *biorthogonal* transformations. For orthogonal transformations, the transformed signal is the same

135

length (N) as the original, and the energy of the signal is unchanged. An example of this is the discrete Fourier transform (DFT) where the same signal is measured along a new set of perpendicular axes corresponding to the coefficients of the Fourier series. In the case of the DFT with $k = M$ frequency vectors, we can write (5.2) as $\mathbf{Y}_k = \sum_{m=1}^{M} \mathbf{W}_{km} \mathbf{X}_m$ where $\mathbf{W}_{km} = e^{-j2\pi km/M}$, or equivalently

$$
\mathbf{W} = \begin{bmatrix} e^{-j2\pi} & e^{-j4\pi} & \cdots & e^{-j2\pi M} \\ e^{-j4\pi} & e^{-j8\pi} & \cdots & e^{-j4\pi M} \\ \vdots & \vdots & & \vdots \\ e^{-j2\pi N} & e^{-j4\pi N} & \cdots & e^{-j2\pi NM} \end{bmatrix} \tag{5.3}
$$

For biorthogonal transforms, the angles between the axes may change and the new axes are not necessarily perpendicular. However, no information is lost, and perfect reconstruction of the original signal is still possible (using $\mathbf{X}^T = \mathbf{W}^{-1}\mathbf{Y}^T$).

Transformations can be further categorized as as either lossless (so that the transformation can be reversed and the original data restored exactly) or as lossy. When a signal is filtered or compressed (through downsampling, for instance), information is often lost and the transformation is not invertible. In general, lossy transformations involve a noninvertible transformation of data using a transformation matrix that has at least one column set to zero. This is an irreversible removal of data that corresponds to a mapping of data to a lower number of dimensions ($p < M$).

5.2 Wiener Filtering

Noncausal frequency-domain Wiener filtering is a lossy transformation in the Fourier domain using orthogonal axes (Fourier coefficients). For the application of filtering additive noise, the optimal (noncausal) Wiener filter is given by

$$
H(f) = \frac{S_y(f)}{S_y(f) + S_d(f)} \tag{5.4}
$$

where $S_y(f)$ is the power spectrum of the desired (or ideal postfiltered) signal, $y[n]$, and $S_d(f)$ is the power spectrum of the noise component, $d[n]$. Note that $S_y(f) + S_d(f)$ is in fact $S_x(f)$, the power spectrum of the observed signal, $x[n]$. Figure 5.1 illustrates the assumptions made in this type of filter; $S_d(f)$ begins at one end of the spectrum (where the signal is assumed to be entirely noise) and is extrapolated into the signal region. The removal of this part of the spectrum leads to an estimate, $S_y(f)$, of the underlying signal (albeit in a slightly attenuated form, as some of the power in the pass-band region is removed).

By studying (5.4) we see that we either need a good model of the noise spectrum S_d, or a good model of the ECG itself, such as the ideal underlying source signal, $S_x = S_y + S_d$. The noise component in an ECG is highly unpredictable and often driven by exogenous impulses, such as electrode motion, that have little or no correlation

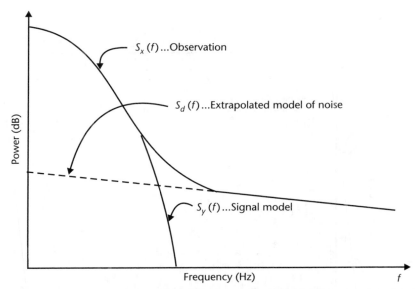

Figure 5.1 A log-log representation of the power spectral components of a signal for the noncausal Wiener filter. $S_y(f)$ is the power spectrum of the required (filtered) signal, $y(n)$, $S_d(f)$ is the power spectrum of the noise component, $d(t)$, and $S_x(f) = S_y(f) + S_d(f)$ is the power spectrum of the observed signal, $x(t)$.

with the current ECG source.[1] Therefore, in the application of the Wiener filter to ECG filtering, it is more practical to make an approximate model of the ECG and use this model to estimate the power spectrum of the signal.

Figure 5.2 illustrates the application of the Wiener filter to noise on the ECG. The left column illustrates the effect of Wiener filtering after a 50 Hz notch filter is applied. The signal model (upper trace, dash-dotted line) is formed by averaging approximately 1,200 R-peak aligned beats on the same lead (as per Section 5.4.1). The observation contains a small quantity of noise mostly around the 100 Hz region (see lower periodogram). Application of the Wiener filter to this observation (solid line) produces the lower plot (dashed line). Note that the noise has been removed, but also the amplitude has been diminished slightly. There is also an additive unit offset for clarity. The lower left plot illustrates the spectral difference between the signals. Note that the filtered signal has a significant dip around 100 Hz and a lower power in the signal band (0.1 to 45 Hz). The right hand column of Figure 5.2 illustrates the same paradigm using an unfiltered signal, which exhibits a large energy peak around 50 Hz (mains noise). The application of the Wiener filter effectively suppresses this peak as well as the 100-Hz peak. Note also the envelope on the mains noise with a frequency of approximately 6 Hz. This signal is also suppressed in both filters, although slightly more effectively when the 50-Hz mains noise is taken out before the Wiener filter is applied. This highlights the effectiveness of applying several filters that target specific components in a signal.

---

1. Of course, such disturbances often lead to an increase in heart rate and/or an increase in sympathetic activity, thus changing the intrabeat and interbeat signal morphology.

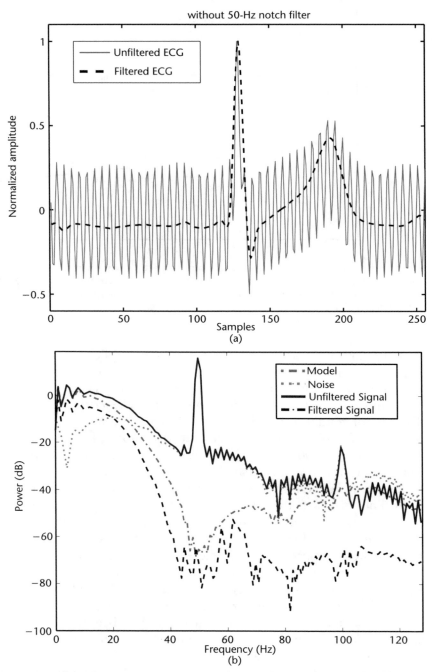

Figure 5.2 (a–d) Application of the Wiener filter to a noisy ECG. Plots (a) and (b) illustrate the application of the Wiener filter after a 50-Hz notch filter. The baseline of the filtered signal and signal model in plot (a) have been shifted for clarity. Plots (c) and (d) illustrate the application of the case for high noise (mostly 50-Hz and 100-Hz) contamination. Note the attenuation in amplitude of the time domain plots (a) and (c).

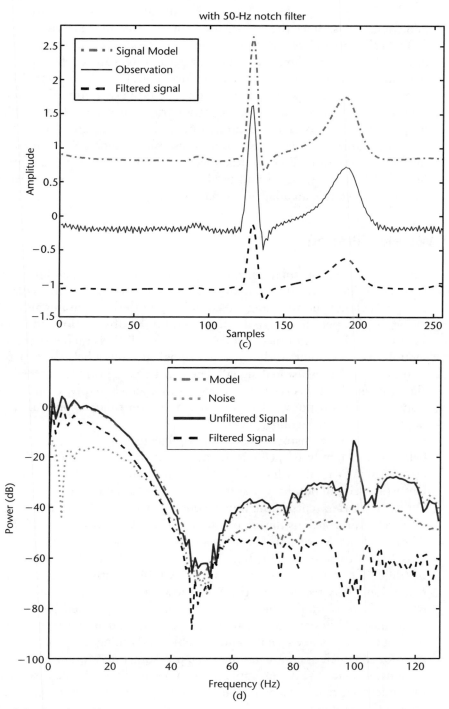

Figure 5.2   (continued.)

For a more mathematical analysis of the Wiener filter with respect to ECG filtering, the reader is referred to Rangayyan [2, Chapter 3.5]. Unfortunately, one of the Wiener filter assumptions is that both the signal and noise are statistical (not deterministic) signals. Since the coordinated ensemble cardiac activity that manifests as an ECG appears to have some deterministic component, the performance of the optimal Wiener filter is diminished. However, this filter can be reformulated in a causal sense and run online. The causal online formulation is closely related to the Kalman filter (KF), a more appropriate method for filtering deterministic signals. The non-causal Wiener filter also assumes stationarity, since the signal is filtered in the frequency domain over the entire segment of ECG. To cope with changes in the system parameters over time, we may use an extended Kalman filter (EKF). In the next chapter, an EKF is described in which an explicit deterministic model of the ECG is constructed and used to track the state space (model parameters) over time to enable an adaptive signal-noise separation.

5.3   Wavelet Filtering

Another method for isolating transient (nonstationary) changes in a time series involves combining the time-domain and frequency-domain analysis of a signal. Such an approach has the advantage of combining both these paradigms to facilitate filtering of both persistent signal sources within the observation, and short transient sources of noise. Joint time-frequency analysis (JTFA) is then essentially a transformation of an N-point M-dimensional signal (usually where $M = 1$ for the ECG) into an $M + 1$-dimensional signal. The short-time Fourier transform (STFT), is a classic example of this type of transformation, which involves repeated FT calculations over small windows that are stacked up over time to construct a spectrogram (a plot of frequency against time).

The wavelet transform (WT) is a popular technique for performing JTFA and belongs to a family of JTFA techniques that include the STFT, the Wigner Ville transform (WVT), the Zhao-Atlas-Marks distribution, and the Hilbert transform.[2] Unfortunately, all but the WT suffer from significant cross-terms which reduce their ability to locate events in the time-frequency plane. Reduced interference distribution techniques such as the exponential or Choi-Williams distribution, the pseudo-WVT, and the Margenau-Hill distribution, have been developed to suppress the cross terms to some extent, but in general, they do not provide the same degree of (time or frequency) resolution as the WT [4]. Furthermore, unlike other fixed resolution JTFA techniques, the WT allows a variable resolution and facilitates better time resolution of high frequencies and better frequency resolution of lower frequencies. Although wavelet analysis has often been quoted as the panacea for analyzing nonstationary signals (and thereby overcoming the problem of the Fourier transform, which assumes stationarity), it is sometimes important to segment data at nonstationarities. An example of such a situation may be a sudden change in dynamics that requires a change in the chosen analysis technique. Of course, JTFA may aid in defining a point of segmentation.

---

2.   All the JTFA techniques have been unified by Cohen [3].

In the following section, a brief overview of some of the key concepts in wavelet denoising are presented. For a more extensive and general overview of the application of wavelets to ECG processing, the reader is referred to the excellent review article by Paul Addison [5], Chapter 4 in Akay et al. [6] on late potentials, and to the relevant publications by Pablo Laguna [7, 8].

5.3.1 The Continuous Wavelet Transform

The continuous wavelet transform (CWT) is a generalization of the STFT that allows for analysis at multiple scales. Similar to the STFT, the CWT makes use of a windowing function to extract signal segments; in this case the window is called a *wavelet*. Unlike the STFT, the analysis window or wavelet is not only translated, but *dilated* and *contracted* depending on the scale of activity under study. Wavelet dilation increases the CWT's sensitivity to long time-scale events, and wavelet contraction increases its sensitivity to short time-scale events. The continuous wavelet transform is given by

$$C(a, \tau) = \int \frac{1}{\sqrt{a}} \Psi^* \left(\frac{t - \tau}{a} \right) x(t) dt \qquad (5.5)$$

where Ψ^* is the complex conjugate of the *mother* wavelet $\Psi(t)$, which is shifted by a time τ and dilated or contracted by a factor a prior to computing its *correlation* with the signal $x(t)$. A wavelet Ψ is finite in length and can be considered as a wavepacket version of the Fourier representation. The correlation between the signal and the wavelet is defined as the integral of their product. The CWT maps $x(t)$ into a bivariate function $C(a, \tau)$ that can be used to determine the similarity between $x(t)$ and a wavelet scaled by a at a given time τ. The correlation is localized in time and is computed over an interval beginning at $t = \tau$ and ending $t = \tau + L$ where L represents the duration of the wavelet. A time plot of the correlation between the signal and the scaled wavelets is called a *scalogram*.

Under contraction ($a < 1$), the wavelet offers high temporal resolution and is well suited for determining the onset of short-time events, such as a spikes and transients. Under dilation, ($a > 1$), the wavelet offers high spectral resolution and is well suited for determining the frequency of sustained, long-term events, such as baseline wander. This time-frequency trade-off provides a practical tool for ECG analysis, since we are often more interested in accurately determining the onset and offset of impulse-like transients, rather than the details of their broad frequency structure. Similarly, knowing the frequency of long-term, sustained activity is often more important than knowledge of the exact onset of the change since it is often a gradual phenomenon. Figure 5.3 illustrates the scalogram (lower plot) produced by the CWT on a segment of ECG (upper plot). Note that the lighter regions of the scalogram correspond to the higher energy regions, such as the QRS complex and the T wave, and are more defined at shorter scales.

In practice, the CWT provides a vast amount of redundancy in the representation (with more than an order of magnitude more wavelet values than original signal components) and therefore effects a decompression rather than a reduction in data. In order to extract information from a wavelet decomposition and remove much of

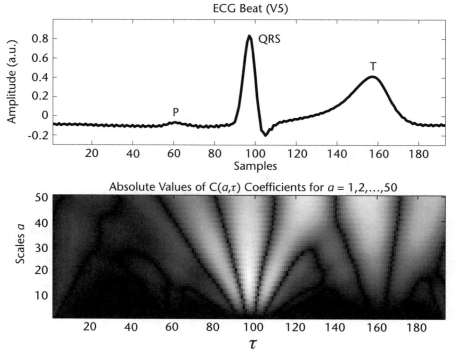

Figure 5.3 A relatively clean 0.75-second segment of lead V5 ECG and its corresponding scalogram form the CWT for scales $0 < a \leq 50$.

the redundancy, we can consider only the local maxima and minima of the transform, such as the wavelet *ridges* and the wavelet *modulus maxima*. Wavelet ridges are used to determine instantaneous frequencies and amplitudes and are defined by

$$\frac{dS(a, \tau)}{da} = 0 \tag{5.6}$$

where $S(a, \tau) = |C(a, \tau)|^2/a$ is the rescaled scalogram. The wavelet modulus maxima are used for locating and characterizing singularities in the signal and are given by

$$\frac{dS(a, \tau)}{d\tau} = 0 \tag{5.7}$$

5.3.2 The Discrete Wavelet Transform and Filter Banks

Another effective way to produce a data reduction is through the discrete wavelet transform (DWT). The DWT operates on wavelets that are discretely sampled and is calculated by passing a signal through a collection of filters (a *filter bank*) in order to decompose a signal into a set of frequency bands. This decomposition allows one to selectively examine or modify the content of a signal within the chosen bands for the purpose of compression, filtering, or signal classification. The STFT and CWT can be computed efficiently using filter banks. Furthermore, the filter bank formulation makes the application of the STFT and CWT in the setting of signal compression, filtering, or classification very natural.

The STFT can be computed using a filter bank known as an *M-channel filter bank*. An *M*-channel filter bank consists of *M* parallel filters all with equal bandwidth but different center frequencies. Perfect reconstruction of the input signal is possible following analysis by an *M*-channel filter bank. The process involves reconstituting the signal's spectrum by adding the frequency content extracted into each channel. The structure of the *M*-channel filter bank offers another perspective on the time-frequency plane tiling associated with the STFT. For any given discrete time n, which corresponds to a column in the time-frequency plane, the impulse response of all channels are of equal length. This implies that the STFT offers the same temporal resolution across all frequencies. Similarly the bandwidth of all the channels are equal, which implies the STFT offers the same spectral resolution across all frequencies. Fixed spectral and temporal resolution across all frequencies leads to the uniform tiling of the time-frequency plane.

A *tree-structured filter bank* can be used to compute the wavelet coefficients $C(a, \tau)$ of the continuous wavelet transform, but only over a dyadic (power of 2) scale of dilations and contractions. A tree-structured filter bank splits an incoming signal into a lowpass channel using the filter $H_0(z)$ and a highpass channel using the filter $H_1(z)$. The lowpass channel can be recursively split N times using the same two filters. Signals extracted from the filter bank at higher iteration levels contain increasingly longer time-scale activity, while those extracted from lower levels contain shorter time-scale activity.

Using only a dyadic scale of wavelet coefficients one can perfectly reconstruct the input signal; this possibility highlights the redundancy of continuously varying the scale parameter a in the CWT. The reconstruction, or synthesis filter bank is a mirror image of the analysis filter bank. The analysis filters $H_0(z)$ and $H_1(z)$ and the reconstruction filters $F_0(z)$ and $F_1(z)$ must be carefully chosen such that the decomposed signal can be perfectly reconstructed. The analysis and reconstruction filters have to satisfy *antialias* and *zero-distortion* conditions. It should be noted that the discrete-time analysis and synthesis filters that satisfy these conditions are not equivalent to the wavelet functions $\Psi(t)$ used in the CWT; they are derived from the wavelet function.

Performing a wavelet decomposition involves the following steps:

1. Select a wavelet appropriate for analyzing the signal of interest. The wavelet should have morphological features that match those to be extracted, highlighted, or detected in the input signal.
2. Derive the filters $H_0(z)$ and $H_1(z)$ so that an efficient filter bank implementation can be used to compute the wavelet coefficients.
3. Derive the filters $F_0(z)$ and $F_1(z)$ so that an efficient inverse filter bank can be used to reconstruct a new version of the signal from the modified wavelet coefficients.

Fortunately, the filters $H_0(z)$, $H_1(z)$, $F_0(z)$, and $F_1(z)$ have already been computed for a large number of wavelet functions, and these filters can be immediately used to study signals of interest. If all the wavelet coefficients produced by the analysis filter bank are preserved and the signal is reconstructed, the synthesized signal will exactly equal the input signal. If some coefficients are selectively preserved, then we are effectively *filtering* in the time or *scale domain* as opposed to the conventional *frequency domain*.

The LP filters produce a set of components, called *approximations*, and the HP filters produce a set of components called *details*. In general, the overall waveform of a signal will be primarily contained in the approximation coefficients, and short-term transients or high-frequency activity (such as spikes) will be contained in the detail coefficients. If we reconstruct the signal only using the approximation coefficients, we will recover the major morphological component. If we reconstruct the signal only using the detail coefficients, we will recover the *spike* components.

5.3.3   A Denoising Example: Wavelet Choice

Figure 5.4 illustrates a selection of biorthogonal wavelets denoted $bior J.K$, where J and K refer to the number of vanishing moments in the LP and HP filters, respectively. Note that in most literature, J refers to the length of the lowpass filter, and K

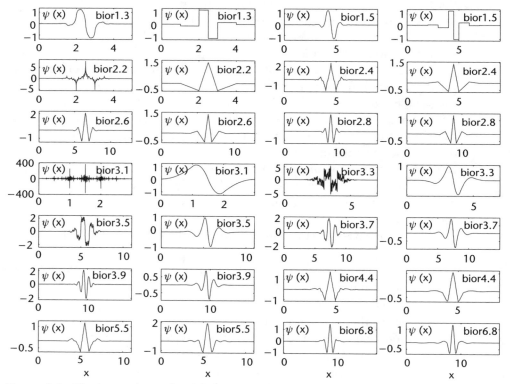

Figure 5.4   Biorthogonal wavelets labeled by their Matlab nomenclature. For each filter, two wavelets are shown; one for signal decomposition (on the left side) and one for signal reconstruction (on the right side). Type *waveinfo*('*bior*') in Matlab for more information. Note how increasing the order of the filter leads to increasing similarity between the mother wavelet and typical ECG morphologies.

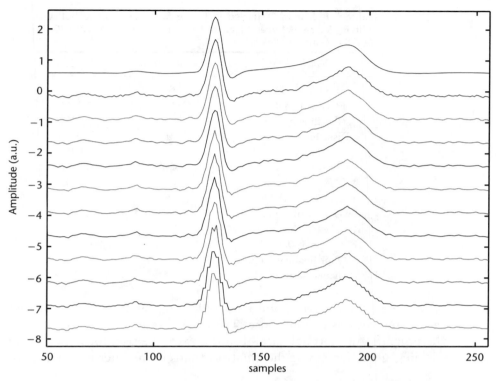

Figure 5.5   The effect of a selection of different wavelets for filtering a section of ECG (using the first approximation only) contaminated by Gaussian pink noise (SNR = 20 dB). From top to bottom; original (clean) ECG, noisy ECG, biorthogonal (8,4) filtered, discrete Meyer filtered, Coiflet filtered, symlet (6,6) filtered, symlet filtered (4,4), Daubechies (4,4) filtered, reverse biorthogonal (3,5), reverse biorthogonal (4,8), Haar filtered, and biorthogonal (6,2) filtered. The zero-noise clean ECG is created by averaging 1,228 R-peak aligned, 1-second-long segments of the author's ECG. RMS error performance of each filter is listed in Table 5.1.

to the length of the highpass filter. Therefore Matlab's *bior4.4* has four vanishing moments[3] with 9 LP and 7 HP coefficients (or taps) in each of the filters.

Figure 5.5 illustrates the effect of using different mother wavelets to filter a section of clean (zero-noise) ECG, using only the first approximation of each wavelet decomposition. The clean (upper) ECG is created by averaging 1,228 R-peak aligned, 1-second-long segments of the author's ECG. Gaussian pink noise is then added with a signal-to-noise ratio (SNR) of 20 dB. The root mean square (RMS) error between the filtered waveform and the original clean ECG for each wavelet is given in Table 5.1. Note that the biorthogonal wavelets with $J, K \geq 8, 4$,

---

3.   If the Fourier transform of the wavelet is J continuously differentiable, then the wavelet has J vanishing moments. Type *waveinfo('bior')* at the Matlab prompt for more information. Viewing the filters using $[lp_{decon}, hp_{decon}, lp_{recon}, hp_{recon}] = wfilters('bior4.4')$ in Matlab reveals one zero coefficient in each of the LP decomposition and HP reconstruction filters, and three zeros in the LP reconstruction and HP decomposition filters. Note that these zeros are simply padded and do not count when calculating the filter size.

Table 5.1 Signals Displayed in Figure 5.5 (from Top to Bottom) with RMS Error Between Clean and Wavelet Filtered ECG with 20-dB Additive Gaussian Pink Noise

Wavelet Family	Family Member	RMS Error
Original ECG	N/A	0
ECG with pink noise	N/A	0.3190
Biorthogonal 'bior'	bior3.3	0.0296
Discrete Meyer 'dmey'	dmey	0.0296
Coiflets 'coif'	coif2	0.0297
Symlets 'sym'	sym3	0.0312
Symlets 'sym'	sym2	0.0312
Daubechies 'db'	db2	0.0312
Reverse biorthogonal 'rbio'	rbio3.3	0.0322
Reverse biorthogonal 'rbio'	rbio2.2	0.0356
Haar 'haar'	haar	0.0462
Biorthogonal 'bior'	bior1.3	0.0472

N/A indicates not applicable.

the discrete Meyer wavelet and the Coiflets appear to produce the best filtering performance in this circumstance. The RMS results agree with visual inspection, where significant morphological distortions can be seen for the other filtered signals. In general, increasing the number of taps in the filter produces a lower error filter.

The wavelet transform can be considered either as a spectral filter applied over many time scales, or viewed as a linear time filter $\Psi[(t - \tau)/a]$ centered at a time τ with scale a that is convolved with the time series $x(t)$. Therefore, convolving the filters with a shape more commensurate with that of the ECG produces a better filter. Figure 5.4 illustrates this point. Note that as we increase the number of taps in the filter, the mother wavelet begins to resemble the ECG's P-QRS-T morphology more closely. The biorthogonal wavelet family members are FIR filters and, therefore, possess a linear phase response, which is an important characteristic for signal and image reconstruction. In general, biorthogonal spline wavelets allow exact reconstruction of the decomposed signal. This is not possible using orthogonal wavelets (except for the Haar wavelet). Therefore, $bior$ 3.3 is a good choice for a general ECG filter. It should be noted that the filtering performance of each wavelet will be different for different types of noise, and an adaptive wavelet-switching procedure may be appropriate. As with all filters, the wavelet performance may also be application-specific, and a sensitivity analysis on the ECG feature of interest is appropriate (e.g., QT interval or ST level) before selecting a particular wavelet.

As a practical example of comparing different common filtering types to the ECG, observe Figure 5.6. The upper trace illustrates an unfiltered recording of a V5 ECG lead from a 30-year-old healthy adult male undergoing an exercise test. Note the presence of high amplitude 50-Hz (mains) noise. The second subplot illustrates the action of applying a 3-tap IIR notch-filter centered on 50 Hz, to reveal the underlying ECG. Note the presence of baseline wander disturbance from electrode motion around $t = 467$ seconds, and the difficulty in discerning the P wave (indicated by a large arrow at the far left). The third trace is a band-pass (0.1 to 45 Hz) FIR filtered version of the upper trace. Note the baseline wander is reduced

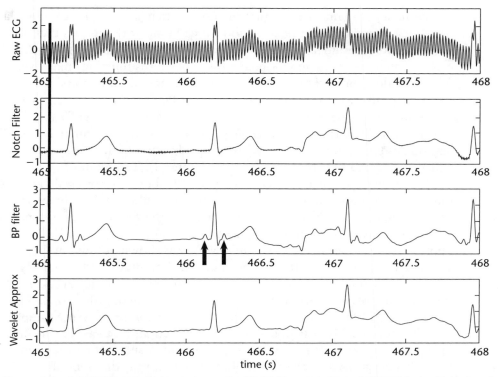

Figure 5.6   Raw ECG with 50 Hz mains noise, IIR 50-Hz notch filtered ECG, 0.1- to 45-Hz band-pass filtered ECG and *bior3.3* wavelet filtered ECG. The left-most arrow indicates the low amplitude P wave. Central arrows indicate Gibbs oscillations in the FIR filter causing a distortion larger than the P wave.

significantly, but a Gibbs[4] ringing phenomena is introduced into the Q and S waves (illustrated by the small arrows), which manifests as distortions with an amplitude larger than the P wave itself. A good demonstration of the Gibbs phenomenon can be found in [9, 10]. This *ringing* can lead to significant problems for a QRS detector (looking for Q wave onset) or any technique for analyzing at QT intervals or ST changes. The lower trace is the first approximation of a biorthogonal wavelet decomposition (*bior3.3*) of the notch-filtered ECG. Note that the P wave is now discernible from the background noise and the Gibbs oscillations are not present.

As mentioned at the start of this section, the number of articles on ECG analysis that employ wavelets is enormous and an excellent overview of many of the key publications in this arena can be found in Addison [5]. Wavelet filtering is a lossless supervised filtering method where the basis functions are chosen a priori, much like the case of a Fourier-based filter (although some of the wavelets do not have orthogonal basis functions). Unfortunately, it is difficult to remove *in-band* noise because the CWT and DWT are signal separation methods that effectively occur in

---

4.   The existence of the ripples with amplitudes independent of the filter length. Increasing the filter length narrows the transition width but does not affect the ripple. One technique to reduce the ripples is to multiply the impulse response of an ideal filter by a tapered window.

the frequency domain[5] (ECG signal and noises often have a significant overlap in the frequency domain). In the next section we will look at techniques that *discover* the basis functions within data, based either on the statistics of the signal's distributions or with reference to a known signal model. The basis functions may overlap in the frequency domain, and therefore, we may separate out in-band noise.

As a postscript to this section, it should be noted that there has been much discussion of the use of wavelets in HRV analysis (see Chapter 3) since long-range beat-to-beat fluctuations are obviously nonstationary. Unfortunately, very little attention has been paid to the unevenly sampled nature of the RR interval time series and this can lead to serious errors (see Chapter 3). Techniques for wavelet analysis of unevenly sampled data do exist [11, 12], but it is not clear how a discrete filter bank formulation with up-down sampling could avoid the inherent problems of resampling an unevenly sampled signal. A recently proposed alternative JTFA technique known as the Hilbert-Huang transform (HHT) [13, 14], which is based upon *empirical mode decomposition* (EMD), has shown promise in the area of nonstationary and nonlinear JFTA (since both the amplitude and frequency terms are a function of time[6]). Furthermore, there is striking similarity between EMD and the least-squares estimation technique used in calculating the Lomb-Scargle Periodogram (LSP) for power spectral density estimation of unevenly sampled signals (see Chapter 3). EMD attempts to find basis functions (such as the sines and cosines in the LSP) by fitting them to the signal and then subtracting them, in much the same manner as in the calculation of the LSP (with the difference being that EMD analyzes the envelope of the signal and does not restrict the basis functions to being sinusoidal). It is therefore logical to extend the HHT technique to fit *empirical modes* to an unevenly sampled times series such as the RR tachogram. If the fit is optimal in a least-squares sense, then the basis functions will remain orthogonal (as we shall discover in the next section). Of course, the basis functions may not be orthogonal, and other measures for optimal fits may be employed. This concept is explored further in Section 5.4.3.2.

5.4   Data-Determined Basis Functions

Sections 5.4.1 to 5.4.3 present a set of transformation techniques for filtering or separating signals without using any prior knowledge of the spectral components of the signals and are based upon a statistical analysis to *discover* the underlying basis functions of a set of signals.

These transformation techniques are principal component analysis[7] (PCA), artificial neural networks (ANNs), and independent component analysis (ICA).

---

5.   The wavelet is convolved with the signal.

6.   Interestingly, the *empirical modes* of the HHT are also determined by the data and are therefore a special case where a JTFA technique (the Hilbert transform) is combined with a data-determined empirical mode decomposition to derive orthogonal basis functions that may overlap in the frequency domain in a nonlinear manner.

7.   This is also known as singular value decomposition (SVD), the Hotelling transform or the Karhunen-Loève transform (KLT).

Both PCA and ICA attempt to find an independent set of vectors onto which we can transform data. Those data that are projected (or mapped) onto each vector *are* the independent sources. The basic goal in PCA is to *decorrelate* the signal by projecting data onto *orthogonal* axes. However, ICA results in a transformation of data onto a set of axes which are not necessarily orthogonal. Both PCA and ICA can be used to perform lossy or lossless transformations by multiplying the recorded (observation) data by a separation or *demixing* matrix. Lossless PCA and ICA both involve projecting data onto a set of axes which are determined by the nature of those data, and are therefore methods of *blind source separation* (BSS). (*Blind* because the axes of projection and therefore the sources are determined through the application of an internal measure and without the use of any prior knowledge of a signal's structure.)

Once we have *discovered* the axes of the independent components in a data set and have separated them out by projecting the data set onto these axes, we can then use these techniques to filter the data set.

5.4.1   Principal Component Analysis

To determine the principal components (PCs) of a multidimensional signal, we can use the method of singular value decomposition. Consider a real $N \times M$ matrix $\mathbf{X}$ of observations which may be decomposed as follows:

$$\mathbf{X} = \mathbf{USV}^T \tag{5.8}$$

where $\mathbf{S}$ is an $N \times M$ nonsquare matrix with zero entries everywhere, except on the leading diagonal with elements $s_i (= S_{nm}, n = m)$ arranged in descending order of magnitude. Each s_i is equal to $\sqrt{\lambda_i}$, the square root of the eigenvalues of $\mathbf{C} = \mathbf{X}^T\mathbf{X}$. A stem-plot of these values against their index i is known as the *singular spectrum*. The smaller the eigenvalues are, the less energy along the corresponding eigenvector there is. Therefore, the smallest eigenvalues are often considered to be associated with the noise in the signal. $\mathbf{V}$ is an $M \times M$ matrix of column vectors which are the eigenvectors of $\mathbf{C}$. $\mathbf{U}$ is an $N \times N$ matrix of projections of $\mathbf{X}$ onto the eigenvectors of $\mathbf{C}$ [15]. If a truncated SVD of $\mathbf{X}$ is performed (i.e. we just retain the most significant p eigenvectors),[8] then the truncated SVD is given by $\mathbf{Y} = \mathbf{US}_p\mathbf{V}^T$, and the columns of the $N \times M$ matrix $\mathbf{Y}$ are the noise-reduced signal (see Figure 5.7).

SVD is a commonly employed technique to compress and/or filter the ECG. In particular, if we align M heartbeats, each N samples long, in a matrix (of size $N \times M$), we can compress it down (into an $N \times p$) matrix, using only the first $p << M$ PCs. If we then reconstruct the set of heartbeats by inverting the reduced rank matrix, we effectively filter the original ECG.

Figure 5.7(a) illustrates a set of 20 heartbeat waveforms which have been cut into 1-second segments (with a sampling frequency $F_s = 256$ Hz), aligned by their R peaks and placed side by side to form a 256×20 matrix. Therefore, the data set is 20-dimensional, and an SVD will lead to 20 eigenvectors. Figure 5.7(b) is

---

8. In practice choosing the value of p depends on the nature of the data set, but is often taken to be the *knee* in the eigenspectrum or as the value where $\sum_{i=1}^{p} s_i > \alpha \sum_{i=1}^{M} s_i$ and α is some fraction ≈ 0.95.

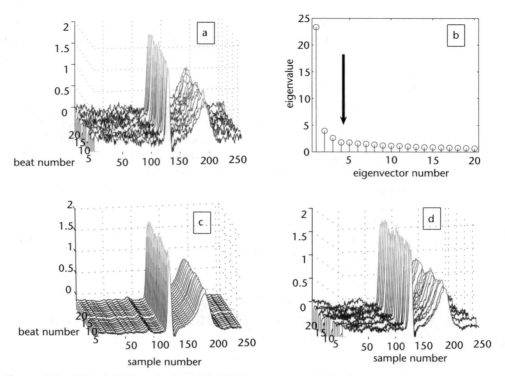

Figure 5.7 SVD of 20 R-peak-aligned P-QRS-T complexes: (a) in the original form with in-band Gaussian pink noise noise (SNR = 14 dB), (b) eigenspectrum of decomposition (with the *knee* indicated by an arrow), (c) reconstruction using only the first principal component, and (d) reconstruction using only the first two principal components.

the eigenspectrum obtained from SVD.[9] Note that the signal/noise boundary is generally taken to be the *knee* of the eigenspectrum, which is indicated by an arrow in Figure 5.7(b). Since the eigenvalues are related to the power, most of the power is contained in the first five eigenvectors (in this example). Figure 5.7(c) is a plot of the reconstruction (filtering) of the data set using just the first eigenvector. Figure 5.7(d) is the same as Figure 5.7(c), but the first five eigenvectors have been used to reconstruct the data set.[10] The data set in Figure 5.7(d) is therefore noisier than that in Figure 5.7(c), but cleaner than that in Figure 5.7(a). Note that although Figure 5.7(c) appears to be extremely clean, this is at the cost of removing some beat-to-beat morphological changes, since only one PC was used.

Note that **S** derived from a full SVD is an *invertible* matrix, and no information is lost if we retain all the PCs. In other words, we recover the original data by performing the multiplication $\mathbf{USV}^T$. However, if we perform a truncated SVD, then the inverse of **S** does not exist. The transformation that performs the filtering is *noninvertible*, and information is lost because **S** is *singular*.

From a data compression point of view, SVD is an excellent tool. If the eigenspace is known (or previously determined from experiments), then the M-dimensions of

---

9.   In Matlab: $[USV] = svd(data); stem(diag(S)^2)$.
10.   In Matlab: $[USV] = svds(data, 5); waterfall(U * S * V')$.

data can in general be encoded in only p-dimensions of data. So for N sample points in each signal, an $N \times M$ matrix is reduced to an $N \times p$ matrix. In the above example, retaining only the first principal component, we achieve a compression ration of 20:1. Note that the data set is encoded in the U matrix, so we are only interested in the first p columns. The eigenvalues and eigenvectors are encoded in S and V matrices, and thus an additional p scalar values are required to encode the relative energies in each column (or signal source) in U. Furthermore, if we wish to encode the *eigenspace* onto which the data set in U is projected, we require an additional p^2 scalar values (the elements of V). Therefore, SVD compression only becomes of significant value when a large number of beats are analyzed. It should be noted that the eigenvectors will change over time since they are based upon the morphology of the beats. Morphology changes both subtly with heart rate–related cardiac conduction velocity changes, and with conduction path abnormalities that produce abnormal beats. Furthermore, the basis functions are lead dependent, unless a multidimensional basis function set is derived and the leads are mapped onto this set. In order to find the global eigenspace for all beats, we need to take a large, representative set of heartbeats[11] and perform SVD upon this *training set* [16, 17]. Projecting each new beat onto these *globally derived* basis vectors leads to a filtering of the signal that is essentially equivalent to passing the P-QRS-T complex through a set of trained weights of a multilayer perceptron (MLP) neural network (see [18] and the following section). Abnormal beats or artifacts erroneously detected as normal beats will have abnormal eigenvalues (or a highly irregular structure when reconstructed by the MLP). In this way, beat classification can be performed. However, in order to retain all the subtleties of the QRS complex, at least $p = 5$ eigenvalues and eigenvectors are required (and another five for the rest of the beat). At a sampling frequency of F_s Hz and an average beat-to-beat interval of RR^{av} (or heart rate of $60/RR^{av}$), the compression ratio is $F_s \cdot RR^{av} \cdot (\frac{N-p}{p})$: 1, where N is the number of samples in each segmented heartbeat. Other studies have used between 10 [19] and 16 [18] free parameters (neurons) to encode (or model) each beat, but these methods necessarily model some noise also.

In Chapter 9 we will see how we can derive a global set of principal eigenvectors V (or KL basis functions) onto which we can project each beat. The strength of the projection along each eigenvector[12] allows us to classify the beat type. In the next section, we will look at an online adaptive implementation of this technique for patient-specific learning, using the framework of artificial neural networks.

5.4.2 Neural Network Filtering

PCA can be reformulated as a neural network problem, and, in fact, a MLP with linear activation functions can be shown to perform singular valued decomposition [18, 20]. Consider an auto-associative multilayered perceptron (AAMLP) neural network, which has as many output nodes as input nodes, illustrated in Figure 5.8. The AAMLP can be trained using an objective cost function measured between the

---

11. That is, $N >> 20$.
12. Derived from a database of test signals.

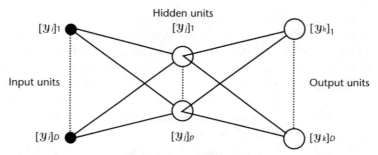

Figure 5.8   Layout of a D-p-D auto-associative neural network.

inputs and outputs; the target data vector is simply the input data vector. Therefore, no labeling of training data is required. An auto-associative neural network
performs dimensionality reduction from D to p dimensions ($D > p$) and then
projects back up to D dimensions. (See Figure 5.8.) PCA, a standard linear dimensionality reduction procedure is also a form of unsupervised learning [20]. In fact,
the number of hidden-layer nodes ($\dim(y_j)$) is usually chosen to be the same as
the number of PCs, p, in the data set (see Section 5.4.1), since (as we shall see later)
the first layer of weights performs PCA if trained with a linear activation function.
The full derivation of PCA shows that PCA is based on minimizing a sum-of-squares
error cost function, as is the case for the AAMLP [20].

The input data used to train the network is now defined as y_i for consistency of
notation. The y_i are fed into the network and propagated through to give an output
y_k given by

$$y_k = f_a \left(\sum_j w_{jk} f_a(\sum_i w_{ij} y_i) \right) \tag{5.9}$$

where f_a is the activation function,[13] $a_j = \sum_{i=0}^{i=N} w_{ij} y_i$, and $D = N$ is the number
of input nodes. Note that the x's from the previous section are now the y_i, our
sources are the y_j, and our filtered data (after training) are the y_k. During training,
the target data vector or desired output, t_k, which is associated with the training
data vector, is compared to the actual output y_k. The weights, w_{jk} and w_{ij} , are then
adjusted in order to minimize the difference between the propagated output and the
target value. This error is defined over all training patterns, M, in the training set as

$$\xi = \frac{1}{2} \sum_{n=1}^{M} \sum_k \left(f_a(\sum_j w_{jk} f_a(\sum_i w_{ij} y_i^p)) - t_k^p \right)^2 \tag{5.10}$$

where $j = p$ is the number of hidden units and ξ is the error to be backpropagated
at each learning cycle. Note that the y_j are the values of the data set after projection

---

13. Often taken to be a *sigmoid* ($f_a(a) = \frac{1}{1+e^{-a}}$), a *tanh*, or a *softmax* function).

onto the p-dimensional ($p < N, D$) hidden layer (the PCs). This is the point at which the dimensionality reduction (and hence filtering) really occurs, since the input dimensionality equals the output dimensionality ($N = D$).

The squared error, ξ, can be minimized using the method of gradient descent [20]. This requires the gradient to be calculated with respect to each weight, w_{ij} and w_{jk}. The weight update equations for the hidden and output layers are given as follows:

$$w_{jk}^{(\tau+1)} = w_{jk}^{(\tau)} - \eta \frac{\partial \xi}{\partial w_{jk}} \tag{5.11}$$

$$w_{ij}^{(\tau+1)} = w_{ij}^{(\tau)} - \eta \frac{\partial \xi}{\partial w_{ij}} \tag{5.12}$$

where τ represents the iteration step and η is a small ($<< 1$) learning term. In general, the weights are updated until ξ reaches some minimum. Training is an iterative process [repeated application of (5.11) and (5.12)], but, if continued for too long,[14] the network starts to fit the noise in the training set and that will have a negative effect on the performance of the trained network on test data. The decision on when to stop training is of vital importance but is often defined when the error function (or its gradient) drops below some predefined level. The use of an independent validation set is often the best way to decide on when to terminate training (see Bishop [20, p. 262] for more details). However, in the case of an auto-associative network, no validation set is required, and the training can be terminated when the ratio of the variance of the input and output data reaches a plateau. (See [21, 22].)

If f_a is set to be linear $y_k = a_k$, $\frac{\partial y_k}{\partial a_k} = 1$, then the expression for δ_k reduces to

$$\delta_k = \frac{\partial \xi}{\partial a_k} = \frac{\partial \xi}{\partial y_k} \cdot \frac{\partial y_k}{\partial a_k} = (y_k - t_k) \tag{5.13}$$

If the hidden layer also contains linear units, further changes must be made to the weight update equations:

$$\delta_j = \frac{\partial \xi}{\partial a_j} = \frac{\partial \xi}{\partial a_k} \cdot \frac{\partial a_k}{\partial y_j} \cdot \frac{\partial y_j}{\partial a_j} = \sum_k \delta_k w_{jk} \tag{5.14}$$

If f_a is linearized (set to unity)—this expression is differentiated with respect to w_{ij} and the derivative is set to zero, the usual equations for least-squares optimization can be given in the form

$$\sum_M^M \left(\sum_{i'=0}^D y_i^m w_{i'j} - t_j^m \right) y_i^m = 0 \tag{5.15}$$

---

14. Note that a momentum term can be inserted into (5.11) and (5.12) to premultiply the weights and increase the speed of convergence of the network.

which is written in matrix notation as

$$(\mathbf{Y}^T\mathbf{Y})\mathbf{W}^T = \mathbf{Y}^T\mathbf{T} \qquad (5.16)$$

$\mathbf{Y}$ has dimensions $M \times D$ with elements y_i^m where M is the number of training patterns and D the number of input nodes to the network (the length of each ECG complex in our examples). $\mathbf{W}$ has dimension $p \times D$ and elements w_{ij} and $\mathbf{T}$ has dimensions $M \times p$ and elements t_j^m. The matrix $(\mathbf{Y}^T\mathbf{Y})$ is a square $p \times p$ matrix which may be inverted to obtain the solution

$$\mathbf{W}^T = \mathbf{Y}^\dagger\mathbf{T} \qquad (5.17)$$

where $\mathbf{Y}^\dagger$ is the $(p \times M)$ pseudo-inverse of $\mathbf{Y}$ and is given by

$$\mathbf{Y}^\dagger = (\mathbf{Y}^T\mathbf{Y})^{-1}\mathbf{Y}^T \qquad (5.18)$$

Note that in practice $(\mathbf{Y}^T\mathbf{Y})$ usually turns out to be near-singular and SVD is used to avoid problems caused by the accumulation of numerical roundoff errors.

Consider M training patterns, each $i = N$ samples long presented to the auto-associative MLP with i input and k output nodes ($i = k$) and $j \leq i$ hidden nodes. For the mth ($m = 1...M$) input vector x_i of the $i \times M$ ($M \geq i$) real input matrix, $\mathbf{X}$, formed by the M (i-dimensional) training vectors, the hidden unit output values are

$$h_j = f_a(\mathbf{W}_1 x_i + w_{1b}) \qquad (5.19)$$

where $\mathbf{W}_1$ is the input-to-hidden layer $i \times j$ weight matrix, w_{1b} is a rank-j vector of biases, and f_a is an activation function. The output of the auto-associative MLP can then be written as

$$y_k = \mathbf{W}_2 h_j + w_{2b} \qquad (5.20)$$

where $\mathbf{W}_2$ is the hidden-to-output layer $j \times k$ weight matrix and w_{2b} is a rank-k vector of biases. Now consider the singular value decomposition of $\mathbf{X}$, such that $\mathbf{X}_i = \mathbf{U}_i\mathbf{S}_i\mathbf{V}_i^T$, where $\mathbf{U}$ is an $i \times i$ column-orthogonal matrix, $\mathbf{S}$ is an $i \times N$ diagonal matrix with positive or zero elements (the singular values) and $\mathbf{V}^T$ is the transpose of an $N \times N$ orthogonal matrix [15]. The best rank-j approximation of $\mathbf{X}$ is $\mathbf{W}_2 h_j = \mathbf{U}_j\mathbf{S}_j\mathbf{V}_j^T$ [23], where

$$h_j = \mathbf{FS}_j\mathbf{V}_j^T \qquad (5.21)$$

$$\mathbf{W}_2 = \mathbf{U}_j\mathbf{F}^{-1} \qquad (5.22)$$

with $\mathbf{F}$ being an arbitrary nonsingular $j \times j$ scaling matrix. $\mathbf{U}_j$ has $i \times j$ elements, $\mathbf{S}_j$ has $j \times j$ elements, and $\mathbf{V}^T$ has $j \times M$ elements. It can be shown that [24]

$$\mathbf{W}_1 = a_1^{-1}\mathbf{FU}_j^T \qquad (5.23)$$

where $\mathbf{W}_1$ are the input-to-hidden layer weights and a is derived from a power series expansion of the activation function, $f_a(x) \approx a_0 + a_1 x$ for small x. For a linear activation function, as in this application, $a_0 = 0$, $a_1 = 1$. The bias weights given in [24] reduce to

$$w_{1b} = -a_1^{-1}\mathbf{F}\mathbf{U}_j^T \mu_X = -\mathbf{U}_j^T \mu_X$$
$$w_{2b} = \mu_X - a_0\mathbf{U}_j\mathbf{F}^{-1} = \mu_X \qquad (5.24)$$

where $\mu_X = \frac{1}{M}\sum_M x_i$, the average of the training (input) vectors and $\mathbf{F}$ is here set to be the $(j \times j)$ identity matrix since the output is unaffected by the scaling. Using (5.19) to (5.24),

$$
\begin{aligned}
y_k &= \mathbf{W}_2 h_j + w_{2b} \\
&= \mathbf{U}_j\mathbf{F}^{-1}h_j + w_{2b} \\
&= \mathbf{U}_j\mathbf{F}^{-1}(\mathbf{W}_1 x_i + w_{1b}) + w_{2b} \\
&= \mathbf{U}_j\mathbf{F}_1^{-1}\mathbf{F}\mathbf{U}_j^T x_i - \mathbf{U}_j\mathbf{F}^{-1}\mathbf{U}_j^T \mu_X + \mu_X
\end{aligned}
\qquad (5.25)
$$

giving the output of the auto-associative MLP as

$$y_k = \mathbf{U}_j\mathbf{U}_j^T(\mathbf{X} - \mu_X) + \mu_X \qquad (5.26)$$

Equations (5.22), (5.23), and (5.24) represent an analytical solution to determine the weights of the auto-associative MLP "in one pass" over the input (training) data with as few as $Mi^3 + 6Mi^2 + \mathcal{O}(Mi)$ multiplications [25]. We can see that $\mathbf{W}_1 = \mathbf{W}_{ij}$ is the matrix that rotates each of the data vectors $x_i^m = y_i^m$ in $\mathbf{X}$ into the hidden data y_i^p, which are our p underlying sources. $\mathbf{W}_2 = \mathbf{W}_{jk}$ is the matrix that transforms our sources back into the observation data; the target data vectors $\sum_N t_i^m = \mathbf{T}$. If $p < N$, we have discarded some of the possible information sources and effected a filtering process. In terms of PCA, $\mathbf{W}_1 = \mathbf{S}\mathbf{V}^T = \mathbf{U}\mathbf{U}^T$.

5.4.2.1   Determining the Network Architecture for Filtering

It is now simple to see how we can derive an heuristic for determining the MLP's architecture: the number of input, hidden, and output units, the activation function, and the cost function. A general method is as follows [26]:

1. Choose the number of input units based upon the type of signal requiring analysis, and reduce the number of them as far as possible. (Downsample the signal as far as possible without removing significant information.)
2. Choose the number of output units based upon how many classes that are to be distinguished. (In the application in this chapter the filtering preserves the sampling frequency of the original signal, so the number of output units must equal the number of input units and hence the input is reconstructed in a filtered form at the output.)
3. Choose the number of hidden units based upon how amenable the data set is to compression. If the activation function is linear, then the choice is obvious; we use the *knee* of the SVD eigenspectrum (see Figure 5.7).

5.4.2.2   ECG Filtering

To reconstruct the ECG (minus the noise component), we set the number of hidden nodes to be the same as the number of PCs required to encode the information in the ECG ($p = 5$ or 6); see Chapter 9 and Moody et al. [16, 17]. Setting the number of output nodes to equal the number of input nodes (i.e., the number of samples in the segmented P-QRS-T wave) results in an auto-associative MLP which reconstructs the ECG with p PCs. That is, the trained neural network filters the ECG. To train the weights of the system we can present a series of patterns to the MLP and back propagate the error between the pattern and the output of the MLP, which should be the same, until the variance of the input over the variance of the output approaches unity. We can also use (5.22), (5.23), (5.24), and SVD to set the values of the weights.

Once an MLP is trained to filter the ECG in this way, we may update the weights periodically with new patterns[15] and continually track the morphology to produce a more generalized filter, as long as we take care to exclude artifacts.[16] It has been suggested [24] that sequential SVD methods [25] can be used to update U. However, at least $12i^2 + \mathcal{O}(i)$ multiplications are required for each new training vector, and therefore, it is only a preferable update scheme when there is a large difference between the new patterns and the old training set (M or i are then large). For normal ECG morphologies, even in extreme circumstances such as increasing ST elevation, this is not the case.

Another approach is to determine a global set of PCs (or KL basis functions) over a range of patients and attempt to classify each beat sequentially by clustering the eigenvalues (KL coefficients) in the KL space. See [16, 17] and Chapter 9 for a more in-depth analysis of this.

Of course, so far there is no advantage to formulating the PCA filtering as a neural network problem (unless the activation function is made nonlinear). The key point we are illustrating by reformulating the PCA approach in terms of the ANN learning paradigm is that PCA and ICA are intimately connected. By using a linear activation function, we are assuming that the *latent variables* that generate our underlying sources are Gaussian. Furthermore, the mean square error–based function leads to orthogonal axes. The reason for starting with PCA is that it offers the simplest computational route, and a direct interpretation of the basis functions; they are the axes of maximal variance in the covariance matrix. As soon as we introduce a nonlinear activation function, we lose an exact interpretation of the axes. However, if the activation function is chosen to be nonlinear, then we are implicitly assuming non-Gaussian sources. Choosing a *tanh*-like function implies heavy-tailed sources, which is probably the case for the cardiac source itself, and therefore is perhaps a better choice for deriving representative basis functions.

Moreover, by replacing the cost function with entropy-based function, we can remove the constraint of second-order (variance-based) independence, and hence

---

15. With just a few (~ 10) iterations through the backpropagation algorithm.
16. Note also that a separate network is required for each beat type on each lead, and therefore a beat classification system is required.

orthogonality between the basis functions. In this way, a more effective filter may be formulated. As we shall see in the next section, it can be shown [27] that if this cost function is changed to become some mutual information-based criterion, then the basis function independence becomes fourth order (in a statistical sense) and the basis-function orthogonality is lost. We are no longer performing PCA, but rather ICA.

5.4.3 Independent Component Analysis for Source Separation and Filtering

Using PCA (or its AAMLP correlate) we have seen how we can separate a signal into a subspace that is *signal* and a subspace that is essentially *noise*. This is done by assuming that only the eigenvectors associated with the p largest eigenvalues represent the signal, and the remaining $(M - p)$ eigenvalues are associated with the noise subspace. We try to maximize the independence between the eigenvectors that span these subspaces by requiring them to be orthogonal. However, orthogonal subspaces may not be the best way to differentiate between the constituent sources (signal and noise) in a set of observations.

In this section, we will examine how choosing a measure of independence other than variance can lead to a more effective method for separating signals. The method will be presented in a gradient-descent formulation in order to illustrate the connections with AANN's and PCA. A detailed description of how ICA can be implemented using gradient descent, which follows closely the work of MacKay [27], is given in the material on the accompanying URLs [28, 29]. Rather than provide this detailed description here, an intuitive description of how ICA separates sources is presented, together with a practical application to noise reduction.

A particularly intuitive illustration of the problem of blind[17] source separation through discovering independent sources is known as the *Cocktail Party Problem*.

5.4.3.1 Blind Source Separation: The Cocktail Party Problem

The Cocktail Party Problem refers to the separation of a set of observations (the mixture of conversations one hears in each ear) into the constituent underlying (statistically independent) source signals. If each of the J speakers (sources) that are talking in a room at a party is recorded by M microphones,[18] the recordings can be considered to be a matrix composed of a set of M vectors,[19] each of which is a (weighted) linear superposition of the J voices. For a discrete set of N samples, we can denote the sources by a $J \times N$ matrix, $\mathbf{Z}$, and the M recordings by an $M \times N$ matrix $\mathbf{X}$. $\mathbf{Z}$ is therefore transformed into the observables $\mathbf{X}$ (through the propagation of sound waves through the room) by multiplying it by an $M \times J$ mixing matrix $\mathbf{A}$, such that $\mathbf{X}^{\mathrm{T}} = \mathbf{A}\mathbf{Z}^{\mathrm{T}}$. [Recall (5.2).]

---

17. Since we *discover*, rather than define, the subspace onto which we project the data set, this process is known as blind source separation (BSS). Therefore, PCA can also be thought of as a BSS technique.
18. In the case of a human, the ears are the $M = 2$ microphones.
19. M is usually required to be greater than or equal to J.

In order for us to pick out a voice from an ensemble of voices in a crowded room, we must perform some type of BSS to recover the original sources from the observed mixture. Mathematically, we want to find a demixing matrix $\mathbf{W}$, which when multiplied by the recordings $\mathbf{X}$, produces an estimate $\mathbf{Y}$ of the sources $\mathbf{Z}$. Therefore, $\mathbf{W}$ is a set of weights (approximately equal[20]) to $\mathbf{A}^{-1}$. One of the key BSS methods is ICA, where we take advantage of (an assumed) linear independence between the sources. In the case of ECG analysis, the independent sources are assumed to be the electrocardiac signal and exogenous noises (such as muscular activity or electrode movement).

5.4.3.2   Higher-Order Independence: ICA

ICA is a general name for a variety of techniques that seek to uncover the (statistically) *independent* source signals from a set of observations that are composed of underlying components that are usually assumed to be mixed in a *linear* and *stationary* manner. Consider $\mathbf{X_{jn}}$ to be a matrix of J observed random vectors: $\mathbf{A}$, an $N \times J$ mixing matrix, and $\mathbf{Z}$, the J (assumed) source vectors, which are mixed such that

$$\mathbf{X}^T = \mathbf{AZ}^T \tag{5.27}$$

Note that here we have chosen to use the transposes of $\mathbf{X}$ and $\mathbf{Z}$ to retain dimensional consistency with the PCA formulation in Section 5.4.1, (5.8). ICA algorithms attempt to find a separating or demixing matrix $\mathbf{W}$ such that

$$\mathbf{Y}^T = \mathbf{WX}^T \tag{5.28}$$

where $\mathbf{W} = \hat{\mathbf{A}}^{-1}$, an approximation of the inverse of the original mixing matrix, and $\mathbf{Y}^T = \hat{\mathbf{Z}}^T$, an $M \times J$ matrix, is an approximation of the underlying sources. These sources are assumed to be statistically independent (generated by unrelated processes) and therefore the joint probability density function (PDF) is the product of the densities for all sources:

$$P(Z) = \prod p(z_i) \tag{5.29}$$

where $p(z_i)$ is the PDF of the ith source and $P(Z)$ is the joint density function.

The basic idea of ICA is to apply operations to the observed data $\mathbf{X}^T$, or the demixing matrix $\mathbf{W}$, and measure the independence between the output signal channels (the columns of $\mathbf{Y}^T$) to derive estimates of the sources (the columns of $\mathbf{Z}^T$). In practice, iterative methods are used to maximize or minimize a given cost function such as *mutual information*, *entropy*, or the fourth-order moment, *kurtosis*, a measure of non-Gaussianity (see Section 5.4.3.3). It can be shown [27] that entropy-based cost functions are related to kurtosis, and therefore, all of the cost functions used in ICA are a measure of non-Gaussianity to some extent.[21]

---

20. Depending on the performance details of the algorithm used to calculate $\mathbf{W}$.
21. The reason for choosing between different entropy-based cost functions is not always made clear, but computational efficiency and sensitivity to outliers are among the concerns. See material on the accompanying URLs [28, 29] for more information.

From the *Central Limit Theorem* [30], we know that the distribution of a sum of independent random variables tends toward a Gaussian distribution. That is, a sum of two independent random variables usually has a distribution that is closer to a Gaussian than the two original random variables. In other words, independence *is* non-Gaussianity. For ICA, if we wish to find *independent* sources, we must find a demixing matrix $\mathbf{W}$, that maximizes the non-Gaussianity of each source. It should also be noted at this point that, for the sake of simplicity, this chapter uses the convention $J \equiv M$, so that the number of sources equals the dimensionality of the signal (the number of independent observations). If $J < M$, it is important to attempt to determine the exact number of sources in a signal matrix. For more information on this topic see the articles on *relevancy determination* [31, 32]. Furthermore, with conventional ICA, we can never recover more sources than the number of independent observations ($J \not> M$), since this is a form of interpolation and a model of the underlying source signals would have to be used. (We have a subspace with a higher dimensionality than the original data.[22])

The essential difference between ICA and PCA is that PCA uses variance, a second-order moment, rather than higher-order statistics (such as the fourth moment, kurtosis) as a metric to separate the signal from the noise. Independence between the projections onto the eigenvectors of an SVD is imposed by requiring that these basis vectors be orthogonal. The subspace formed with ICA is not necessarily orthogonal, and the angles between the axes of projection depend upon the exact nature of the data set used to calculate the sources.

The fact that SVD imposes orthogonality means that the data set has been decorrelated (the projections onto the eigenvectors have zero covariance). This is a much weaker form of independence than that imposed by ICA.[23] Since independence implies noncorrelatedness, many ICA methods also constrain the estimation procedure such that it always gives uncorrelated estimates of the independent components (ICs). This reduces the number of free parameters and simplifies the problem.

5.4.3.3   Gaussianity

To understand how ICA transforms a signal, it is important to understand the metric of independence, non-Gaussianity (such as kurtosis). The first two moments of random variables are well known: the *mean* and the *variance*. If a distribution is Gaussian, then the mean and variance are sufficient to characterize the variable. However, if the PDF of a function is not Gaussian, then many different signals can have the same mean and variance. For instance, all the signals in Figure 5.10 have a mean of zero and unit variance.

The mean (central tendency) of a random variable x is defined to be

$$\mu_x = E\{x\} = \int\limits_{-\infty}^{+\infty} x p_x(x) \mathrm{d}x \qquad (5.30)$$

---

22. In fact, there are methods for attempting this type of analysis; see [33–40].
23. Orthogonality implies independence, but independence does not necessarily imply orthogonality.

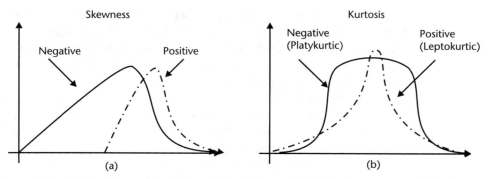

Figure 5.9 Distributions with third and fourth moments [(a) skewness, and (b) kurtosis, respectively] that are significantly different from normal (Gaussian).

where $E\{\}$ is the expectation operator and $p_x(x)$ is the probability that x has a particular value. The variance (second central moment), which quantifies the spread of a distribution is given by

$$\sigma_x^2 = E\{(x - \mu_x)^2\} = \int\limits_{-\infty}^{+\infty} (x - \mu_x)^2 p_x(x) dx \qquad (5.31)$$

and the square root of the variance is equal to the standard deviation, σ, of the distribution. By extension, we can define the Nth central moment to be

$$\upsilon_n = E\{(x - \mu_x)^n\} = \int\limits_{-\infty}^{+\infty} (x - \mu_x)^n p_x(x) dx \qquad (5.32)$$

The third moment of a distribution is known as the *skew*, ζ, and it characterizes the degree of asymmetry about the mean. The skew of a random variable x is given by $\upsilon_3 = \frac{E\{(x-\mu_x)^3\}}{\sigma^3}$. A positive skew signifies a distribution with a tail extending out toward a more positive value and a negative skew signifies a distribution with a tail extending out toward a more negative [see Figure 5.9(a)].

The fourth moment of a distribution is known as *kurtosis* and measures the relative peakedness, or flatness, of a distribution with respect to a Gaussian (normal) distribution. See Figure 5.9(b). Kurtosis is defined in a similar manner to the other moments as

$$\kappa = \upsilon_4 = \frac{E\{(x - \mu_x)^4\}}{\sigma^4} \qquad (5.33)$$

Note that for a Gaussian $\kappa = 3$, whereas the first three moments of a Gaussian distribution are zero.[24] A distribution with a positive kurtosis [> 3 in (5.37)] is

24. The proof of this is left to the reader, but noting that the general form of the normal distribution is $p_x(x) = \frac{e^{-(x-\mu_x^2)/2\sigma^2}}{\sigma\sqrt{2\pi}}$, and $\int_{-\infty}^{\infty} e^{-ax^2} dx = \sqrt{\pi/a}$ should help (especially if you differentiate the integral twice). Note also then, that the above definition of kurtosis [and (5.37)] sometimes has an extra -3 term to make a Gaussian have zero kurtosis, such as in Numerical Recipes in C. Note that Matlab uses the above convention, without the -3 term. This convention is used in this chapter.

termed *leptokurtic* (or super-Gaussian). A distribution with a negative kurtosis [< 3 in (5.37)] is termed *platykurtic* (or sub-Gaussian). Gaussian distributions are termed *mesokurtic*. Note also that skewness and kurtosis are normalized by dividing the central moments by appropriate powers of σ to make them dimensionless.

These definitions are, however, for continuously valued functions. In reality, the PDF is often difficult or impossible to calculate accurately, and so we must make empirical approximations of our sampled signals. The standard definition of the mean of a vector $\mathbf{x}$ with M values ($\mathbf{x} = [x_1, x_2, \ldots, x_M]$) is

$$\hat{\mu}_x = \frac{1}{M} \sum_{i=1}^{M} x_i \tag{5.34}$$

the variance of $\mathbf{x}$ is given by

$$\hat{\sigma}^2(\mathbf{x}) = \frac{1}{M} \sum_{i=1}^{M} (x_i - \hat{\mu}_x)^2 \tag{5.35}$$

and the skewness is given by

$$\hat{\zeta}(\mathbf{x}) = \frac{1}{M} \sum_{i=1}^{M} \left[\frac{x_i - \hat{\mu}_x}{\hat{\sigma}} \right]^3 \tag{5.36}$$

The empirical estimate of kurtosis is similarly defined by

$$\hat{\kappa}(x) = \frac{1}{M} \sum_{i=1}^{M} \left[\frac{x_i - \hat{\mu}_x}{\hat{\sigma}} \right]^4 \tag{5.37}$$

This estimate of the fourth moment provides a measure of the non-Gaussianity of a PDF. Large positive values of kurtosis indicate a highly peaked PDF that is much narrower than a Gaussian. A negative value of kurtosis indicates a broad PDF that is much wider than a Gaussian (see Figure 5.9).

In the case of PCA, the measure we use to discover the axes is *variance*, and this leads to a set of orthogonal axes. This is because the data set is decorrelated in a second-order sense and the dot product of any pair of the newly discovered axes is zero. For ICA, this measure is based on non-Gaussianity, such as kurtosis, and the axes are not necessarily orthogonal.

Our assumption is that if we maximize the non-Gaussianity of a set of signals, then they are maximally independent. This assumption stems from the central limit theorem; if we keep adding independent signals together (which have highly non-Gaussian PDFs), we will eventually arrive at a Gaussian distribution. Conversely, if we break a Gaussian-like observation down into a set of non-Gaussian mixtures, each with distributions that are as non-Gaussian as possible, the individual signals will be independent. Therefore, kurtosis allows us to separate non-Gaussian independent sources, whereas variance allows us to separate independent Gaussian noise sources.

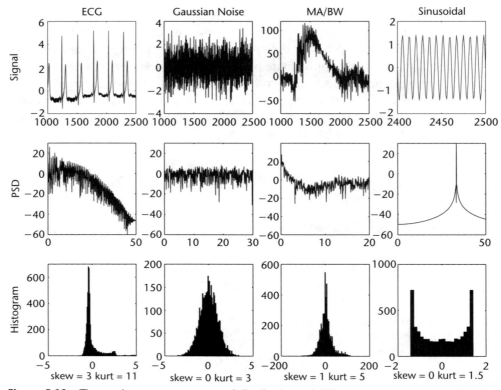

Figure 5.10 Time series, power spectra and distributions of different signals and noises found on the ECG. From left to right: (1) the underlying electrocardiogram signal, (2) additive (Gaussian) observation noise, (3) a combination of muscle artifact (MA) and baseline wander (BW), and (4) power-line interference, sinusoidal noise with $f \approx 33$ Hz ± 2 Hz.

Figure 5.10 illustrates the time series, power spectra, and distributions of different signals and noises found in an ECG recording. Note that all the signals have significant power contributions within the frequency of interest (< 40 Hz) where there exists clinically relevant information in the ECG. Traditional filtering methods, therefore, cannot remove these noises without severely distorting the underlying ECG.

5.4.3.4   ICA for Removing Noise on the ECG

For the application of ICA for noise removal from the ECG, there is an added complication; the sources (that correspond to cardiac sources) have undergone a context-dependent transformation that depends on the signal within the analysis window. Therefore, the sources are not clinically relevant ECGs, and the transformation must be inverted (after removing the noise sources) to reconstruct the clinically meaningful observations. That is, after identifying the sources of interest we can discard those that we do not want by altering the inverse of the demixing matrix to have columns of zeros for the unwanted sources, and reprojecting the data set back from the IC space into the *observation space* in the following manner:

$$\mathbf{X}_{filt}^{T} = \mathbf{W}_{p}^{-1}\mathbf{Y}^{T} \qquad (5.38)$$

where $\mathbf{W}_{p}^{-1}$ is the altered inverse demixing matrix. The resultant data $\mathbf{X}_{filt}$ is a filtered version of the original data $\mathbf{X}$.

The sources that we discover with PCA have a specific ordering according to the energy along each axis for a particular source. This is because we look for the axis along which the data vector has maximum variance, and, hence, energy or power.[25] If the SNR is large enough, the signal of interest is confined to the first few components. However, ICA allows us to discover sources by measuring a relative cost function between the sources that is dimensionless. Therefore, there is no relevance to the order of the columns in the separated data, and often we have to apply further signal-specific measures, or heuristics, to determine which sources are interesting.

Any projection onto another set of axes (or into another space) is essentially a method for separating data out into separate components, or *sources*, which will hopefully allow us to see important structure in a particular projection. For example, by calculating the power spectrum of a segment of data, we hope to see peaks at certain frequencies. Thus, the power (amplitude squared) along certain frequency vectors is high, meaning we have a strong component in the signal at that frequency. By discarding the projections that correspond to the unwanted sources (such as the noise or artifact sources) and inverting the transformation, we effectively perform a filtering of the signal. This is true for both ICA and PCA, as well as Fourier-based techniques. However, one important difference between these techniques is that Fourier techniques *assume* that the projections onto each frequency component are independent of the other frequency components. In PCA and ICA, we attempt to *find* a set of axes that are independent of one another in some sense. We assume there are a set of independent sources in the data set, but do not assume their exact properties. Therefore, in contrast to Fourier techniques, they may overlap in the frequency domain. We then define some measure of independence to facilitate the *decorrelation* between the assumed sources in the data set. This is done by maximizing this independence measure between projections onto each axis of the new space into which we have transformed the data set. The *sources* are the data set projected onto each of the new axes.

Figure 5.11 illustrates the effectiveness of ICA in removing artifacts from the ECG. Here we see 10 seconds of three leads of ECG before and after ICA decomposition (upper and lower graphs, respectively). Note that ICA has separated out the observed signals into three specific sources: (1) the ECG, (2) high kurtosis transient (movement) artifacts, and (3) low kurtosis continuous (observation) noise. In particular, ICA has separated out the *in-band* QRS-like spikes that occurred at 2.6 and 5.1 seconds. Furthermore, time-coincident artifacts at 1.6 seconds that distorted the QRS complex were extracted, leaving the underlying morphology intact.

Relating this back to the cocktail party problem, we have three "speakers" in three locations. First and foremost, we have the series of cardiac depolarization/

---

25. All the projections are proportional to $\mathbf{x}^{2}$.

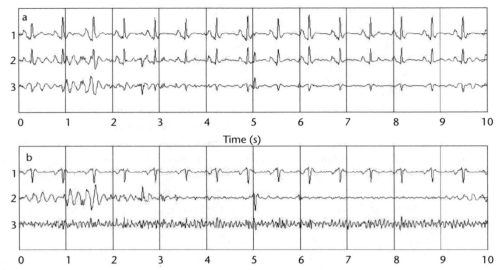

Figure 5.11   Ten seconds of three-channel ECG: (a) before ICA decomposition and (b) after ICA decomposition. Note that ICA has separated out the observed signals into three specific sources: (1) the ECG, (2) high kurtosis transient (movement) artifacts, and (3) low kurtosis continuous (observation) noise.

repolarization events corresponding to each heartbeat, located in the chest. Each electrode is roughly equidistant from each of these. Note that the amplitude of the third lead is lower than the other two, illustrating how the cardiac activity in the heart is not spherically symmetrical. Another source (or speaker) is the perturbation of the contact electrode due to physical movement. The third speaker is the Johnson (thermal) observation noise.

However, we should not assume that ICA is a panacea to remove all noise. In most situations, complications due to lead position, a low SNR, and positional changes in the sources cause serious problems. The next section addresses many of the problems in employing ICA, using the ECG as a practical illustrative guide. Moreover, since an ICA decomposition does not necessarily mean the relevant clinical characteristics of the ECG have been preserved (since our interpretive knowledge of the ECG is based upon the observations, not the sources). In order to reconstruct the original ECGs in the absence of noise, we must set to zero the columns of the demixing matrix that correspond to artifacts or noise, then invert it and multiply by the decomposed data set to "restore" the original ECG observations.

An example of this procedure using the data set in Figure 5.11 is presented in Figure 5.12. In terms of our general ICA formalism, the estimated sources $\hat{\mathbf{Z}}$ [Figure 5.11(b)] are recovered from the observation $\mathbf{X}$ [Figure 5.11(a)] by estimating a de-mixing matrix $\mathbf{W}$. It is no longer obvious to which lead the underlying source [signal 1 in Figure 5.11(b)] corresponds. In fact, this source does not correspond to any clinical lead, just some transformed combination of leads. In order to perform a diagnosis on this lead, the source must be projected back into the observation domain by inverting the demixing matrix $\mathbf{W}$. It is at this point that we can perform a removal of the noise sources. Columns of $\mathbf{W}^{-1}$ that correspond to noise and/or artifact [signal 2 and signal 3 on Figure 5.11(b) in this case] are set to

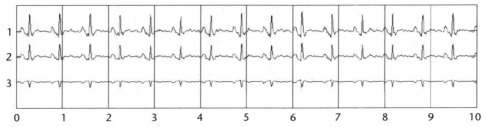

Figure 5.12 Ten seconds of data after ICA decomposition (see Figure 5.11), and reconstruction with noise channels set to zero.

zero ($\mathbf{W}^{-1} \rightarrow \mathbf{W}_p^{-1}$) where the number of nonnoise sources is $p = 1$. The filtered version of each clinical lead of $\mathbf{X}$ is then reconstructed in the observation domain using (5.38) to reveal a cleaner three-lead ECG (Figure 5.12).

5.4.3.5 Practical Problems with ICA

There are two well-known issues with standard ICA which makes filtering problematic. Since we can premultiply the mixing matrix $\mathbf{A}$ by any other matrix with the same properties, we can arbitrarily scale and permute the filtered output, Y. The *scaling problem* is overcome by inverting the transformation (after setting the relevant columns of W^{-1} to zero). However, the *permutation problem* is a little more complicated since we need to apply a set of heuristics to determine which ICs are signal and which are noise. (Systems to automatically select such channels are not common and are specific to the type of signal and noise being analyzed. He et al. [41] devised a system to automatically select channels using a technique based upon kurtosis and variance.) However, caution in the use of ICA is advised, since the linear stationary mixing paradigm does not always hold, even approximately. This is because the noise sources tend to originate from relatively static locations (such as muscles or the electrodes) while the cardiac source is rotating and translating through the abdomen with respiration. For certain electrode placements and respiratory activity, the ICA paradigm holds, and demixing is possible. However, in many instances the assumptions break down, and a method for tracking the changes in the mixing matrix is needed. Possibilities include the Kalman filter, hidden Markov models, or particle filter–based formulations [42–44].

To summarize, a useful ICA-based ECG filtering algorithm must be able to:

- Track nonstationarities in the mixing between signal and noise sources;
- Separate noise sources from signals for the given set of ECG leads;
- Identify which ICs are signal related and which ICs are noise related;
- Remove the ICs corresponding to noise and invert the transformation without causing significant clinical distortion in the ECG.[26]

Even if a robust ICA-based algorithm for tracking the nonstationarities in the ECG signal-noise mixing is developed, it is unclear whether it is possible to develop

---

26. "Clinical distortion" refers to any distortion of the ECG that leads to a significant change in the clinical features (such as QT interval and ST level).

a robust system to distinguish between the ICs and identify which are noise related. Furthermore, since the ICA mixing/demixing matrix must be tracked over time, the filter response is constantly evolving, and thus, it is unclear if ICA will lead to significant distortions in the derived clinical parameters from the ECG. Other problems include the possibility that the noise sources can sometimes be correlated to the cardiac source (such as for drug injections that change the dynamics of the heart and simultaneously agitate the patient causing electrode noise). Finally, the lack of high quality data in more than one or two leads can severely restrict the effectiveness of ICA.

There is, however, an interesting connection between ICA and wavelet analysis. In restricted circumstances (two-dimensional image analysis) ICA can be shown to produce Gabor wavelet-like basis functions [45]. The use of ICA as a post-processing step after construction of a scalogram or spectrogram may provide a more effective way of identifying interesting components in the signal. Furthermore, wavelet basis functions do not necessarily have to be orthogonal and therefore offer more flexibility in separating correlated, yet independent, transient sources.

5.4.3.6   Measuring Clinical Distortion in Signals

Although a variety of filtering techniques have been presented in this chapter, no method for systematically analyzing the effect of a filter on the ECG has been described. Unfortunately, simple measures based on RMS error and similar metrics do not tell us how badly a technique distorts the ECG in terms of the useful clinical metrics (such as the QT interval and the ST level). In order to do this, a sensitivity analysis to calibrate the evaluation metric against each clinical parameter is required. Furthermore, since simple mean square error-based metrics such as those presented above can give different values for equal power signals with different colorations (or autocorrelations), it is important to perform a separate analysis of the signal over a wide range of correlated noises. This, of course, presents another question: how may we measure the coloration of the noise in the ECG?

One approach to this problem is to pass a QRS detector across the ECG, align all the beats in the window (ensuring it is large enough, say, 60 beats), and perform SVD using only the first five components (which encode all the information and very little noise). If we then calculate the residual (the reconstructed signal minus the observation) and plot the spectrum of this signal, we will observe a $1/f^\beta$-like slope in the $\log - \log$ plot. Performing a regression on this line gives us our value of β, which corresponds to the the color of the noise. ($\beta = 0$ is white noise, $\beta = 1$ is pink nose, $\beta = 2$ is brown noise, and $\beta > 2$ is black noise.) See [46] for more details of this method. It should be noted, however, that simple colored noise models may be insufficient to capture the nonstationary nature of many noises, and an autoregressive moving average model (ARMA) may be more appropriate for categorizing noise types. This, of course, is a more complex and less intuitive approach.

If we have calculated the performance of a filter in terms of the distortion of a clinical parameter as a function of SNR and color, then this SVD-based and least-squares fitting method allows us to know exactly the form of the error surface in the power-color plane. Therefore, we can assess how likely our chosen filtering method is causing a clinically significant amount of distortion. If different filters lead to large difference in the distortion levels for different colors and/or SNRs, then a mechanism for switching between filters may help optimize filtering performance and minimize clinical distortion. Furthermore, we are able to obtain a beat-by-beat evaluation of whether we should trust the filtered signal in a particular circumstance. The derivation of confidence limits on the output of an algorithm for a particular signal are extremely important, and this concept will be discussed further in Chapter 11.

5.5 Summary and Conclusions

Linear filtering has been presented from the generalized viewpoint of matrix transformations to project observations into a new subspace whose axes are either a priori defined (as in Fourier-like decompositions) or discovered from the structure of the observations themselves. The new projections hopefully reveal different underlying sources of information in the observations. The sources are then correlated with either the signal or the noise. If the subspace dimensionality is less than the original observation space, then the matrix transformation is lossy.

If the sources are discovered from the structure of the data, it is possible to separate sources, which may overlap in the frequency domain. It has been shown that the method for discovering this type of subspace can be cast in terms of a neural network learning paradigm where the difference between the axes depends on the activation function and the cost function used in the error back propagation update. If the underlying sources are assumed to have Gaussian PDFs, then a linear activation function should be used. Nonlinear activation functions should be used for non-Gaussian sources. (A *tanh* function, for example, implies heavy tailed latent variables.) Additionally, the use of a mean-square error cost function provides second-order decorrelation and leads to orthogonal basis functions. A mutual information-based cost function performs a fourth-order decorrelation and leads to a set of nonorthogonal basis functions. By projecting the observations onto these basis functions, using the discovered demixing matrix to provide the transformation, the estimated source signals are revealed.

To improve the robustness of the separation of partially or completely unknown underlying sources, either a statistically constructed model (as with learning algorithms in this chapter), or an explicit parameterized model of the ECG can be used. However, since the ECG is obviously nonlinear and nonstationary, the chosen signal processing technique must be appropriately adapted. Nonlinear ECG model-based techniques are therefore presented in the next chapter, together with an overview of how to apply nonlinear systems theory and common pitfalls encountered with such techniques.

References

[1]   Sörnmo, L., and P. Laguna, *Bioelectric Signal Processing in Cardiac and Neurological Applications*, Amsterdam: Elsevier (Academic Press), 2005.

[2]   Rangayyan, R. M., *Biomedical Signal Analysis: A Case-Study Approach*, Series on Biomedical Engineering, New york: Wiley-IEEE Press, 2002.

[3]   Cohen, R., and A. Ryan, *Wavelets and Multiscale Signal Processing*, London, U.K.: Chapman and Hall, 1995.

[4]   Williams, W., "Recent Advances in Time-Frequency Representations: Some Theoretical Foundation," in M. Akay, (ed.), *Time Frequency and Wavelets in Biomedical Signal Processing*, Chapter 1, New York: Wiley-IEEE Press, 1997.

[5]   Addison, P. S., "Wavelet Transforms and the ECG: A Review," *Physiological Measurement*, Vol. 26, No. 5, 2005, pp. R155–R199.

[6]   Dickhaus, H., and H. Heinrich, "Analysis of ECG Late Potentials Using Time-Frequency Methods," in M. Akay, (ed.), *Time Frequency and Wavelets in Biomedical Signal Processing*, Chapter 4, New York: Wiley-IEEE Press, 1997.

[7]   Martínez, J. P., et al., "A Wavelet-Based ECG Delineator: Evaluation on Standard Database," *IEEE Trans. Biomed. Eng.*, Vol. 51, No. 4, 2004, pp. 570–581.

[8]   Laguna, P., http://diec.unizar.es/~laguna/, 2006.

[9]   Grinfeld, P., "The Gibbs Pheonomenon — Java Applet Demo," 1999, http://www.math.drexel.edu/~pg/fb//java/la_applets/Gibbs/index.html.

[10]   Greenberg, J., HST.582J/6.555J/16.456J, "Design of FIR Filters by Windowing," 1999, http://web.mit.edu/6.555/www/fir.html.

[11]   Antoniadis, A., and J. Fan, "Regularization of Wavelet Approximations," *Journal of the American Statistical Association*, Vol. 96, No. 455, 2001, pp. 939–967.

[12]   Hilton, M. F., et al., "Evaluation of Frequency and Time-Frequency Spectral Analysis of Heart Rate Variability as a Diagnostic Marker of the Sleep Apnoea Syndrome," *Med. Biol. Eng. Comput.*, Vol. 37, No. 6, November 1999, pp. 760–769.

[13]   Huang, N. E., et al., "The Empirical Mode Decomposition and the Hilbert Spectrum for Nonlinear and Non-Stationary Time Series Analysis," *Proc. R. Soc. Lond. A*, Vol. 454, 1998, pp. 903–995.

[14]   Huang, N. E., and S. S. Shen, *The Hilbert-Huang Transform and Its Applications*, Singapore: World Scientific Publishing Company, 2005, http://www.worldscibooks.com/mathematics/etextbook/5862/.

[15]   Golub, G. H., and C. F. Van Loan, *Matrix Computations*, 2nd ed., Oxford, U.K.: North Oxford Academic, 1989.

[16]   Moody, G. B., and R. G. Mark, "QRS Morphology Representation and Noise Estimation Using the Karhunen-Loève Transform," *Computers in Cardiology*, 1989, pp. 269–272.

[17]   Mark, R. G., and G. B. Moody, "ECG Arrhythmia Analysis: Design and Evaluation Strategies," Chapter 18 in I. Gath and G. F. Inbar, (eds.), *Advances in Processing and Pattern Analysis of Biological Signals*, New York: Plenum Press, 1996, pp. 251–272.

[18]   Clifford, G. D., and L. Tarassenko, "One-Pass Training of Optimal Architecture Auto-Associative Neural Network for Detecting Ectopic Beats," *IEE Electronic Letters*, Vol. 37, No. 18, August 2001, pp. 1126–1127.

[19]   Gao, D., et al., "Bayesian ANN Classifier for ECG Arrhythmia Diagnostic System: A Comparison Study," *International Joint Conference on Neural Networks*, Montreal, July 2005.

[20]   Bishop, C., *Neural Networks for Pattern Recognition*, New York: Oxford University Press, 1995.

[21]   Clifford, G. D., L. Tarassenko, and N. Townsend, "Fusing Conventional ECG QRS Detection Algorithms with an Auto-Associative Neural Network for the Detection of Ectopic Beats," *5th International Conference on Signal Processing*, Beijing, China, August 2000, IFIP, World Computer Congress, pp. 1623–1628.

[22]   Tarassenko, L., G. D. Clifford, and N. Townsend, "Detection of Ectopic Beats in the Electrocardiogram Using an Auto-Associative Neural Network," *Neural Processing Letters*, Vol. 14, No. 1, 2001, pp. 15–25.

[23]   Golub, G. H., "Least Squares, Singular Values and Matrix Approximations," *Applikace Matematiky*, No. 13, 1968, pp. 44–51.

[24]   Bourlard, H., and Y. Kamp, "Auto-Association by Multilayer Perceptrons and Singular Value Decomposition," *Biol. Cybern.*, No. 59, 1988, pp. 291–294.

[25]   Bunch, J. R., and C. P. Nielsen, "Updating the Singular Value Decomposition," *Numer. Math.*, No. 31, 1978, pp. 111–129.

[26]   Tarassenko, L., *A Guide to Neural Computing Applications*, Oxford, U.K.: Oxford University Press, 1998.

[27]   MacKay, D. J. C., "Maximum Likelihood and Covariant Algorithms for Independent Component Analysis," http://www.inference.phy.cam.ac.uk/mackay/abstracts/ica.html, 1996, updated 2002.

[28]   Clifford, G. D., http://alum.mit.edu/www/gari, 2003, updated June 2006.

[29]   Greenberg, J., et al., HST.582J/6.555J/16.456J, "Biomedical Signal and Image Processing: Course Notes," http://web.mit.edu/6.555/www/, 2006.

[30]   Trotter, H. F., "An Elementary Proof of the Central Limit Theorem," *Arch. Math.*, Vol. 10, 1959, pp. 226–234.

[31]   Penny, W., S. Roberts, and R. Everson, "ICA: Model Order Selection and Dynamic Source Models," Chapter 12 in S. Roberts and R. Everson, (eds.), *Independent Component Analysis: Principles and Practice*, Cambridge, U.K.: Cambridge University Press, 2001.

[32]   Choudrey, R. A., and S. J. Roberts, "Bayesian ICA with Hidden Markov Model Sources," *International Conference on Independent Component Analysis*, Nara, Japan, 2003, pp. 809–814.

[33]   Joho, M., H. Mathis, and R. Lambert, "Overdetermined Blind Source Separation: Using More Sensors than Source Signals in a Noisy Mixture," *Proc. International Conference on Independent Component Analysis and Blind Signal Separation*, Helsinki, Finland, June 19–22, 2000, pp. 81–86.

[34]   Lee, T., et al., "Blind Source Separation of More Sources than Mixtures Using Overcomplete Representations," *IEEE Sig. Proc. Lett.*, Vol. 6, No. 4, 1999, pp. 87–90.

[35]   Lewicki, M. S., and T. J. Sejnowski, "Learning Overcomplete Representations," *Neural Computation*, Vol. 12, No. 2, 2000, pp. 337–365.

[36]   Benaroya, L., et al., "Non Negative Sparse Representation for Wiener Based Source," *Proc. ICASSP,* Hong Kong, 2003, pp. 613–616.

[37]   Clifford, G. D., and P. E. McSharry, "A Realistic Coupled Nonlinear Artificial ECG, BP, and Respiratory Signal Generator for Assessing Noise Performance of Biomedical Signal Processing Algorithms," *Proc. of SPIE International Symposium on Fluctuations and Noise*, Vol. 5467, No. 34, 2004, pp. 290–301.

[38]   McSharry, P. E., and G. D. Clifford, "A Comparison of Nonlinear Noise Reduction and Independent Component Analysis Using a Realistic Dynamical Model of the Electrocardiogram," *Proc. of SPIE International Symposium on Fluctuations and Noise*, Vol. 5467, No. 9, 2004, pp. 78–88.

[39]   James, C. J., and D. Lowe, "Extracting Multisource Brain Activity from a Single Electromagnetic Channel," *Artificial Intelligence in Medicine*, Vol. 28, No. 1, May 2003, pp. 89–104.

[40]   Broomhead, D. S., and G. P. King, "Extracting Qualitative Dynamics from Experimental Data," *Physica D*, Vol. 20, 1986, pp. 217–236.

[41]   He, T., G. D. Clifford, and L. Tarassenko, "Application of ICA in Removing Artifacts from the ECG," *Neural Comput. and Applic.*, Vol. 15, No. 2, 2006, pp. 105–116.

[42]   Penny, W., S. Roberts, and R. Everson, "Hidden Markov Independent Components Analysis," Chapter 1 in M. Grolami, (ed.), *Advances in Independent Component Analysis*, New York: Springer-Verlag, 2000.

[43]   Penny, W., S. Roberts, and R. Everson, "Hidden Markov Independent Components for Biosignal Analysis," *Proc. of MEDSIP-2000*, 2000.

[44]   Everson, R., and S. Roberts, "Particle Filters for Nonstationary ICA," in S. Roberts and
        R. Everson, (eds.), *Independent Component Analysis: Principles and Practice*, Cambridge,
        U.K.: Cambridge University Press, 2001, pp. 280–298.

[45]   Hyvärinen, A., R. Cristescu, and E. Oja, "Fast Algorithm for Estimating Overcomplete
        ICA Bases for Image Windows," *Proc. IJCNN99*, 1999.

[46]   Clifford, G. D., and P. E. McSharry, "Method to Filter ECGs and Evaluate Clinical Param-
        eter Distortion Using Realistic ECG Model Parameter Fitting," *Computers in Cardiology*,
        Vol. 32, 2005.

CHAPTER 6

Nonlinear Filtering Techniques

Patrick E. McSharry and Gari D. Clifford

6.1 Introduction

The ECG is routinely used to provide important clinical information. In practice, the utility of any diagnosis based on the ECG relies on the quality of the available signal. A typical ECG recorded in a clinical environment may be corrupted by one or more of the following: (1) electrical interference from surrounding equipment such as the effect of the electrical mains supply; (2) analog-to-digital conversion; and (3) movement and muscle artifacts. In order to employ the ECG signal for facilitating medical diagnosis, filtering techniques may be employed to *clean* the signal, thereby attempting to remove the distortions caused by these various sources of noise.

Many techniques for filtering are based on a spectral decomposition of the signal (see [1]). Such techniques include notch filters for removing the effect of the electrical mains supply, and both low and high bandpass filters for removing noise that is localized in particular regions of the frequency spectrum. These techniques all rely on the principle of linear superposition and there is a fundamental assumption that the underlying signal and the noise are active in different parts of the frequency spectrum. Section 3.1 provides a description of these techniques.

Linear filtering techniques are of limited use in cases where both the noise and signal occupy similar regions of the frequency domain. This restriction motivates the use of nonlinear filtering methods that do not rely on the linear assumptions underlying spectral analysis. In this chapter, three nonlinear techniques are described. These are (1) nonlinear noise reduction (NNR) [2], (2) independent component analysis (ICA) [3], and (3) model-based filtering [4]. For simplicity, these methods are demonstrated using univariate signals. Each of these techniques can easily be extended to multivariate signals arising from multiple leads and this will generally provide better performance.

Accurate metrics for evaluating the effectiveness of filtering techniques applied to the ECG are difficult to define due to the inherently complicated structure of the noise and the absence of knowledge about the underlying dynamical processes. Without having access to a noise-free ECG signal, the fact that the true underlying dynamics of a real ECG can never be known implies that one cannot distinguish between the clean ECG signal and the many sources of noise that can occur during recording in a clinical environment. While the availability of biomedical databases [5] provides a useful benchmark for comparing different techniques, this approach can never truly distinguish between noise and signal. ECGSYN, a dynamical model for generating ECG signals with known temporal and spectral characteristics and prespecified average morphology [6] is used to compare and evaluate these techniques under a range of different conditions (see Section 4.3.2 for further details of ECGSYN).

The layout of the chapter is as follows. Section 6.2 provides an overview of nonlinear dynamics and the application of this theory to signals known as nonlinear time series analysis or nonlinear signal processing. This section describes how to reconstruct a multidimensional state space using a univariate signal and calculate nonlinear descriptive statistics such as Lyapunov exponents, correlation dimension, and entropy. The associated discussion also describes how to test the significance of these statistics and how failure to do so can lead to erroneous conclusions. Section 6.3 discusses the different forms of noise that affect the ECG and suggests different metrics for evaluating filtering techniques. Section 6.4 describes and compares two empirical filtering techniques, NNR and a state space implementation of ICA. Section 6.5 gives details of two model-based filtering approaches using ECGSYN to provide constraints on the underlying ECG signal; the first uses a nonlinear least squares parameter estimation technique and the second uses an extended Kalman filter.

These approaches illustrate different paradigms for utilizing nonlinear methods for filtering the ECG. Statistical techniques such as PCA and ICA make statistical assumptions about the relationship between the signal and the noise in a reconstructed state space. In contrast, the model-based approach makes an explicit assumption concerning the underlying structure of the ECG signal and this is encoded in a dynamical model such as ECGSYN. Nonlinear techniques are then used to find an optimal fit of this model to the data. For this reason, the model-based approach is tailor-made for ECG signals.

6.2 Nonlinear Signal Processing

Chaotic dynamics provide one possible explanation for the different complex and erratic patterns that appear in a large number of observed signals. Chaos refers to the existence of behavior so unpredictable as to appear random because of the inherent sensitivity to small perturbations in the initial conditions. This suggests that many complex systems could possibly be described by low-dimensional deterministic mathematical models. Although many real-world systems are undoubtedly nonlinear (a necessary but not sufficient condition for chaos), in practice, the quality of recorded signals is usually better suited to traditional linear analyses. Despite the fact that there is very little evidence of chaos in real systems, the field of nonlinear dynamics can help improve our understanding of many complicated systems [7]. The recent proliferation of high-speed computers and cheap storage for large databases suggests that the construction of data-driven nonlinear models is now feasible and that such developments have the potential to make a substantial contribution to science. Nonlinear signal processing relates to the data analysis that is required to construct, estimate, and evaluate these nonlinear models. The decision to pursue nonlinear models brings many challenges. As traditional techniques based on normal distributions and least squares are no longer valid, new techniques for parameter estimation [8] and model evaluation [9] are required.

6.2.1 State Space Reconstruction

Reconstructing a state space using an observed time series is usually the first step in building a model for describing nonlinear dynamics. Suppose that the underlying system dynamics of the ECG evolve on an attractor $\mathbf{A}$ according to $\mathbf{G} : \mathbf{A} \to \mathbf{A}$. Let τ_s be the sampling time of the recorded signal $s(t)$ that provides discrete observations, $s_n = s(n\tau_s)$. It is possible to construct a replica state space using a delay vector reconstruction [10–12] of the observations s_n defined by

$$\mathbf{s}_n = \left[s_n, s_{n+d} \ldots, s_{n+(m-1)d} \right] \in \Re^m \tag{6.1}$$

where m is the reconstruction dimension and $\tau_d = d\tau_s$ is the time delay. In order to reconstruct the dynamics, $\mathbf{G}$, of the system state space using a data-driven model, $\mathbf{F} : \mathbf{\Phi}(\mathbf{A}) \to \mathbf{\Phi}(\mathbf{A})$, it is necessary to ensure that the mapping $\mathbf{\Phi} : \mathbf{A} \to \mathbf{\Phi}(\mathbf{A})$ provides a faithful representation of the system's attractor.

Mathematical theory can be used to describe the conditions under which it should be possible to obtain a faithful representation of the underlying dynamics. This states that the reconstruction dimension, m, should satisfy $m > 2D_0$ where D_0 is the box-counting dimension [11, 13]. Unfortunately this theory is of little help when faced with noisy data of finite duration—the challenge of most interesting signal processing problems. For example, while the choice of τ_d is irrelevant in the theory, it is extremely important in practice. One approach for selecting τ_d is to identify the first minimum in the mutual information of the signal [14]. Another approach is based on a geometric interpretation of the reconstruction [15].

The fact the value of D_0 is unknown a priori implies that m must also be estimated. One technique for estimating m is known as the method of *false nearest neighbors* [16]. This method determines a sufficient value for m by varying the size of m and monitoring the number of false nearest neighbors associated with areas of the reconstructed state space that have self-intersections. Unfortunately, the detection of false nearest neighbors is subject to the choice of an arbitrary constant that varies with location in state space. By testing for consistency between the model dynamics and the observational uncertainty while incorporating the variation of the local instabilities of the nonlinear dynamics throughout state space, it is possible to calculate a robust estimate for the minimum value of m [9]. In practice, if the state space reconstruction is one component of a technique with an obvious application, such as the case of filtering, then it is advisable to determine values for τ_d and m by optimizing the accuracy of the filtering technique. This is possible when using the synthetic ECG signals generated by ECGSYN.

6.2.2 Lyapunov Exponents

The best known hallmark of chaotic dynamics is perhaps the inherent unpredictability of the future despite the fact that the underlying system has to obey deterministic equations of motion. This unpredictability may be quantified through the increasing average forecast error that results from larger prediction lead times. Such *sensitive dependence on initial condition* describes the inherent instability of the solutions that generate this unpredictability; two nearby initial conditions will, on average, diverge over time. Although many linear systems give rise to a slow rate of divergence, it is the exponential divergence in nonlinear systems that is characteristic of chaotic systems.

A deterministic dynamical system may be described by a discrete map, $\mathbf{x}_{n+1} = \mathbf{F}(\mathbf{x}_n)$ where $\mathbf{x}_n \in \Re^m$. The evolution of an infinitesimal uncertainty, ε_0, in the initial condition, $\mathbf{x}_0$, over a finite number of time steps, k, is given by $\varepsilon_k = \mathbf{M}(\mathbf{x}_0, k)\varepsilon_0$, where $\mathbf{M}(\mathbf{x}_0, k)$ is the linear tangent propagator formed by the product of the Jacobians along the k steps of the trajectory $\mathbf{M}(\mathbf{x}_0, k) = \mathbf{J}(\mathbf{x}_{k-1})\mathbf{J}(\mathbf{x}_{k-2}) \ldots \mathbf{J}(\mathbf{x}_0)$.

The linear dynamics that describe the evolution of the uncertainty quantified by ε_k may be analyzed using the singular value decomposition (SVD), $\mathbf{M} = \mathbf{U}\mathbf{\Sigma}\mathbf{V}^T$, where the columns of the orthogonal matrix $\mathbf{U}(\mathbf{V})$ are the left (right) singular vectors, respectively, and the entries of the diagonal matrix $\mathbf{\Sigma}$ are the singular values, $\sigma_i(\mathbf{x}_0, k)$, which are usually ranked in decreasing order [17]. The *finite time* Lyapunov exponents [18, 19] are defined as

$$\lambda_i^{(k)}(\mathbf{x}_0) = \frac{1}{k} \log_2 \sigma_i(\mathbf{x}_0, k), \quad i = 1, 2, \ldots, m \tag{6.2}$$

and depend on both the initial condition, $\mathbf{x}_0$, and the number of steps, k. The first finite time Lyapunov exponent $\lambda_1^{(k)}(\mathbf{x}_0)$ describes the maximum possible linear growth over the time k for which the linear propagator was defined. The Lyapunov exponents, Λ_i, are defined by taking the limit as k goes to infinity,

$$\Lambda_i = \lim_{k \to \infty} \lambda_i^{(k)}(\mathbf{x}_0), \quad i = 1, 2, \ldots, m \tag{6.3}$$

A system is said to be chaotic if the leading Lyapunov exponent, Λ_1, is positive, whereas a negative value indicates the existence of a stable fixed point. Indeed, the Lyapunov spectrum provides a means of classifying the dynamics of a system which could be useful for diagnosing *dynamical diseases* where transitions between stable and oscillatory behavior can indicate changes from health to illness or vice versa [20].

A number of approaches are available for estimating Lyapunov exponents [21–24]. By calculating the finite time Lyapunov exponents, one can monitor the convergence as a function of the amount of data available [19]. Confidence intervals should be calculated if one wishes to establish whether or not a system is chaotic [25]. In the case of an observed signal, it is advisable to first check for the existence of exponential growth. The combined effects of small data sets and noisy observations mean that it is difficult to calculate reliable estimates from signals. Techniques which specifically aim to calculate the maximal Lyapunov exponent for real signals [26, 27] are available from the TISEAN package [28].

6.2.3   Correlation Dimension

A number of different approaches, both dynamical and geometrical, exist for estimating the number of *active* degrees of freedom in a given system. Techniques for estimating fractal dimensions have received a lot of attention. The motivation for this has been the realization that if a system is governed by low-dimensional deterministic dynamics, then a model with only a few degrees of freedom exists.

The ability to obtain accurate estimates has proven difficult. It is advisable that such dimension estimates should be supported by a quantification of the confidence in the estimate. In practice, it may be easier to construct a low-dimensional model from the data than to obtain a direct estimate of the underlying system's dimension.

The *box-counting dimension* of a self-similar point set is calculated by counting the number of hyper-cubes $M(\epsilon)$ of side ϵ required to cover the set, then for a self-similar set $M(\epsilon) \propto \epsilon^{-D_0}$ as $\epsilon \to 0$ and

$$D_0 = \lim_{\epsilon \to 0} \frac{\ln M(\epsilon)}{\ln(1/\epsilon)} \qquad (6.4)$$

Renyi [29] defined a family of generalized dimensions which differ in the way regions with different densities are weighted, thereby giving more weight to regions which are visited more frequently and thus contain larger fractions of the measure. These *Renyi dimensions*, D_q, are a decreasing function of q: $D_{q_1} \leq D_{q_2}$ if $q_1 > q_2$. A measure for which D_q varies with q is called a *multifractal* measure [30].

The *correlation dimension*, D_2, may be estimated from experimental data and used to suggest a suitable reconstruction dimension, m, since $D_2 \leq D_0$. D_2 reflects how the probability that the distance between two randomly chosen points will be less than ε, scales as a function of ε. For a finite sequence of points $\{x_i\}_{i=1}^N$, a quantify known as the correlation integral measures the fraction of pairs of points (x_i, x_j) whose distance is smaller than ε [31],

$$C(\varepsilon, N) = \frac{2}{N(N-1)} \sum_{i=1}^{N-1} \left[\sum_{j=i+1}^{N} \Theta(\epsilon - ||x_i - x_j||) \right] \qquad (6.5)$$

where Θ is the Heaviside step function: $\Theta(x) = 0$ if $x \leq 0$ and $\Theta(x) = 1$ if $x > 0$. If this correlation integral scales as a power law, $C \sim \varepsilon^{D_2}$, then

$$D_2 = \lim_{\varepsilon \to 0} \lim_{N \to \infty} \frac{d \ln C(\varepsilon, N)}{d \ln \varepsilon} \qquad (6.6)$$

For recorded signals, it is generally difficult to identify a scaling region since the finite sample size, N, places a lower bound on ε. Furthermore the finite accuracy of the measurements and the sparseness of near neighbors limits the calculation of C when ε is small.

Interpreting estimates of D_2 is also complicated by the fact that infinite dimensional stochastic signals can lead to finite and low-dimensional dimension estimates [32]. In addition, estimates for C can be biased by temporal correlations as small spatial distances between pairs of points may arise simply because the difference between their times of observation was small. Restricting attention to pairs of points separated by a specific temporal window may help to reduce this problem [32]. In practice, this problem of spatio-temporal correlations will always be present and the best approach is to use a space-time-separation diagram to test when sufficient data are not available [33].

An alternative approach employs a maximum likelihood estimate of D_2 without estimating the slope of the correlation integral directly [34]. This approach has been extended to provide a coherent estimate of D_2, which is consistent with measures at all smaller length scales [35]. When estimating D_2 from recorded signals, it is useful to know the rate of convergence of the estimate with the quantity of data, N, so as to determine confidence intervals. There have been numerous attempts at deriving a formula for determining the minimum length of the time series, N_{min}, required to obtain accurate dimension estimates, ranging from $N_{min} = 10^{D_2/2}$ [36] to $N_{min} = D_2^{42}$ [37]; see [25] for a discussion. For $D_2 = 10$, approximations of the amount of data required vary from 10^5 to 10^{42}.

In practice, estimation of D_2 is complicated by the fact that it is extremely difficult to maintain suitable experimental conditions in order to collect a sufficient quantity of data during a period when the underlying data generating process is stationary. In addition, measurement errors also restrict the estimation of D_2.

6.2.4 Entropy

Information theory provides a probabilistic approach to measuring the statistical dependence between random variables. Let X be a random variable with probability density function $p(x)$. The information corresponding to a particular probability $p(x)$ is defined as $-\log p(x)$. This essentially implies that the more probable an event, the less information it contains. The entropy of the distribution of X, a measure of the uncertainty or disorder, is given as the average information in X:

$$H = -\int p(x) \log p(x) dx \qquad (6.7)$$

The more erratic the observations of the variable X, the higher the entropy.

For example, consider a distribution such that X is uniformly distributed between 0 and 1. The integral in (6.7) may be evaluated by dividing the interval [0, 1] into n segments of length $\varepsilon = 1/n$ giving $H(\varepsilon) = -\sum_{i=1}^{n} \frac{1}{n} \log \varepsilon = -\log \varepsilon = \log n$. This demonstrates that the larger n is, the more information is gained by knowing that the variable X takes a value in some interval of length $1/n$. Alternatively, if the variable X always falls into one of the n intervals, all the probabilities will be zero except for one which will be unity. In this case the entropy is given by $H(\varepsilon) = 0$. The small value for the entropy indicates the certainty that the variable X will always land in the same interval.

Similarly, for a sequence of n random variables, $X_1, \ldots, X_n$, the joint entropy is given by

$$H_n = \int \cdots \int p(x_1, \ldots, x_n) \log p(x_1, \ldots, x_n) dx_1 \ldots dx_n \qquad (6.8)$$

where $p(x_1, \ldots, x_n)$ is the joint probability for the n variables $X_1, \ldots, X_n$. The Kolmogorov-Sinai (KS) entropy measures the mean rate of creation of information by measuring how much information each new observation brings. In practice, given a signal recorded with a sampling time τ_s and a state space with dimension n partitioned using a grid size ε, the KS entropy can be expressed as

$$H_{KS} = \lim_{\tau_s \to 0} \lim_{\varepsilon \to 0} \lim_{n \to \infty} (H_{n+1} - H_n) \qquad (6.9)$$

In the case of a deterministic periodic systems, the KS entropy is zero because the initial condition specifies all future states. In contrast, the KS entropy is maximum for uncorrelated random processes because each new state is totally independent of the previous states [38].

The estimation of entropy for recorded signals is complicated by the usual problems of small data and noisy signals. Approximate entropy (ApEn) was proposed as a measure of system complexity and quantifies the unpredictability of fluctuations in a time series [39]. The difficulty in estimating the entropy of short noisy time series has motivated an alternative approach, known as sample entropy [40], with the advantage of being less dependent on the length of the time series.

6.2.5 Nonlinear Diagnostics

Although the concept of using nonlinear statistics, such as D_2 or Λ_1, to categorize the state of an observed system is appealing, one should be aware that this is complicated by the previously discussed problems of obtaining accurate estimates. The ability to measure the complexity of an observed system may be useful for classifying states of health and disease and could form the basis of a diagnostic tool.

For clinical applications it is important to rule out simple linear statistics before inventing complicated nonlinear measures. The possible existence of strong correlations between simple linear statistics and their nonlinear counterparts suggests that newly proposed statistics based on nonlinear dynamics should be tested against simple traditional benchmarks. Indeed, published results using the correlation integral to forecast epileptic seizures from the electroencephalogram EEG were reproduced using the variance of the EEG signal [41]. The fact that an increase in variance produces a decrease in the value of correlation integral implies that carefully designed statistical tests with clinical relevance are required [42].

In practice, nonlinear statistics should only be evaluated on segments of data that arise when the underlying dynamics are stationary. Application of a test for stationarity to RR intervals [43] using 48-hour Holter recordings from 23 healthy subjects during sinus rhythm demonstrated that while it was relatively easy to find stationary periods containing 1,024 RR intervals, only a few stationary segments of between 8,192 and 32,768 RR intervals were found [44]. Using statistical tests based on the correlation dimension, the authors were able to reject the hypothesis that the RR intervals represented a static transformation of a linear process and found evidence for time irreversibility. These results suggest that heart rate variability is driven by nonlinear processes and that the RR intervals may contain more information than can be extracted by linear analyses in the time and frequency domains.

Despite the drawbacks caused by the difficulty in estimating nonlinear statistics, a number of techniques have been proposed in the field of biomedical research. Both an effective correlation dimension [45] and a method based on the convergence and divergence of short-term maximum Lyapunov exponents from adaptively selected electrodes [46] have been used to provide predictions of epileptic seizures. Approximate entropy has been used to discern changing complexity from relatively small amounts of data arising from RR intervals [47]. Sample entropy [40] has also been employed to explore the multiple time scales involved in physiological dynamics.

A technique, known as multiscale entropy [48], can distinguish between RR intervals from subjects within healthy and pathologic groups such as atrial fibrillation and congestive heart failure.

Nonlinear dynamics has proven useful for constructing improved methods for predictive recognition of patients threatened by sudden cardiac death [49]. Such nonlinear methods have shown promise in classifying fatal cardiac arrhythmias such as ventricular tachycardia (VT) and ventricular fibrillation (VF). In a study of 17 chronic heart failure patients before the onset of a life-threatening arrhythmia and at a control time (without either VT or VF events), neither time nor frequency domain statistics showed significant differences between the VT-VF and the control time series, whereas methods based on symbolic dynamics and finite-time growth rates were able to discriminate significantly between both groups [50].

6.3 Evaluation Metrics

Noise usually describes the uncertainty in the data resulting from measurement errors or specifically the part of the data that does not directly reflect the underlying system of interest. Sources of noise commonly encountered in the ECG include (1) electrical interference, (2) analog-to-digital conversion, and (3) movement or muscle artifacts. There is an important difference between *observational uncertainty* and *dynamical uncertainty*. Observational uncertainty refers to measurement errors which are independent of the dynamics. Sources include finite precision measurements, truncation errors, and missing data (both temporal and spatial). In contrast, dynamical uncertainty refers to external fluctuations interacting with and changing internal variables in the underlying system. Dynamical uncertainty includes parametrical and structural uncertainty, both of which lead to model error. An example of dynamical uncertainty is where a parameter value, assumed constant in the equations describing the underlying dynamics, was actually varying during the time when the data were being recorded. In short, observational uncertainty obscures the state vectors whereas dynamical uncertainty changes the actual dynamics.

In the following, only the effects of noise due to observational uncertainty are considered. Let τ_s be the sampling time of the recorded signal so that the observed time series is $y_n = y(n\tau_s)$. A simple description of observational uncertainty is provided by additive measurement error where the observed time series is

$$y_n = x_n + \epsilon_n \tag{6.10}$$

x_n is the true state vector and ϵ_n represents the unobserved measurement error. This measurement error term is usually described by a random variable, for example an identically and normally distributed (IND) process, $\epsilon \sim N(0, \sigma_{noise}^2)$, where σ_{noise}^2 is the variance of the noise. If the variance of the signal is σ_{signal}^2, then the SNR is defined as

$$\gamma = \frac{\sigma_{signal}}{\sigma_{noise}} \tag{6.11}$$

After employing a particular technique for *cleaning* a noisy dataset, a performance metric is required to assess its failure or success. Let the cleaned signal be z_n. Following Schreiber and Kaplan [2], a *noise reduction factor* is defined as

$$\chi = \sqrt{\frac{\langle y_n - x_n \rangle^2}{\langle z_n - x_n \rangle^2}} \tag{6.12}$$

where $\langle \cdot \rangle$ denotes the average calculated by summing over the observed time series, indexed by n. The value of χ provides a measure of the degree by which the RMS error is reduced. Unlike the investigation of Schreiber and Kaplan [2], the ECG model may be used to obtain a truly noise-free signal x_n so that the value of χ may be viewed as the actual noise reduction factor and not merely a lower bound. The higher the value of χ, the better the noise reduction procedure, whereas $\chi = 1$ indicates no improvement since similar accuracy could have been achieved by using the noisy signal, y_n, instead of z_n.

An alternative measure of noise reduction performance is given by a measure of the linear correlation between the cleaned signal, z_n, and the original noise-free signal, x_n. The cross-correlation coefficient ρ between x_n and z_n is given by [51]

$$\rho = \frac{\langle [x_n - \mu_x][z_n - \mu_z] \rangle}{\sigma_x \sigma_z} \tag{6.13}$$

where μ_x and σ_x are the mean and standard deviation of x_n, and μ_z and σ_z are the mean and standard deviation of z_n. A value of $\rho \sim 1$ reflects a strong correlation, $\rho \sim -1$ implies a strong anticorrelation, and $\rho \sim 0$ indicates that x_n and z_n are uncorrelated. This means that a value of $\rho = 1$ suggests that the noise reduction technique has removed all the noise from the observed signal.

6.4 Empirical Nonlinear Filtering

The ability to reconstruct a multidimensional state spaces from a univariate signal means that a number of multivariate techniques can now be applied. In the following, nonlinear noise reduction and independent component analysis are described. The two techniques are then employed to filter a synthetic ECG signal with known characteristics produced by ECGSYN. The performance is measured as a function of the SNR using both the noise reduction factor and the correlation between the cleaned signal and the original noise-free signal.

6.4.1 Nonlinear Noise Reduction

The ECG signal cannot be classified as either periodic or deterministically chaotic. Although the dynamics of the cardiac interbeat interval time series is similar to a $1/f$-like noise process [52, 53], midway between the complete randomness of white noise and the much smoother Brownian motion, the ECG signal displays limited predictability over times less than one heartbeat since each beat contains the familiar

P wave, QRS complex, and T wave. Schreiber and Kaplan [2] successfully applied a technique, originally constructed for removing noise from chaotic signals [54], to ECG signals. This short-term predictability may be used to reduce measurement errors by a local geometric method. The basic idea behind nonlinear noise reduction (NNR) is to use the manifold of the underlying dynamical system to project out the noise. This may be achieved by using a local linear model to predict a particular point in the state space while using its neighbors to construct a local linear map.

Following [2], consider a state space reconstruction with dimension m and time delay d, such that the underlying noise-free time series x_n is described by the evolution of a deterministic dynamical system,

$$x_n = f(x_{n-md}, \ldots, x_{n-2d}, x_{n-d}) \qquad (6.14)$$

By rewriting the dynamics represented by (6.14) in the implicit form of

$$g(x_{n-md}, \ldots, x_{n-d}, x_n) = 0 \qquad (6.15)$$

it is apparent that the noise-free dynamics are constrained to an m-dimensional hypersurface. While this is only approximately true for the observed noisy time series, $y_n = x_n + \epsilon_n$, one can still attempt to estimate the noise-free value x_n from the noisy y_n by projecting them onto the subspace spanned by the filtered data expressed through (6.15). The objective is to estimate this subspace from the noisy data while assuming that the observed time series lies close to a low-dimensional manifold. NNR relies on the assumption that the signal lies on a manifold with dimension less than $m + 1$, and that the variance of the noise is smaller than that of the signal.

In order to calculate a noise-free estimate for a particular reconstructed state vector, $\mathbf{y}_n$, its local neighborhood is defined; let $\mathcal{B}_n$ denote the indices of the set of points that form this neighborhood, y_j, $j \in \mathcal{B}_n$, and $|\mathcal{B}_n|$ be the number of neighbors. The mean value, μ_{y_i}, of each coordinate, $i = 0, \ldots, m$, is given by

$$\mu_{y_i} = \frac{1}{|\mathcal{B}_n|} \sum_{k \in |\mathcal{B}_n|} y_{k-(m+i)d} \qquad (6.16)$$

The covariance matrix, C_{ij}, of the points in the neighborhood, $\mathcal{B}_n \in \Re^{m+1}$, is

$$C_{ij} = \frac{1}{|\mathcal{B}_n|} \sum_{k \in |\mathcal{B}_n|} y_{k-(m+i)d} \, y_{k-(m+j)d} - \mu_{y_i} \mu_{y_j} \qquad (6.17)$$

and its eigenvectors give the principal axes of an ellipsoid that approximates this cloud of neighbors. Corrections based on the first and last coordinates in the delay vector may be penalized by using a diagonal weight matrix, $\mathbf{R}$, to transform the covariance matrix, $\Gamma_{ij} = R_{ii} C_{ij} R_{jj}$, where $R_{00} = R_{mm} \gg 1$ and all other diagonal values are equal to one [7]. The Q orthonormal eigenvectors of the matrix, Γ_{ij}, with the smallest eigenvectors are called e_q for $q = 1, \ldots, Q$. A projection matrix, P_{ij}, may be defined as

$$P_{ij} = \sum_{q=1}^{Q} e_{q,i} e_{q,j} \qquad (6.18)$$

so that the ith component of the correction vector, c_n, is given by

$$c_{n,i} = \frac{1}{R_{ii}} \sum_{j=0}^{m} P_{ij} R_{jj} (\mu_{y_i} - y_{n-(m+j)d}) \qquad (6.19)$$

This correction vector can then be added to each reconstructed state vector in order to move it towards the manifold spanned by the $m + 1 - Q$ largest eigenvectors. The role of the penalty matrix, $\mathbf{R}$, is to force the two largest eigenvalues to lie in the subspace spanned by the first and second coordinates of the reconstructed state space and ensures that the correction vector will not have any components in these directions. Following this procedure, given that each scalar observation occurs in $m + 1$ different reconstructed state vectors, this will provide as many suggested corrections. Taking the average of all these corrections gives the overall correction used for filtering the time series.

In the case of data from a deterministic system, it may be beneficial to iterate this process a number of times to clean the time series. For the ECG, where the signal is only expected to lie close to a manifold, the best results are obtained using only one iteration [2]. This type of filtering is nonlinear in the sense that the effective filter given by the local linear map varies throughout state space depending on the local dynamics. In particular it has the ability to remove noise from the recorded signal, even in cases when the underlying signal and the noise overlap in the frequency domain.

This NNR technique is available as *nrlazy* from the TISEAN software package [28, 55], and it requires the choice of various parameters such as the reconstruction dimension, m, the time delay, d, and the neighborhood radius, r. Using ECGSYN, it is possible to generate noise-free artificial ECG signals such that the correct answer is known a priori. Within this setting, it is possible to optimize the filtering procedure by performing a thorough search of the parameter space required to implement NNR.

6.4.2 State Space Independent Component Analysis

ICA is a statistical technique for decomposing a dataset into independent subparts [3, 56]. Using the delay reconstruction described in Section 6.2.1, the observed univariate ECG signal, $y_i = y(i\tau_s)$, is transformed into an $m \times n$ matrix,

$$\mathbf{Y} = \begin{bmatrix} y_1 & y_2 & \cdots & y_n \\ y_{1+d} & y_{2+d} & \cdots & y_{n+d} \\ \vdots & \vdots & & \vdots \\ y_{1+(m-1)d} & y_{2+(m-1)d} & \cdots & y_{n+(m-1)d} \end{bmatrix} \qquad (6.20)$$

where each column of $\mathbf{Y}$ contains one reconstructed state vector as defined by (6.1) with reconstruction dimension m and delay d. Note that the observed ECG signal, y_i, is assumed to have a mean of 0 and a standard deviation of 1, achieved by removing the mean, μ_y, of y and dividing by its standard deviation, σ_y. After application of the ICA algorithm, the resulting cleaned signal is rescaled by multiplying by σ_y and adding μ_y so that it is compatible with y_i.

In mathematical terms, the problem may be expressed as

$$\mathbf{Y} = \mathbf{BX} \tag{6.21}$$

where $\mathbf{X}$ is an $m \times n$ matrix containing the independent source signals, $\mathbf{B}$ is the $m \times m$ mixing matrix, and $\mathbf{Y}$ is an $m \times n$ matrix containing the observed (mixed) signals. ICA algorithms attempt to find a separating or demixing matrix $\mathbf{W}$ such that

$$\mathbf{X} = \mathbf{WY} \tag{6.22}$$

In practice, iterative methods are used to maximize or minimize a given cost function such as mutual information, entropy, or the kurtosis (fourth-order cumulant), which is given by

$$kurt(\mathbf{Y}) = E\{\mathbf{Y}^4\} - 3(E\{\mathbf{Y}^2\})^2 \tag{6.23}$$

where $E\{\mathbf{Y}\}$ is the expectation of $\mathbf{Y}$. The following analysis uses Cardoso's multidimensional ICA algorithm *jadeR* [3], which is based upon the joint diagonalization of cumulant matrices, because it combines the benefits of both PCA and ICA to provide a stable deterministic solution. (ICA suffers from a scaling and column ordering problem due to the indeterminacy of solution to scalar multipliers to and column permutations of the mixing matrix.)

Most ICA methods assume there are at least as many independent measurement sensors as the number of sources that one wishes to separate. Following James et al. [56], ICA was applied to the embedding matrix $\mathbf{Y}$, with the assumption of one signal and one noise source. Cardoso's *jadeR* algorithm was used for the ICA. An estimate $\hat{\mathbf{X}}$ of the sources $\mathbf{X}$ was obtained from

$$\hat{\mathbf{X}} = \mathbf{WY} \tag{6.24}$$

where $\hat{\mathbf{X}}$ is the ICA estimate of $\mathbf{X}$. Note that due to the scaling and inversion indeterminacy problem of ICA, both $\pm$ each row of $\mathbf{X}$ must be considered. The scaling problem is addressed by multiplying by σ_y and adding μ_y. The row with the highest correlation with the original noise-free signal is chosen as the best estimate, $z(t)$, of noise-free signal $x(t)$.

6.4.3 Comparison of NNR and ICA

The performance of NNR and ICA was compared using a synthetic ECG signal generated by ECGSYN. Both techniques were used to remove the distortions arising from a stochastic noise source. The noise was assumed to result from additive measurement errors represented by a normal distribution with zero mean. Signal to noise ratios of $\gamma = 10, 5, 2.5$ were considered. The effect of IND additive measurement errors with $\gamma = 10$ on the ECG signal is shown in Figure 6.1.

The NNR technique produced optimal results for a delay of $d = 1$. For a signal to noise ratio of $\gamma = 10$, NNR was first applied to a coarse range of values of

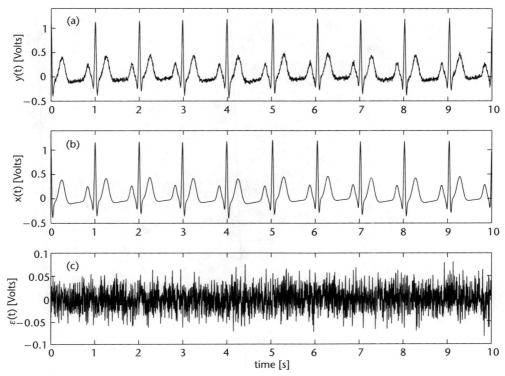

Figure 6.1   ECG signal generated by ECGSYN using additive IND measurement errors with a signal-to-noise ratio of $\gamma = 10$: (a) synthetic ECG signal with additive measurement noise, $y(t)$; (b) noise-free synthetic ECG signal, $x(t)$; and (c) measurement errors $\epsilon(t)$.

m and r in order to illustrate how the performance of the technique varied with these two parameters. This gave an optimal noise reduction factor of $\chi = 2.09$ for $m = 16$ and $r = 0.08$ (Figure 6.2). A closer examination of the dependence of χ on m was obtained by taking a cross-section of the surface shown in Figure 6.2 at $r = 0.08$ where m was sampled at all integer values between 1 and 120. As shown in Figure 6.3(a) there is a maximum noise reduction factor of $\chi = 2.2171$ at $m = 20$. The various time series and the error involved in the noise reduction process are illustrated in Figure 6.4. This shows that while the cleaned signal, $z(t)$, [Figure 6.4(c)] closely resembles the original noise-free signal, $x(t)$, [Figure 6.4(b)], there still remains considerable structure in the error, $z(t) - x(t)$, [Figure 6.4(d)]. This structure is particularly evident and appears larger around the QRS complex. As pointed out by Schreiber and Kaplan [2], the NNR technique attempts to minimize the resulting RMS error and does not directly aim to recover other key characteristics of the ECG that may be of more clinical relevance to the physician. Despite this, NNR does recover the peaks and troughs that define the morphology of the ECG. Both the P waves and T waves are clearly visible in Figure 6.4(c) and their positions and magnitudes remain faithful to that of the original noise free ECG shown in Figure 6.4(b).

The NNR technique gave optimal results for neighborhoods of different sizes depending on the signal to noise ratio: (1) $r = 0.08$ for $\gamma = 10$, (2) $r = 0.175$ for $\gamma = 5$, and (3) $r = 0.4$ for $\gamma = 2.5$. Figure 6.3 shows both the noise reduction

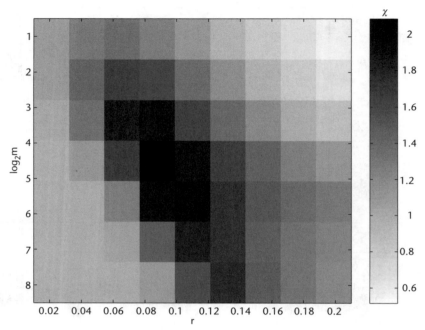

Figure 6.2 Noise reduction factor, χ, for different values of the reconstruction dimension, m, and neighborhood size, r, using NNR applied to data with a signal-to-noise ratio of $\gamma = 10$.

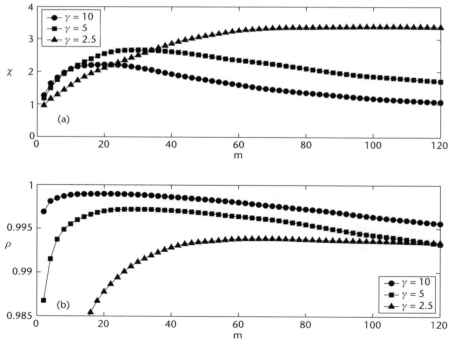

Figure 6.3 Variation in (a) noise reduction factor, χ, and (b) correlation, ρ, with reconstruction dimension, m, for NNR applied to data with signal to noise ratios of $\gamma = 10$ (•), $\gamma = 5$ (■), and $\gamma = 2.5$ (▲), having neighborhood sizes of $r = 0.08, 0.175, 0.4$, respectively.

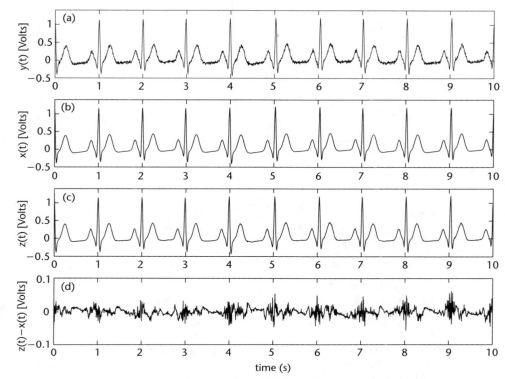

Figure 6.4 Illustration of NNR: (a) original noisy ECG signal, $y(t)$; (b) underlying noise-free ECG, $x(t)$; (c) noise-reduced ECG signal, $z(t)$; and (d) remaining error, $z(t)-x(t)$. The signal-to-noise ratio was $\gamma = 10$ and the NNR used parameters $m = 20$, $d = 1$, and $r = 0.08$.

factor, χ, and the correlation, ρ, as a function of the reconstruction dimension, m, for signals having $\gamma = 10, 5, 2.5$. For $\gamma = 10$, maxima occur at $\chi = 2.2171$ and $\rho = 0.9990$, both with $m = 20$. For the intermediate signal to noise ratio, $\gamma = 5$, maxima occur at $\chi = 2.6605$ and $\rho = 0.9972$ with $m = 20$. In the case of $\gamma = 2.5$, the noise reduction factor has a maximum, $\chi = 3.3996$ at $m = 100$, whereas the correlation, $\rho = 0.9939$, has a maximum at $m = 68$.

ICA gave best results for all signal to noise ratios for a delay of $d = 1$. As may be seen from Figure 6.5, optimizing the noise reduction factor, χ, or the correlation, ρ, gave maxima at different values of m. For $\gamma = 10$, the maxima were $\chi = 26.7265$ at $m = 7$ and $\rho = 0.9980$ at $m = 9$. For the intermediate signal to noise ratio, $\gamma = 5$, the maxima are $\chi = 18.9325$ at $m = 7$ and $\rho = 0.9942$ at $m = 9$. Finally for $\gamma = 2.5$, the maxima are $\chi = 10.8842$ at $m = 8$ and $\rho = 0.9845$ at $m = 11$. A demonstration of the effect of optimizing the ICA algorithm over either χ or ρ is illustrated in Figure 6.6. While both the χ-optimized cleaned signal [Figure 6.6(b)] and the ρ-optimized cleaned signal [Figure 6.6(d)] are similar to the original noise-free signal [Figure 6.6(a)], an inspection of their respective errors, [Figure 6.6(c)] and [Figure 6.6(e)], emphasizes their differences. The χ-optimized outperforms the ρ-optimized in recovering the R peaks.

A summary of the results obtained using both the NNR and ICA techniques are presented in Table 6.1. These results demonstrate that NNR performs better in terms of providing a cleaned signal which is maximally correlated with the original

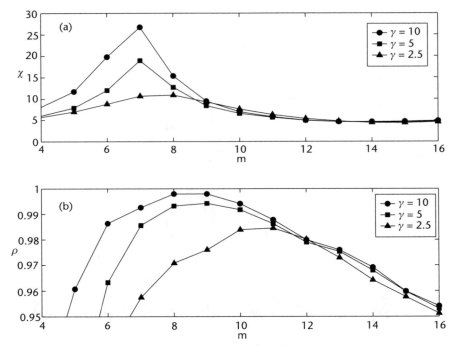

Figure 6.5 Variation in (a) noise reduction factor, χ, and (b) correlation, ρ, for ICA with reconstruction dimension, m, and delay, $d = 1$. The signal-to-noise ratios are $\gamma = 10$ (•), $\gamma = 5$ (■), and $\gamma = 2.5$ (▲).

Table 6.1 Noise Reduction Performance in Terms of Noise Reduction Factor, χ, and Correlation, ρ, for Both NNR and ICA for Three Signal-to-Noise Ratios, $\gamma = 10, 5, 2.5$

Method	Measure	$\gamma = 10$	$\gamma = 5$	$\gamma = 2.5$
NNR	χ	2.2171	2.6605	3.3996
ICA	χ	26.7265	18.9325	10.8842
NNR	ρ	0.9990	0.9972	0.9939
ICA	ρ	0.9980	0.9942	0.9845

noise-free signal, whereas ICA performs better in terms of yielding a cleaned signal which is closer to the original noise-free signal, as measured by an RMS metric.

The decision between seeking an optimal χ or ρ depends on the actual application of the ECG signal. If the morphology of the ECG is of importance and the various waves (P, QRS, T) are to be detected, then perhaps a large value of ρ is of greater relevance. In contrast, if the ECG is to be used to derive RR intervals for generating an RR tachogram, then the location in time of the R peaks are required. In this latter case, the noise reduction factor, χ, is preferable since it penalizes heavily for large squared deviations and therefore will favor more accurate recovery of extrema such as the R peak.

6.5 Model-Based Filtering

The majority of the filtering techniques presented so far involve little or no assumptions about the nature of either the underlying dynamics that generated the signal or the noise that masks it. These techniques generally proceed by attempting to

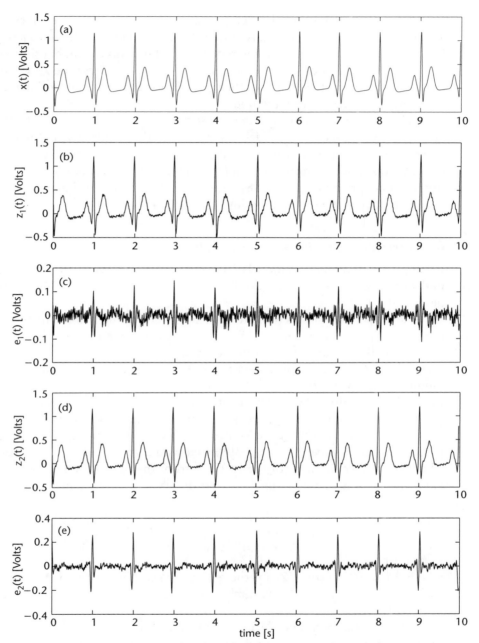

Figure 6.6 Demonstration of ICA noise reduction for $\gamma = 10$: (a) original noise-free ECG signal, $x(t)$; (b) χ-optimized noise-reduced signal, $z_1(t)$, with $m = 7$; (c) error, $e_1(t) = z_1(t) - x(t)$; (d) ρ-optimized noise-reduced signal, $z_2(t)$, with $m = 8$; and (e) error, $e_2(t) = z_2(t) - x(t)$.

separate the signal and noise using the statistics of the data and often rely on a set of assumed heuristics; there is no explicit modeling of any of the underlying sources. If, however, a known model of the signal (or noise) can be built into the filtering scheme, then it is likely that a more effective filter can be constructed.

The simplest model-based filtering is based upon the concept of Wiener filtering, presented in Section 3.1. An extension of this approach is to use a more realistic model for the dynamics of the ECG signal that can track changes over time. The advantage of such an approach is that once a model has been fitted to a segment of ECG, not only can it produce a filtered version of the waveform, but the parameters can also be used to derive wave onsets and offsets, compress the ECG, or classify beats. Furthermore, the quality of the fit can be used to obtain a confidence measure with respect to the filtering methods.

Existing techniques for filtering and segmenting ECGs are limited by the lack of an explicit patient-specific model to help isolate the required signal from contaminants. Only a vague knowledge of the frequency band of interest and almost no information concerning the morphology of an ECG are generally used. Previously proposed adaptive filters [57, 58] require another reference signal or some ad hoc generic model of the signal as an input.

6.5.1 Nonlinear Model Parameter Estimation

By employing a dynamical model of a realistic ECG, known as ECGSYN (described in detail in Section 4.3.2), a tailor-made approach for filtering ECG signals is now described.

The model parameters that are fit basically constitute a nondynamic version of the model described in [6, 59] and add an extra parameter for each asymmetric wave (only the T wave in the example given here). Each symmetrical feature of the ECG (P, Q, R, and S) is described by three parameters incorporating a Gaussian (amplitude a_i, width b_i) and the phase $\theta_i = 2\pi/t_i$ (or relative position with respect to the R peak). Since the T wave is often asymmetric, it is described by the sum of two Gaussians (and hence requires six parameters) and is denoted by a superscripted $-$ or $+$ to indicate that they are located at values of θ (or t) slightly to either side of the peak of the T wave (the original θ_T that would be used for a symmetric model). The vertical displacement of the ECG, z, from the isoelectric line (at an assumed value of $z = 0$) is then described by an ordinary differential equation,

$$\dot{z}(a_i, b_i, \theta_i) = -\sum_{i \in \{P, Q, R, S, T^-, T^+\}} a_i \Delta\theta_i \exp\left(\frac{-\Delta\theta_i^2}{2b_i^2}\right) \qquad (6.25)$$

where $\Delta\theta_i = (\theta - \theta_i)mod(2\pi)$ is the relative phase. Numerical integration of (6.25) using an appropriate set of parameter values, a_i, b_i, and θ_i, leads to the familiar ECG waveform.

One efficient method of fitting the ECG model described above to an observed segment of the signal $s(t)$ is to minimize the squared error between $s(t)$ and $z(t)$. This can be achieved using an 18-dimensional nonlinear gradient descent in the parameter space [60]. Such a procedure has been implemented using two different libraries, the Gnu Scientific Libraries (GSL) in C, and in Matlab using the function *lsqnonlin.m*.

To minimize the search space for fitting the parameters, (a_i, b_i, and θ_i), a simple peak-detection and time-aligned averaging technique is performed to form an average beat morphology using at least the first 60 beats centred on their R peaks. The template window length is unimportant, as long as it contains all the $PQRST$ features and does not extend into the next beat. This method, including outlier

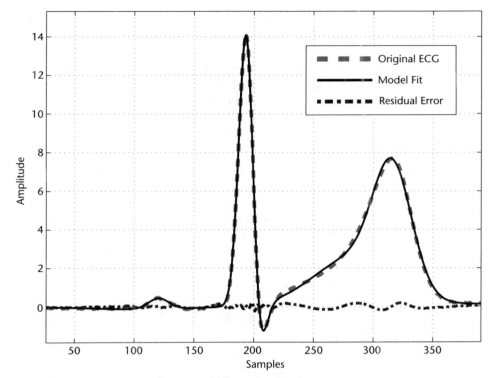

Figure 6.7 Original ECG, nonlinear model fit, and residual error.

rejection, is detailed in [61]. T^- and T^+ are initialized ± 40 ms either side of θ_T. By measuring the heights, widths, and positions of each peak (or trough), good initial estimates of the model parameters can be made. Figure 6.7 illustrates an example of a template ECG, the resulting model fit, and the residual error.

Note that it is important that the salient features that one might wish to fit (the P wave and QRS segment in the case of the ECG) are sampled at a high enough frequency to allow them to contribute sufficiently to the optimization. In empirical tests it was found that when $F_s < 450$ Hz, upsampling is required (using an appropriate antialiasing filter). With $F_s < 450$ Hz there are often fewer than 30 sample points in the QRS complex and this can lead to some unrealistic fits that still fulfill the optimization criteria.

One obvious application of this model-fitting procedure is the segmentation of ECG signals and feature location. The model parameters explicitly describe the location, height, and width of each point (θ_i, a_i, and b_i) in the ECG waveform, in terms of a well-known mathematical object, a Gaussian. Therefore, the feature locations and parameters derived from these (such as the P, Q, and T onset and hence the PR and QT interval) are easily extracted. Onsets and offsets are conventionally difficult to locate in the ECG, but using a Gaussian descriptor, it is trivial to locate these points as two or three standard deviations of b_i from the θ_i in question. Similarly, for ECG features that do not explicitly involve the P, Q, R, S, or T points (such as the ST segment), the filtering aspect of this method can be applied.

Furthermore, the error in the fitting procedure can be used to provide a confidence measure for the estimates of any parameters extracted from the ECG signal.

A related application domain for this model-based approach is (lossy) compression with a rate of $(F_s/3k : 1)$ per beat, where $k = n + 2m$ is the number of features or turning points used to fit the heartbeat morphology (with n symmetric and m asymmetric turning points). For a low F_s (≈ 128 Hz), this translates into a compression ratio greater than 7:1 at a heart rate of 60 bpm. However, for high sampling rates ($F_s = 1,024$) this can lead to compression rates of almost 60:1.

Although classification of each beat in terms of the values of a_i, b_i, and θ_i is another obvious application for this model, it is still unclear if the clustering of the parameters is sufficiently tight, given the sympathovagal and heart-rate induced changes typically observed in an ECG. It may be necessary to normalize for heart-rate dependent morphology changes at least. This could be achieved by utilizing the heart rate modulated compression factor α, which was introduced in [59]. However, clustering for beat typing is dependent on population morphology averages for a *specific* lead configuration. Not only would different configurations lead to different clusters in the 18-dimensional parameter space, but small differences in the exact lead placement relative to the heart would cause an offset in the cluster. A method for determining just how far from the standard position the recording is, and a transformation to project back onto the correct position would be required. One possibility could be to use a procedure designed by Moody and Mark [62] for their ECG classifier *Aristotle*. In this approach, the beat clusters are defined in a space resulting from a Karhunen-Loève (KL) decomposition and therefore an estimate of the difference between the classified KL-space and the observed KL-space is made. Classification is then made after transforming from the observation to classification space in which the training was performed. By measuring the distance between the fitted parameters and pretrained clusters in the 18-dimensional parameter space, classification is possible. It should be noted that, as with all classifiers, if an artifact closely resembles a known beat, a good fit to the known beat will obviously arise. For this reason, setting tolerances on the acceptable error magnitude may be crucial and testing on a set of labeled databases is required.

By fitting (6.25) to small segments of the ECG around each QRS-detection fiducial point, an idealistic (zero-noise) representation of each beat's morphology may be derived. This leads to a method for filtering and segmenting the ECG and therefore accurately extracting clinical parameters even with a relatively high degree of noise in the signal. It should be noted that since the model is a compact representation of oscillatory signals with few turning points compared to the sampling frequency and it therefore has a bandpass filtering effect leading to a lossy transformation of the data into a set of integrable Gaussians distributed over time. This approach could therefore be used on any band-limited waveform. Moreover, the error in each fit can provide beat-by-beat confidence levels for any parameters extracted from the ECG and each fit can run in real time (0.1 second per beat on a 3-GHz P4 processor).

The real test of the filtering properties is not the residual error, but how distorted the clinical parameters of the ECG are in each fit. In Section 3.1, an analysis of the sensitivity of clinical parameters to the color of additive noise and the SNR is given together with an independent method for calculating the noise color and SNR. An online estimate of the error in each derived fit can therefore be made. By titrating colored noise into real ECGs, it has been shown that errors in clinical parameters derived from the model-fit method presented here are clinically insignificant in the presence of high amounts of colored noise. However, clinical features that include low-amplitude features such as the P wave and the ST level are more sensitive to noise power and color. Future research will concentrate on methods to constrain the fit for particular applications where performance is substandard.

An advantage of this method is that it leads to a high degree of compression and may allow classification in the same manner as in the use of KL basis functions (see Chapter 9). Although the KL basis functions offer a similar degree of compression to the Gaussian-based method, the latter approach has the distinct advantage of having a direct clinical interpretation of the basis functions in terms of feature location, width, and amplitude. Using a Gaussian representation, onsets and offsets of waves are easily located in terms of the number of standard deviations of the Gaussian away from the peak of the wave.

6.5.2 State Space Model-Based Filtering

The extended Kalman filter (EKF) is an extension of the traditional Kalman filter that can be applied to a nonlinear model [63, 64]. In the EKF, the full nonlinear model is employed to evolve the states over time while the Kalman filter gain and the covariance matrix are calculated from the linearized equations of motion. Recently, Sameni et al. [65] used an EKF to filter noisy ECG signals using the realistic artificial ECG model, ECGSYN described earlier in Section 2.2. The equations of motion were first transformed into polar coordinates:

$$\dot{r} = r(1 - r)$$
$$\dot{\theta} = \omega \qquad\qquad (6.26)$$
$$\dot{z} = -\sum_i a_i \Delta\theta_i \exp\left(-\frac{\Delta\theta_i^2}{2b_i^2}\right) - (z - z_0)$$

Using this representation, the phase, θ, is given as an explicit state variable and r is no longer a function of any of the other parameters and can be discarded. Using a time step of size δt, the two-dimensional equations of motion of the system, with discrete time evolution denoted by n, may be written as

$$\theta(n + 1) = \theta(n) + \omega\delta t$$
$$z(n + 1) = z(n) - \sum_i \delta t a_i \Delta\theta_i \exp\left(-\frac{\Delta\theta_i^2}{2b_i^2}\right) + \eta\delta t \qquad (6.27)$$

where $\Delta\theta_i = (\theta - \theta_i)mod(2\pi)$ and η is a random additive noise. Note that η replaces the previous baseline wander term and describes all the additive sources of process noise.

In order to employ the EKF, the nonlinear equations of motion must first be linearized. Following [65], one approach is to consider θ and z as the underlying state variables and the model parameters, $a_i, b_i, \theta_i, \omega, \eta$ as process noises. Putting all these together gives a process noise vector,

$$\mathbf{w}_n = [a_P, \ldots, a_T, b_P, \ldots, b_T, \theta_P, \ldots, \theta_T, \omega, \eta]^\dagger \qquad (6.28)$$

with covariance matrix $\mathcal{Q}_n = E\{\mathbf{w}_n\mathbf{w}_n{}^\dagger\}$ where the subscript $\dagger$ denotes the transpose.

The phase of the observations ψ_n, and the noisy ECG measurements s_n are related to the state vector by

$$\begin{bmatrix} \psi_n \\ s_n \end{bmatrix} = \begin{bmatrix} 1 & 0 \\ 0 & 1 \end{bmatrix} \begin{bmatrix} \theta_n \\ z_n \end{bmatrix} + \begin{bmatrix} v_n^{(1)} \\ v_n^{(2)} \end{bmatrix} \tag{6.29}$$

where $\boldsymbol{\nu}_n = [v_n^{(1)}, v_n^{(2)}]^\dagger$ is the vector of measurement noises with covariance matrix $\mathbf{R}_n = E\{\boldsymbol{\nu}_n\boldsymbol{\nu}_n{}^\dagger\}$.

The variance of the observation noise in (6.29) represents the degree of uncertainty associated with a single observation. When $\mathbf{R}_n$ is high, the EKF tends to ignore the observation and rely on the underlying model dynamics for its output. When $\mathbf{R}_n$ is low, the EKF's gain adapts to incorporate the current observations. Since the 17 noise parameters in (6.28) are assumed to be independent, $\mathcal{Q}_k$ and $\mathbf{R}_n$ are diagonal. The process noise η is a measure of the accuracy of the model, and is assumed to be a zero-mean Gaussian noise process.

Using this EKF formulation, Sameni et al. [65] successfully filtered a series of ECG signals with additive Gaussian noise. An example of this can be seen in Figure 6.8. Future developments of this model are therefore very promising, since the

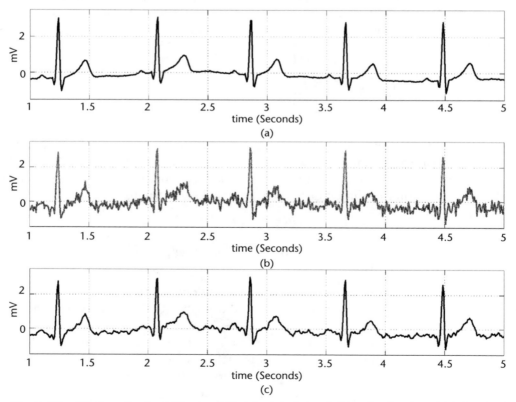

Figure 6.8 Filtering of noisy ECG using EKF: (a) original signal; (b) noisy signal; and (c) denoised signal.

combination of a realistic model and a robust tracking mechanism make the concept of online signal tracking in real time feasible. A combination of an initialization with the nonlinear gradient descent method from Section 6.5.1 to determine initial model parameters and noise estimates, together with subsequent online tracking, may lead to an optimal ECG filter (for normal morphologies). Furthermore, the ability to relate the parameters of the model to each PQRST morphology may lead to fast and accurate online segmentation procedures.

6.6 Conclusion

This chapter has provided a summary of the mathematics involved in reconstructing a state space using a recorded signal so as to apply techniques based on the theory of nonlinear dynamics. Within this framework, nonlinear statistics such as Lyapunov exponents, correlation dimension, and entropy were described. The importance of comparing results with simple benchmarks, carrying out statistical tests and using confidence intervals when conveying estimates was also discussed. This is important when employing nonlinear dynamics as the basis of any new biomedical diagnostic tool.

An artificial electrocardiogram signal, ECGSYN, with controlled temporal and spectral characteristics was employed to illustrate and compare the noise reduction performance of two techniques, nonlinear noise reduction and independent components analysis. Stochastic noise was used to create data sets with different signal-to-noise ratios. The accuracy of the two techniques for removing noise from the ECG signals was compared as a function of signal-to-noise ratio. The quality of the noise removal was evaluated by two techniques: (1) a noise reduction factor and (2) a measure of the correlation between the cleaned signal and the original noise-free signal. NNR was found to give better results when measured by correlation. In contrast, ICA outperformed NNR when compared using the noise reduction factor. These results suggest that NNR is superior at recovering the morphology of the ECG and is less likely to distort the shape of the P, QRS, and T waves, whereas ICA is better at recovering specific points on the ECG such as the R peak, which is necessary for obtaining RR intervals.

Two model-based filtering approaches were also introduced. These methods use the dynamical model underlying ECGSYN to provide constraints on the filtered signal. A nonlinear least squares parameter estimation procedure was used to estimate all 18 parameters required to specify the morphology of the ECG waveform. In addition, an approach using the extended Kalman filter applied to a discrete two-dimensional adaptation of ECGSYN in polar coordinates was also employed to filter an ECG signal.

The correct choice of filtering technique depends not only on the characteristics of the noise and signal in the time and frequency domains, but also on the application. It is important to test a candidate filtering technique over a range of possible signals (with a range of signal to noise ratios and different noise processes) to determine the filter's effect on the clinical parameter or attribute of interest.

References

[1]   Papoulis, P., *Probability, Random Variables, and Stochastic Processes*, 3rd ed., New York: McGraw-Hill, 1991.

[2]   Schreiber, T., and D. T. Kaplan, "Nonlinear Noise Reduction for Electrocardiograms," *Chaos*, Vol. 6, No. 1, 1996, pp. 87–92.

[3]   Cardoso, J. F., "Multidimensional Independent Component Analysis," *Proc. ICASSP'98*, Seattle, WA, 1998.

[4]   Clifford, G. D., and P. E. McSharry, "Method to Filter ECGs and Evaluate Clinical Parameter Distortion Using Realistic ECG Model Parameter Fitting," *Computers in Cardiology*, September 2005.

[5]   Moody, G. B., and R. G. Mark, "Physiobank: Physiologic Signal Archives for Biomedical Research," MIT, Cambridge, MA, http://www.physionet.org/physiobank, updated June 2006.

[6]   McSharry, P. E., et al., "A Dynamical Model for Generating Synthetic Electrocardiogram Signals," *IEEE Trans. Biomed. Eng.*, Vol. 50, No. 3, 2003, pp. 289–294.

[7]   Kantz, H., and T. Schreiber, *Nonlinear Time Series Analysis*, Cambridge, U.K.: Cambridge University Press, 1997.

[8]   McSharry, P. E., and L. A. Smith, "Better Nonlinear Models from Noisy Data: Attractors with Maximum Likelihood," *Phys. Rev. Lett.*, Vol. 83, No. 21, 1999, pp. 4285–4288.

[9]   McSharry, P. E., and L. A. Smith, "Consistent Nonlinear Dynamics: Identifying Model Inadequacy," *Physica D*, Vol. 192, 2004, pp. 1–22.

[10] Packard, N., et al., "Geometry from a Time Series," *Phys. Rev. Lett.*, Vol. 45, 1980, pp. 712–716.

[11] Takens, F., "Detecting Strange Attractors in Fluid Turbulence," in D. Rand and L. S. Young, (eds.), *Dynamical Systems and Turbulence*, New York: Springer-Verlag, Vol. 898, 1981, p. 366.

[12] Broomhead, D. S., and G. P. King, "Extracting Qualitative Dynamics from Experimental Data," *Physica D*, Vol. 20, 1986, pp. 217–236.

[13] Sauer, T., J. A. Yorke, and M. Casdagli, "Embedology," *J. Stats. Phys.*, Vol. 65, 1991, pp. 579–616.

[14] Fraser, A. M., and H. L. Swinney, "Independent Coordinates for Strange Attractors from Mutual Information," *Phys. Rev. A*, Vol. 33, 1986, pp. 1134–1140.

[15] Rosenstein, M. T., J. J. Collins, and C. J. De Luca, "Reconstruction Expansion as a Geometry-Based Framework for Choosing Proper Time Delays," *Physica D*, Vol. 73, 1994, pp. 82–98.

[16] Kennel, M. B., R. Brown, and H. D. I. Abarbanel, "Determining Embedding Dimension for the Phase-Space Reconstruction Using a Geometrical Construction," *Phys. Rev. A*, Vol. 45, No. 6, 1992, pp. 3403–3411.

[17] Strang, G., *Linear Algebra and Its Applications*, San Diego, CA: Harcourt College Publishers, 1988.

[18] Lorenz, E. N., "A Study of the Predictability of a 28-Variable Atmospheric Model," *Tellus*, Vol. 17, 1965, pp. 321–333.

[19] Abarbanel, H. D. I., R. Brown, and M. B. Kennel, "Local Lyapunov Exponents Computed from Observed Data," *Journal of Nonlinear Science*, Vol. 2, No. 3, 1992, pp. 343–365.

[20] Glass, L., and M. Mackey, *From Clocks to Chaos: The Rhythms of Life*, Princeton, NJ: Princeton University Press, 1988.

[21] Wolf, A., et al., "Determining Lyapunov Exponents from a Time Series," *Physica D*, Vol. 16, 1985, pp. 285–317.

[22] Sano, M., and Y. Sawada, "Measurement of the Lyapunov Spectrum from a Chaotic Time Series," *Phys. Rev. Lett.*, Vol. 55, 1985, pp. 1082–1085.

[23]   Eckmann, J. P., et al., "Liapunov Exponents from Time Series," *Phys. Rev. A*, Vol. 34, No. 6, 1986, pp. 4971–4979.

[24]   Brown, R., P. Bryant, and H. D. I. Abarbanel, "Computing the Lyapunov Spectrum of a Dynamical System from an Observed Time Series," *Phys. Rev. A*, Vol. 43, No. 6, 1991, pp. 2787–2806.

[25]   McSharry, P. E., "The Danger of Wishing for Chaos," *Nonlinear Dynamics, Psychology, and Life Sciences*, Vol. 9, No. 4, October 2005, pp. 375–398.

[26]   Rosenstein, M.T., J. J. Collins, and C.J. De Luca, "A Practical Method for Calculating Largest Lyapunov Exponents from Small Data Sets," *Physica D*, Vol. 65, 1994, pp. 117–134.

[27]   Kantz, H., "Quantifying the Closeness of Fractal Measures," *Phys. Rev. E*, Vol. 49, No. 6, 1994, pp. 5091–5097.

[28]   Hegger, R., H. Kantz, and T. Schreiber, "TISEAN: Nonlinear Time Analysis Software," Max-Planck-Institut für Physik Komplexer System, http://www.mpipks-dresden.mpg.de/~tisean/, December 2005.

[29]   Renyi, A., *Probability Theory*, Amsterdam: North Holland, 1971.

[30]   Ott, E., T. Sauer, and J. A. Yorke, *Coping with Chaos*, New York: John Wiley & Sons, 1994.

[31]   Grassberger, P., and I. Procaccia, "Characterization of Strange Attractors," *Phys. Rev. Lett.*, Vol. 50, 1983, pp. 346–349

[32]   Theiler, J. T., "Spurious Dimension from Correlation Algorithms Applied to Limited Time-Series Data," *Phys. Rev. A*, Vol. 34, 1986, pp. 2427–2432.

[33]   Provenzale, A., et al., "Distinguishing Between Low-Dimensional Dynamics and Randomness in Measured Time Series," *Physica D*, Vol. 58, 1992, pp. 31–49.

[34]   Takens, F., "On the Numerical Determination of the Dimension of an Attractor," in B. L. J. Braaksma, H. W. Broer, and F. Takens, (eds.), *Dynamical Systems and Bifurcations*, Volume 1125 of *Lecture Notes in Mathematics*, Berlin, Germany: Springer, 1985, pp. 99–106.

[35]   Guerrero, A., and L. A. Smith, "Towards Coherent Estimation of Correlation Dimension," *Phys. Lett. A*, Vol. 318, 2003, pp. 373–379.

[36]   Ruelle, D., "Deterministic Chaos: The Science and the Fiction," *Proc. R. Soc. Lond. A.*, Vol. 427, 1990, pp. 241–248.

[37]   Smith, L. A., "Intrinsic Limits on Dimension Calculations," *Phys. Lett. A*, Vol. 133, 1988, pp. 283–288.

[38]   Eckmann, J. P., and D. Ruelle, "Ergodic Theory of Chaos and Strange Attractors," *Rev. Mod. Phys.*, Vol. 57, 1985, pp. 617–656.

[39]   Pincus, S. M., "Approximate Entropy as a Measure of System Complexity," *Proc. Natl. Acad. Sci.*, Vol. 88, 1991, pp. 2297–2301.

[40]   Richman, J. S., and J. R. Moorman, "Physiological Time Series Analysis Using Approximate Entropy and Sample Entropy," *Am. J. Physiol.*, Vol. 278, No. 6, 2000, pp. H2039–H2049.

[41]   McSharry, P. E., L. A. Smith, and L. Tarassenko, "Prediction of Epileptic Seizures: Are Nonlinear Methods Relevant?" *Nature Medicine*, Vol. 9, No. 3, 2003, pp. 241–242.

[42]   McSharry, P. E., L. A Smith, and L. Tarassenko, "Comparison of Predictability of Epileptic Seizures by a Linear and a Nonlinear Method," *IEEE Trans. Biomed. Eng.*, Vol. 50, No. 5, 2003, pp. 628–633.

[43]   Isliker, H., and J. Kurths, "A Test for Stationarity: Finding Parts in Time Series APT for Correlation Dimension Estimates," *Int. J. Bifurcation Chaos*, Vol. 3, 1993, pp. 1573–1579.

[44]   Braun, C., et al., "Demonstration of Nonlinear Components in Heart Rate Variability of Healthy Persons," *Am. J. Physiol. Heart Circ. Physiol.*, Vol. 275, 1998, pp. H1577–H1584.

[45] Lehnertz, K., and C. E. Elger, "Can Epileptic Seizures Be Predicted? Evidence from Non-linear Time Series Analysis of Brain Electrical Activity," *Phys. Rev. Lett.*, Vol. 80, No. 22, 1998, pp. 5019–5022.

[46] Iasemidis, L. D., et al., "Adaptive Epileptic Seizure Prediction System," *IEEE Trans. Biomed. Eng.*, Vol. 50, No. 5, 2003, pp. 616–627.

[47] Pincus, S. M., and A. L. Goldberger, "Physiological Time-Series Analysis: What Does Regularity Quantify?" *Am. J. Physio. Heart Circ. Physiol.*, Vol. 266, 1994, pp. H1643–H1656.

[48] Costa, M., A. L. Goldberger, and C. K. Peng, "Multiscale Entropy Analysis of Complex Physiologic Time Series," *Phys. Rev. Lett.*, Vol. 89, No. 6, 2002, p. 068102.

[49] Voss, A., et al., "The Application of Methods of Non-Linear Dynamics for the Improved and Predictive Recognition of Patients Threatened by Sudden Cardiac Death," *Cardiovascular Research*, Vol. 31, No. 3, 1996, pp. 419–433.

[50] Wessel, N., et al., "Short-Term Forecasting of Life-Threatening Cardiac Arrhythmias Based on Symolic Dynamics and Finite-Time Growth Rates," *Phys. Rev. E*, Vol. 61, 2000, pp. 733–739.

[51] Chatfield, C., *The Analysis of Time Series*, 4th ed., London, U.K.: Chapman and Hall, 1989.

[52] Kobayashi, M., and T. Musha, "1/f Fluctuation of Heartbeat Period," *IEEE Trans. Biomed. Eng.*, Vol. 29, 1982, p. 456.

[53] Goldberger, A. L., et al., "Fractal Dynamics in Physiology: Alterations with Disease and Ageing," *Proc. Natl. Acad. Sci.*, Vol. 99, 2002, pp. 2466–2472.

[54] Schreiber, T., and P. Grassberger, "A Simple Noise Reduction Method for Real Data," *Phys. Lett. A.*, Vol. 160, 1991, p. 411.

[55] Hegger, R., H. Kantz, and T. Schreiber, "Practical Implementation of Nonlinear Time Series Methods: The Tisean Package," *Chaos*, Vol. 9, No. 2, 1999, pp. 413–435.

[56] James, C. J., and D. Lowe, "Extracting Multisource Brain Activity from a Single Electromagnetic Channel," *Artificial Intelligence in Medicine*, Vol. 28, No. 1, 2003, pp. 89–104.

[57] "Filtering for Removal of Artifacts," Chapter 3 in R. M. Rangayyan, *Biomedical Signal Analysis: A Case-Study Approach*, New York: IEEE Press, 2002, pp. 137–176.

[58] Barros, A., A. Mansour, and N. Ohnishi, "Removing Artifacts from ECG Signals Using Independent Components Analysis," *Neurocomputing*, Vol. 22, No. 1–3, 1998, pp. 173–186.

[59] Clifford, G. D., and P. E. McSharry, "A Realistic Coupled Nonlinear Artificial ECG, BP and Respiratory Signal Generator for Assessing Noise Performance of Biomedical Signal Processing Algorithms," *Proc. of Intl. Symp. on Fluctuations and Noise 2004*, Vol. 5467-34, May 2004, pp. 290–301.

[60] More, J. J., "The Levenberg-Marquardt Algorithm: Implementation and Theory," *Lecture Notes in Mathematics*, Vol. 630, 1978, pp. 105–116.

[61] Clifford, G., L. Tarassenko, and N. Townsend, "Fusing Conventional ECG QRS Detection Algorithms with an Auto-Associative Neural Network for the Detection of Ectopic Beats," *Proc. of 5th International Conference on Signal Processing, 16th IFIP WorldComputer Congress*, Vol. III, 2000, pp. 1623–1628.

[62] Moody, G. B., and R. G. Mark, "QRS Morphology Representation and Noise Estimation Using the Karhunen-Loève Transform," *Computers in Cardiology*, Vol. 16, 1989, pp. 269–272.

[63] Kay, S. M., *Fundamentals of Statistical Signal Processing: Estimation Theory*, Englewood Cliffs, NJ: Prentice-Hall, 1993.

[64] Grewal, M. S., and A. P. Andrews, *Kalman Filtering: Theory and Practice Using Matlab*, 2nd ed., New York: John Wiley & Sons, 2001.

[65] Sameni, R., et al., "Filtering Noisy ECG Signals Using the Extended Kalman Filter Based on a Modified Dynamic ECG Model," *Computers in Cardiology*, Vol. 32, 2005, pp. 1017–1020.

CHAPTER 7

The Pathophysiology Guided Assessment of T-Wave Alternans

Sanjiv M. Narayan

7.1   Introduction

Sudden cardiac arrest (SCA) causes more than 400,000 deaths per year in the United States alone, largely from ventricular arrhythmias [1]. T-wave alternans (TWA) is a promising ECG index that indicates risk for SCA from beat-to-beat alternations in the shape, amplitude, or timing of T waves. Decades of research now link TWA clinically with inducible [2–4] and spontaneous [5–7] ventricular arrhythmias, and with basic mechanisms leading to their initiation [8, 9].

This bench-to-bedside foundation makes TWA a very plausible predictor of susceptibility to SCA, and motivates the need to define optimal conditions for its detection that are tailored to its pathophysiology. TWA has become a prominent risk stratification method over the past 5 to 10 years, with recent approval for reimbursement, and the suggestion by the U.S. Centers for Medicare and Medicaid Services (CMS) for the inclusion of TWA analysis in the proposed national registry for SCA management [10].

7.2   Phenomenology of T-Wave Alternans

Detecting TWA from the surface ECG exemplifies a bench-to-bedside bioengineering solution to tissue-level and clinical observations. *T-wave alternans* refers to alternation of the ECG ST segment [3, 11], T wave and U wave [12], and has also been termed *repolarization alternans* [4, 13]. Visible TWA was first reported in the early 1900s by Hering [14] and Sir Thomas Lewis [15] and was linked with ventricular arrhythmias. Building upon reports of increasingly subtle TWA on visual inspection [16], contemporary methods use signal processing to extract microvolt-level T-wave fluctuations that are invisible to the unaided eye [17].

7.3   Pathophysiology of T-Wave Alternans

TWA is felt to reflect a combination of spatial [18] and temporal [8] dispersion of repolarization (Figure 7.1), both of which may be mechanistically implicated in the initiation of ventricular tachyarrhythmias [19, 20].

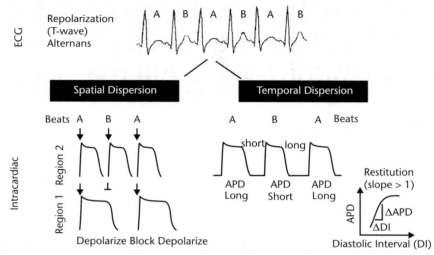

Figure 7.1 Mechanisms underlying TWA. Left: spatial dispersion of repolarization. Compared to region 2, region 1 has longer APD and depolarizes every other cycle (beats 1 and 3). Right: temporal dispersion of repolarization. APD alternates between cycles, either from alternans of cytosolic calcium (not shown), or steep APD restitution. APD restitution (inset) is the relationship of APD to diastolic interval (DI), the interval separating the current action potential from the prior one. If restitution is steep (slope >1), DI shortening abruptly shortens APD, which abruptly lengthens the next DI and APD, leading to APD alternans.

Spatial variations in action potential duration (APD) or shape [18], or conduction velocity [21, 22], may prevent depolarization in myocytes still repolarizing from their last cycle (Figure 7.1, left, Region 1) and cause 2:1 behavior (alternans) [8]. Moreover, this mechanism may allow unidirectional block at sites of delayed repolarization and facilitate reentrant arrhythmias.

Temporal dispersion of repolarization (alternans of APD; Figure 7.1, right) may also contribute to TWA [18]. APD alternans has been reported in human atria [23] and ventricles [24, 25] and in animal ventricles [8], and under certain conditions, it has been shown to lead to conduction block and arrhythmias [8, 9].

APD alternans is facilitated by *steep restitution*. APD restitution expresses the relationship between the APD of one beat and the diastolic interval (DI) separating its upstroke from the preceding action potential [24] the bottom right of Figure 7.1, bottom right). If APD restitution is steep (maximum slope >1), slight shortening of the DI from a premature beat can significantly shorten APD, which lengthens the following DI and APD and so on, leading to alternans [26]. By analogy, steep restitution in conduction velocity [21, 22] can also cause APD alternans. Under certain conditions [27], both may lead to wavefront fractionation and ventricular fibrillation (VF) [20] or, in the presence of structural barriers, ventricular tachycardia (VT) [9]. At an ionic level, alternans of cytosolic calcium [28, 29] may underlie APD alternans [30] and link electrical with mechanical alternans [29, 31].

TWA may be perturbed by abrupt changes in heart rate [24] or ectopic beats [8, 24]. Depending on the timing of the perturbation relative to the phase of alternation, alternans magnitude may be enhanced or attenuated and its phase (ABA versus BAB; see Figure 7.2, top) maintained or reversed [8, 31, 32]. Under critical

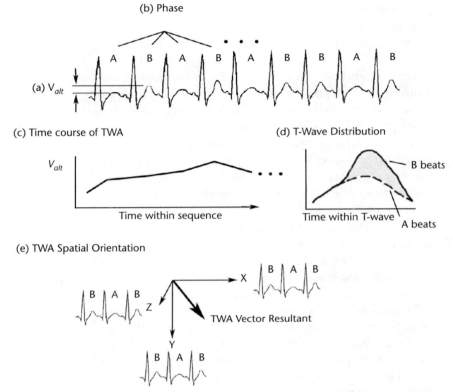

Figure 7.2   Measurable indices of TWA include: (a) TWA magnitude; (b) TWA phase, which shows reversal (ABBA) towards the right of the image; (c) distribution of TWA within the T wave, that is, towards the distal T wave in this example; (d) time-course of TWA that clearly varies over several beats; and (e) TWA spatial orientation.

conditions, ischemia [33] or extrasystoles [31, 33] may reverse the phase of alternans in only one region, causing alternans that is out of phase between tissue regions (discordant alternans), leading to unidirectional block and ventricular fibrillation [8].

7.4   Measurable Indices of ECG T-Wave Alternans

Several measurable indices of TWA have demonstrated clinical relevance, as shown in Figure 7.2. First, TWA magnitude is reported by most techniques and is the pivotal index [Figure 7.2(a)]. In animal studies, higher TWA magnitudes reflect greater repolarization dispersion [9, 34] and increasing likelihood for ventricular arrhythmias [11, 35]. Clinically, TWA magnitude above a threshold (typically 1.9 mCV measured spectrally) is generally felt to reflect increased arrhythmia susceptibility [3, 6]. However, this author [36] and others [37] have recently shown that the susceptibility to SCA may rise with increasing TWA magnitude.

The second TWA index is its phase [Figure 7.2(b)]. This may be detected by methods to quantify sign-change between successive pairs of beats, or spectrally as a sudden fall in TWA magnitude that often coincides with an ectopic beat or other perturbation [38]. As discussed in Section 7.3, regional phase reversal of tissue alternans (discordant alternans) heralds imminent ventricular arrhythmias in animal models [8, 9]. Clinically, we recently reported that critically timed ectopic beats may reverse ECG TWA phase, and that this reflects heightened arrhythmic susceptibility. In 59 patients with left ventricular systolic dysfunction from prior myocardial infarction, TWA phase reversal was most likely in patients with sustained arrhythmias at electrophysiologic study (EPS) and with increasingly premature ectopic beats [13]. On a long-term 3-year follow-up, logistic regression analysis showed that TWA phase reversal better predicted SCA than elevated TWA magnitude, sustained arrhythmias at EPS, or left ventricular ejection fraction [36]. TWA phase reversal may therefore help in SCA risk stratification, particularly if measured at times of elevated arrhythmic risk such as during exercise, psychological stress, or early in the morning.

Third, the temporal evolution of TWA has been reported using time- and frequency-domain methods [Figure 7.2(c)]. At present, it is unclear whether specific patterns of TWA evolution, such as a sudden rise or fall, oscillations, or constant magnitude, add clinical utility to the de facto approach of dichotomizing TWA magnitude at some threshold. Certainly, transient peak TWA following abrupt changes in heart rate [4] is less predictive of clinical events than steady-state values attained after the perturbation. Because of restitution, APD alternans is a normal response to abrupt rate changes in control individuals *as well as* patients at risk for SCA [24]. However, at-risk patients may exhibit a steeper slope and different shape of restitution (Figure 7.1, bottom right) [39], leading to prolonged TWA decay after transient rises in heart rate compared to controls. Moreover, we recently reported prolonged TWA decay leading to hysteresis, such that TWA magnitude remains elevated after heart rate deceleration from a faster rate, in at-risk patients but not controls [4]. This has been supported by animal studies [40]. Finally, TWA magnitude may oscillate at any given rate, yet the magnitude of oscillations may be inversely related to TWA magnitude [41]. Theoretically, therefore, the analysis of TWA could be considerably refined by exploiting specific temporal patterns of TWA at steady-state and during perturbations.

Fourth, the distribution of TWA within the T wave also indicates arrhythmic risk [Figure 7.2(d)], and is most naturally detected with time-domain techniques [42]. Theoretically, the terminal portions of the T wave reflect the trailing edge of repolarization, which, if spatially heterogeneous, may enable unidirectional conduction block and facilitate reentrant ventricular arrhythmias. Indeed, pro-arrhythmic interventions in animals cause APD alternans predominantly in phase III, corresponding with the T-wave terminus. In preliminary clinical studies, we reported that pro-arrhythmic heart rate acceleration [42] and premature ectopic beats caused TWA to distribute later within the T wave [13], particularly in individuals with inducible arrhythmias at EPS [13]. One potentially promising line of investigation would be to develop methods to quantify whether TWA distribution within the T wave indicates specific pathophysiology and different outcomes. For example, data suggests that acute ischemia in dogs causes "early" TWA (in the ST segment) [11], which may portend a different prognosis than "late" TWA (distal T wave) in patients with substrates for VT or VF but without active ischemia [42].

Fifth, the spatial distribution of TWA has recently been studied by analyzing TWA vector between ECG leads [Figure 7.2(e)]. Pathophysiologically, alternans of tissue APD is distributed close to scar in animal hearts [9], and ECG TWA during clinical coronary angioplasty overlies regional ischemic zones [43]. We recently reported that ECG TWA magnitude, in patients with prior MI but without active ischemia, is greatest in leads overlying regions of structural disease defined by echocardiographic wall motion abnormalities [44]. In addition, Verrier et al. reported that TWA in lateral ECG leads best predicted spontaneous clinical arrhythmias in patients with predominantly lateral prior MI [45], while Klingenheben et al. reported that patients with nonischemic cardiomyopathy at the greatest risk for events were those in whom TWA was present in the largest number of ECG leads [37]. Methods to more precisely define the regionality of TWA may improve the specificity of TWA for predicting SCA risk.

7.5 Measurement Techniques

Several techniques have been applied to measure TWA from the surface ECG. Each technique poses theoretical advantages and disadvantages, and the optimal method for extracting TWA may depend upon the clinical scenario. TWA may be measured during controlled sustained heart rate accelerations, during exercise testing, controlled heart rate acceleration during pacing, uncontrolled or transient exercise-related heart rate acceleration in ambulatory recordings, and from discontinuities in rhythm such as ectopic beats. At the present time, few studies have compared methods for their precision to detect TWA between these conditions, or the predictive value of their TWA estimates for meaningful clinical endpoints.

Martinez and Olmos recently developed a comprehensive "unified framework" for computing TWA from the surface ECG [17], in which they classified TWA detection into preprocessing, data reduction, and analysis stages. This section focuses upon the strengths and limitations of TWA analysis methods, broadly comprising short-term Fourier transform (STFT)–based methods (highpass linear filtering), sign-change counting, and nonlinear filtering methods.

7.5.1 Requirements for the Digitized ECG Signal

The amplitude resolution of digitized ECG signals must be sufficient to measure TWA as small as 2 mcV (the spectrally defined threshold [38]). Assuming a dynamic range of 5 mV, 12-bit and 16-bit analog-to-digital converters provide theoretical resolutions of 1.2 mcV and < 0.1 mcV, respectively, lower than competing noise sources. The ECG sampling frequency of most applications, ranging from 250 to 1,000 Hz, is also sufficient for TWA analysis. Some time-domain analyses for TWA found essentially identical results for sampling frequencies of 250 to 1,000 Hz, with only slight deterioration with 100-Hz sampling [46]. For ambulatory ECG detection, frequency-modulated (FM) and digital recorders show minimal distortion for heart rates between 60 to 200 bpm, and a bandpass response between 0.05 and 50 Hz has been recommended [47].

7.5.2   Short-Term Fourier Transform–Based Methods

These methods compute TWA from the normalized row-wise STFT of the beat-to-beat series of coefficients at the alternans frequency (0.5 cycle per beat). Examples include the spectral [2, 32, 48] and complex demodulation [11] methods. The spectral method is the basis for the widely applied commercial CH2000 and HeartWave systems (Cambridge Heart Inc., Bedford, Massachusetts) and, correspondingly, has been best validated (under narrowly defined conditions).

In general, STFT methods compute the detection statistics using a preprocessed and data reduced matrix of coefficients $\mathbf{Y} = \{y_i(p)\}$ as $\mathbf{Y}_w[p, l]$:

$$\mathbf{Y}_w[p, l] = \sum_{i=-\infty}^{\infty} y_i[p]w[i - l](-1)^i \tag{7.1}$$

where $\mathbf{Y}_w[p, l]$ is the alternans statistic of length l, $\mathbf{Y} = \{y_i(p)\}$ is the reduced coefficient matrix derived from the ECG beat series, and $w(i)$ is the L-beat analysis window of beat-to-beat periodicity (periodogram). This is equivalent to highpass linear filtering [17].

For the spectral method, the TWA statistic z can be determined by applying STFT to voltage time series [2, 32] or derived indices such as coefficients of the Karhunen-Loève (KL) transform (see Chapter 9 in this book) [49]. The statistic is the 0.5 cycle per beat bin of the periodogram, proportion to the squared modulus of the STFT:

$$z_l[p] = \frac{1}{L} |Y_w[p, l]|^2 \tag{7.2}$$

For complex demodulation (CD), the TWA statistic z can also be determined from voltage time series [11] or coefficients of the KL transform (KLCD) [17] as the magnitude of the lowpass filtered demodulated 0.5 cycle/beat component:

$$z_l[p] = |y_l[p] * h_{hpf}[l]| \tag{7.3}$$

where $h_{hpf}[k] = h_{lpf}[k] \cdot (-1)^k$ is a highpass filter resulting from frequency translation of the lowpass filter. Complex demodulation results in a new detection statistic for each beat.

The spectral method is illustrated in Figure 7.3. In Figure 7.3(a), ECGs are preprocessed prior to TWA analysis. Beats are first aligned because TWA may be localized to parts of the T wave, and therefore lost if temporal jitter occurs between beats. We and others have shown that beat alignment for TWA analysis is best accomplished by QRS cross-correlation [17, 32]. Beat series are then filtered and baseline corrected to provide an isoelectric baseline (typically the T-P segment) [17]. Successive beats are then segmented to identify the analysis window, typically encompassing the entire JT interval (shown) [32]. Unfortunately, the literature is rather vague on how the T-wave terminus is defined, largely because several methods exist for this purpose yet none has emerged as the gold standard [50]. After preprocessing, alternans at each time point [arrow in Figure 7.3(a)] is manifest as oscillations over successive T waves. Fourier analysis then results in a large amplitude spectral peak at 0.5 cycle/beat (labeled ΣT). Time-dependent analysis separates

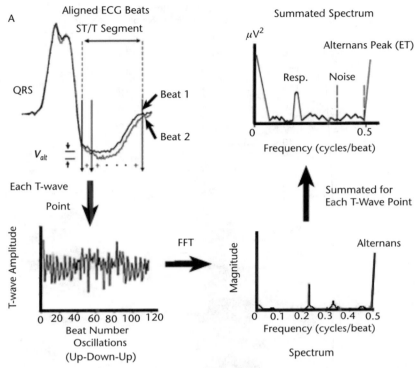

Figure 7.3 (a) Spectral computation of TWA. In aligned ECG beats, alternans at each time point within the T wave (vertical arrows) results in down-up-down oscillations. Fourier transform yields a spectrum in which alternans is the peak at 0.5 cycle/beat peak (ΣT). In the final spectrum (summated for all time points), ΣT is related to spectral noise to compute V_{alt} and k-score [see part (b)]. (b) Positive TWA (from HeartWave system, Cambridge Heart, Inc.) shows (i) $V_{alt} \leq 1.9$ mcV in two precordial or one vector lead (here $V_{alt} \approx 46$ mcV in V3-V6) with (ii) k-score ≥ 3 (gray shading) for > 1 minute (here ≈ 5 minutes), at (iii) onset rate < 110 bpm (here 103 bpm), with (iv) $< 10\%$ bad beats and < 2 mcV noise, without (v) artifactual alternans. Black horizontal bars indicate periods when conditions for positive TWA are met.

time points within the T wave (illustrated), and allows TWA to be temporally lo-calized within the T wave. However, to provide a summary statistic, spectra are summated across the T wave (detection window L). Finally, TWA is quantified by its (1) voltage of alternation (V_{alt}) equal to (ΣT-spectral noise)/T wave duration; and (2) k-score (TWA ratio), equal to ΣT/noise standard deviation.

7.5.3 Interpretation of Spectral TWA Test Results

Since TWA is rate related, it is measured at accelerated rates during exercise or pacing, while maintaining heart rate below the threshold at which false-positive TWA may occur in normal individuals from restitution (traditionally, 111 bpm) [42, 51]. Criteria for interpreting TWA from the most widely used commercial system (Cambridge Heart, Bedford, Massachusetts) are well described [38]. *Positive TWA*, illustrated in Figure 7.3(b), is defined as TWA sustained for > 1 minute with amplitude (V_{alt}) ≥ 1.9 mcV in any vector ECG lead (X, Y, Z) or two adjacent precordial leads, with k-score > 3.0 and onset heart rate < 110 bpm, meeting noise

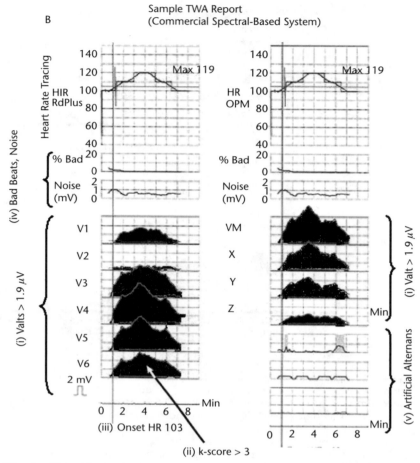

Figure 7.3   (continued.)

criteria of < 10 % ectopic beats, < 2 mcV spectral noise, and *absence* of artifactual alternans from respiratory rate or RR interval alternans.

Notably, the optimal TWA magnitude cutpoint for predicting sudden death risk has been questioned. We authors [4] and others [52] have used custom and commercial spectral methods, respectively, to show that higher cutpoints of 2.6 and 3 mcV better predict clinical endpoints. A recent study confirmed that TWA magnitude ≥ 2.9 mcV was more specific for predicting sudden death [53].

7.5.4   Controversies of the STFT Approach

The major strength of STFT is its sensitivity for stationary signals. Indeed, in simulations [32] and subsequent clinical reports during pacing [3, 13, 36, 54], spectral methods can detect TWA of amplitudes ≤ 1 mcV [3, 13, 36, 54]. It has yet to be demonstrated whether alternative techniques including time-domain nonlinear filtering (described below) achieve this sensitivity on stationary signals.

However, STFT also has several drawbacks. Primarily, the linear filtering involved in STFT methods is sensitive to nonstationarity of the TWA signal within the detection window. The detection window (L) ranges in duration from 30 [55] to 128 [3] beats, which represents 16 to 77 seconds at rates of 100 to 110 bpm. Nonstationarity over this time course may reflect changing physiology at constant heart rate, rate-related fluctuations, or noise. Although it has been suggested that alternative STFT methods such as complex demodulation may better track transient TWA [55], all linear filtering methods have theoretical limitations for nonstationary signals, and differences in their ability to track TWA "transients" can be minimized as demonstrated by Martinez and Olmos [17].

By extension, STFT methods are also adversely influenced by rhythm discontinuities, including abrupt changes in heart rate, or atrial or ventricular ectopy. Not only can ectopy reverse the true phase of TWA, as described in Sections 7.3 and 7.4, but an ectopic beat may technically degrade the STFT computation of TWA, depending upon its phase relationship, by introducing an impulse to the power spectrum as we have shown [32]. Beat deletion and substitution are typically used to eliminate ectopy [56], yet the best strategy requires knowledge of the phase TWA relative to the position of the ectopic beat. Deletion is preferred if the ectopic reverses TWA phase, while substitution is preferred if phase is maintained [32]. We have demonstrated both types of behavior following premature beats in patients at risk for ventricular arrhythmias [13] (see Figure 7.4), in whom phase reversal indicated a worse outcome [36].

7.5.5 Sign-Change Counting Methods

These methods use a strategy that counts sign-changes or zero-crossings from beat to beat. The Rayleigh test [57] measures the regularity of the phase reversal pattern to

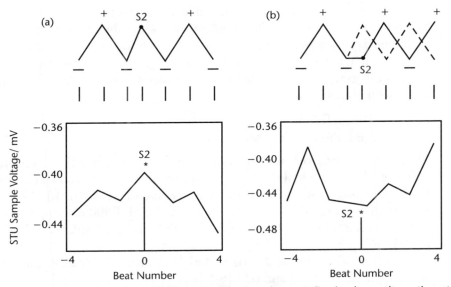

Figure 7.4 Extrasystoles (S_2) and TWA phase. The top shows stylized voltage alternation at one time point within the STU segment. Extrasystoles (S_2) may leave phase (a) unaltered or (b) reversed in the subsequent oscillation. Inset panels depict each case using actual mid-STU data for three beats preceding and following S_2.

determine if a beat series is better explained by a random distribution or a periodic pattern, with sign reversal indicating alternate-beat periodicity.

The ECG or derived parameter series is analyzed using a sliding window of beats. In each data block, the number of deviations relative to alternation (i.e., $y_i > y_{i+1}$; $y_{i+1} < y_{i+2}$ ..., or the opposite phase) is measured, and a significance is assigned that reflects the probability of obtaining such a pattern from a random variable. A given significance value is associated with a fixed threshold λ_Z in the number of beats following one of the patterns. Therefore, TWA is deemed present if

$$Z_l = \frac{1}{2} \left(L + | \sum_{i=l-L+1}^{l} sign(\Delta y_i)(-1)^i | \right) \geq \lambda_Z \qquad (7.4)$$

where $\{\Delta y_i\} = \{y_i - y_{i-1}\}$. STFT can now be applied to the sign of the series, although the nonlinearity of sign analysis limits the effect of outliers in the detection statistic, unlike true STFT-based methods. Notably, however, amplitude information is lost in sign analysis [17].

The correlation method modifies sign-counting in that the alternans correlation index y_i [in (7.4)] is usually near one, since ST-T complexes are similar to the template. When TWA is present, the correlation alternates between values > 1 and < 1. Burattini et al. [58] used consecutive sign changes in the series to decide the presence of TWA.

The Rayleigh test and the correlation method are highly dependent upon the length of the analysis window. In their favor, short counting windows (as in the correlation method) facilitate the detection of brief TWA episodes, enabling TWA to be detected from short ECG recordings, or its time course to be defined sequentially within ambulatory ECGs. However, short windows increase the likelihood that random sequences will falsely be assigned as alternans [17]. Moreover, the reliability of both methods requires the signal to have a dominant frequency (the alternans component) and a high signal-to-noise ratio. Unfortunately, high amplitude components such as respiration, baseline wander, or slow physiological variations can seriously degrade their performance. These observations may limit the applicability of these methods [17].

7.5.6 Nonlinear Filtering Methods

Nonlinear filtering methods have recently been described that likely improve the ability to detect TWA in the presence of nonstationarities and ectopic beats. These methods include the modified moving average method (MMA) [59], which was recently incorporated commercially into the CASE-8000 electrophysiology system (GE Marquette, Inc., Milwaukee, Wisconsin), and the Laplacian Likelihood Ratio (LLR) [60].

Verrier et al. [45] have described the MMA method that creates parallel averages for designated even (A) and odd (B) "beats" (JT segments), defined as

$$\text{ECG beat A}_n (i) = \text{ECG beat}_{2n}(i) \qquad (7.5)$$
$$\text{ECG beat B}_n (i) = \text{ECG beat}_{2n-1}(i) \qquad (7.6)$$

where $i = 1, \ldots$ is the number of samples per beat, $n = 1, 2, \ldots N/2$, and N is the total number of beats in the data segment.

Modified moving average complexes A and B are initialized with the first even and odd ECG beats in the sequence, respectively. The next modified moving average computed beat is formed using the present MMA beat and the next ECG beat. If the next ECG beat has larger amplitude than the present MMA computed beat, the next MMA computed beat value is made higher than the present MMA computed beat value; the reverse occurs if the next ECG beat is smaller than the present MMA computed beat. Increment and decrements are nonlinear, to minimize the effects of outlying beats. As described by the authors [45]:

$$\text{Computed beat } A_n(i) = \text{Computed beat } A_{n-1}(i) + \Delta_A \tag{7.7}$$

where

$$
\begin{aligned}
\Delta_A &= -32 & \text{if} && \eta \leq -32 \\
\Delta_A &= -\eta & \text{if} && -1 \geq \eta > -32 \\
\Delta_A &= -1 & \text{if} && 0 > \eta > -1 \\
\Delta_A &= 0 & \text{if} && \eta = 0 \\
\Delta_A &= 1 & \text{if} && 1 \geq \eta > 0 \\
\Delta_A &= \eta & \text{if} && 32 \geq \eta > 1 \\
\Delta_A &= 32 & \text{if} && \eta > 32
\end{aligned}
$$

where $\eta = [\text{ECG beat } A_{n-1}(i) - \text{Computed beat } A_{n-1}(i) / 8]$ and n is the beat number within series A. The parallel computation is performed for beats of type B. TWA is then computed as

$$\text{TWA} = \max_{i=J\,point}^{i=Twaveend} |Beat\,B_n(i) - Beat\,A_n(i)| \tag{7.8}$$

When beat differences are small, the method behaves linearly. However, nonlinearity limits the effect of abrupt changes, artifacts, and anomalous beats. In a recent modeling study, MMA effectively determined TWA in signals with premature beats, while spectral methods attenuated TWA at points of discontinuity reflecting detection artifact and TWA phase reversal (Figure 8 in [17]).

Other nonlinear methods are based upon the median beat, including the LLR [60], in which the individual statistic is proportional to the absolute sum of values of the demodulated series lying between 0 and the maximum likelihood estimator of the alternating amplitude (described in detail in [17]). This computation takes the form of an STFT with a rectangular window, where some extreme elements are discarded. Again, the nonlinearity inherent in this approach makes it robust in the face of outliers and noise from discontinuities and ectopic beats.

7.6   Tailoring Analysis of TWA to Its Pathophysiology

Despite the many approaches described to compute TWA [17], few studies have compared methods for the same clinical dataset, or validated them against clinical endpoints. Moreover, TWA varies with physiologic conditions, yet it is presently unclear which measurement approach—or physiologic milieu—optimally enables TWA to stratify SCA risk. This is true whether measuring TWA magnitude, TWA phase, the distribution of TWA within the T wave, or the temporal evolution and spatial distribution of TWA.

7.6.1   Current Approaches for Eliciting TWA

Early studies showed that TWA magnitude rises with heart rate in all individuals, but at a lower threshold in patients at presumed risk for SCA than controls [4, 42, 54]. As a result, TWA is typically measured during acceleration while maintaining heart rates < 111 bpm [38] to minimize false-positive TWA from normal rate-responsiveness. It remains unclear whether the onset heart rate criterion < 111 bpm is optimal [38], since studies suggest that TWA at lower onset heart rates (90 to 100 bpm) better predicts SCA [53, 61]. Studies that define receiver operating characteristics of onset heart rate of TWA for predicting SCA would be helpful.

An exciting recent development has been to detect TWA from ambulatory ECG recordings [45] at times of maximum spontaneous heart rate (likely reflecting exercise or psychological stress), times of maximum ST segment shift (possibly reflecting clinical or subclinical coronary ischemia), and early morning (8 a.m.), when the SCA risk is elevated [45]. The investigators showed that TWA identified patients at risk for SCA when analyzed at maximum spontaneous heart rate and at 8 a.m., but not during maximum ST segment shift. Intuitively, ambulatory recordings provide a satisfying, continuous, and convenient approach for analyzing TWA, and should perhaps become the predominant scenario for detecting nonstationary TWA.

7.6.2   Steady-State Rhythms and Stationary TWA

This is the simplest clinical scenario that may apply during cardiac pacing, and it lends itself readily to spectral analysis. The seminal clinical reports of Smith et al. [2] and Rosenbaum et al. [3] determined TWA in this fashion, while subsequent reports confirmed that elevated TWA magnitude correlates with induced [2, 3, 13, 54] and spontaneous [3, 36] ventricular arrhythmias, particularly if measured at heart rates of 100 to 120 bpm [4].

Moreover, we demonstrated that TWA magnitude exhibits rate-hysteresis [4], and is therefore higher after deceleration to a particular rate than on acceleration to it. This has been supported by mechanistic studies [40] and suggests that TWA magnitude should be measured during constant heart rate.

Rosenbaum et al. compared spectral with complex demodulation methods for steady-state TWA and showed that TWA better predicted the results of EPS when measured spectrally [62]. In recent preliminary studies, we compared TWA using spectral and MMA methods in 224 ECG lead recordings during constant pacing at a rate of 110 bpm in 43 patients with mean LVEF $32 \pm 9\%$ and coronary disease. In ECGs where TWA was measurable by both methods ($n = 102$), MMA amplified TWA magnitude (V_{alt}) by approximately three-fold compared to the spectral method in all axes (for example, 13.4 ± 10.0 versus 4.3 ± 7.5 mcV in the x-axis, $p = 0.004$; see Figure 7.5). This supports recent reports by Verrier et al. [45] that TWA

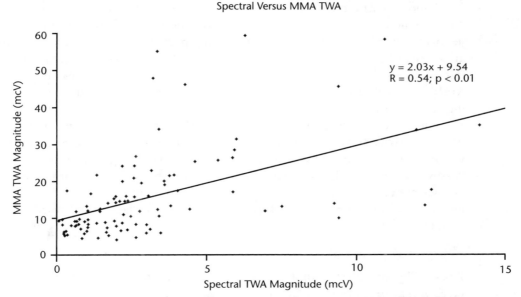

Figure 7.5   Relationship of MMA and spectral TWA in the same ECGs. Both metrics were correlated but MMA increased TWA amplitude compared to spectral TWA ($n = 102$ ECGs). Not shown are $n = 122$ ECGs where MMA yielded alternans yet TWA was spectrally undetectable.

magnitude from MMA ($V_{alt} \approx 45$ mcV) is larger than from spectral methods (typical V_{alt} 2 to 6 mcV [13, 42, 54]).

However, MMA in our studies also yielded TWA in an additional 122 ECG leads in which TWA was undetectable using the spectral method. We are performing long-term follow-up on these patients to determine whether signal amplification by MMA reduces the specificity of TWA for clinical events compared to spectral TWA.

Importantly, it is now recognized that TWA amplitude oscillates even during constant rate pacing, by up to 10 mcV in a quasi-periodic fashion with a period of approximately 2 to 3 minutes [41]. Thus, TWA is likely nonstationary under all measurement conditions. This has significant implications for the selection and development of optimal measurement techniques.

7.6.3   Fluctuating Heart Rates and Nonstationary TWA

Analysis of time-varying TWA poses several problems. First, STFT methods are less robust than nonlinear filtering (and sign change) approaches for nonstationary TWA.

Second, it is unclear at which time period TWA should be analyzed. Certainly, TWA should be measured below heart rates likely to cause false-positive TWA in normal controls (< 111 bpm [38]). However, it is unclear what rates of acceleration or deceleration are acceptable. We have shown that TWA magnitude rises faster, and decays slower, in patients at risk for SCA than controls [4], and these dynamics may have prognostic significance. Indeed, measuring TWA during deceleration may lead to elevated TWA estimates due to hysteresis [4, 40], yet current practice measures TWA at any time without abrupt heart rate change, and largely disregard differences between acceleration and deceleration [38].

A more central question is: Under what (patho)physiologic conditions is TWA most predictive for SCA? TWA has traditionally been measured during controlled heart rate changes, at exercise test, or during pacing [16], yet spontaneous fluctuations may better reflect autonomic and hemodynamic conditions leading to the initiation of spontaneous arrhythmias and SCA. TWA was recently computed using MMA in fluctuating conditions during ambulatory ECGs, and successfully predicted SCA risk [45].

Therefore, the robustness of MMA and other nonlinear filtering approaches to nonstationarity and ectopic beats may make them more suitable than spectral analysis for detecting nonstationarities in TWA, such as during heart rate acceleration versus deceleration, during fluctuations in heart rate, and from ambulatory ECGs. Studies are required to validate these methods comparatively against intracardiac indices of repolarization dispersion, and to compare their utility for clinical risk prediction.

7.6.4   Rhythm Discontinuities, Nonstationary TWA, and TWA Phase

Despite the extensive literature describing action potential duration restitution and alternans [24, 39] following ectopic beats and abrupt heart rate changes, it remains unclear how TWA and its clinical utility are affected by discontinuities in rhythm.

Ectopic beats (during native rhythm) or extrastimuli (during pacing) alter the pathophysiology of TWA (Sections 7.3 and 7.4) and therefore influence the choice of detection method. Detection of TWA phase is best achieved by sign-change methods, although signal degradation of the spectral method (and other linear filters) from ectopy allows them to infer TWA phase reversal. For example, phase reversal is inferred if spectral TWA extinguishes at the time of an ectopic beat then reappears rapidly, although traditional interpretation paradigms ignore this effect [38]. Paradoxically, the very fact that nonlinear filtering methods including MMA are largely unaffected by ectopy [17] makes them less attractive for detecting phase reversal.

Abrupt changes in heart rate affect action potential duration [24, 39] and, in a sense, the first beat at a new rate represents a premature or postmature beat and would be expected to influence TWA because of restitution. Increased TWA magnitude from rate acceleration, and hysteretic decay in magnitude with deceleration, are described above and are best detected using nonlinear rather than linear methods [17]. However, the time-evolution of TWA can be detected spectrally using overlapping windows [4, 41], retaining the frequency resolution of the original segment length to which STFT is applied [17]. However, overlap introduces correlation between consecutive TWA estimates that must be factored into interpretation schemes.

One special case of abrupt heart rate changes is the recent description of *resonant pacing*, where shortened cycle lengths are applied repeatedly to augment TWA magnitude [63]. In preliminary studies, 11 patients with congestive heart failure were paced using repeating 4-beat patterns of cycle lengths 535, 555, 555, 555 ms (resonant pacing, mean 550 ms) versus conventional pacing at cycle length 550 ms. TWA magnitude (V_{alt}) correlated closely for resonant and conventional pacing, yet resonant pacing significantly increased TWA magnitude and SNR. In this small series, resonant pacing also eliminated TWA phase reversals induced by premature beats. The investigators speculated that enhanced TWA magnitude may result from perturbed calcium cycling by the premature cycle. Further studies are required to determine whether resonant pacing may better augment TWA using an interposed long cycle (e.g., 565, 545, 545, 545 ms), to exploit TWA hysteresis [4, 40], whether resonant pacing reduces TWA phase reversal in a larger series, whether such TWA should be measured nonlinearly rather than spectrally, and how resulting TWA augmentation affects its clinical utility for predicting SCA.

7.7 Conclusions

Of the numerous methods described to measure TWA, few have been applied to clinical datasets or validated against clinically meaningful endpoints. During steady-state, many methods may be similarly effective for computing TWA. However, TWA analysis should increasingly focus upon its nonstationarities. Not only does TWA fluctuate even at constant heart rate, but TWA may better predict SCA if transients are measured during extreme physiologic milieu or at times of ectopic beats. Non-linear methods to compute TWA are likely more robust to nonstationarity than linear (spectral) methods, and should therefore be developed and validated further.

Notably, the optimal detection of TWA may require combinations of approaches for differing scenarios. Thus, linear approaches may be appropriate at relatively stable heart rate, nonlinear filtering may be preferred during rate fluctuations in ambulatory ECGs, and sign-change methods may be required to examine TWA phase. Future work should also investigate the value of examining TWA in preferred spatial orientations, and how this may change with varying conditions. By tailoring TWA measurement to a more detailed understanding of its pathophysiology, the role of TWA is likely to broaden towards providing a more continuous assessment of arrhythmic susceptibility.

Acknowledgments

This chapter was supported, in part, by a grant to Dr. Narayan from the National Heart, Lung, and Blood Institute (HL 70529).

References

[1] Zheng, Z.-J., et al., "Sudden Cardiac Death in the United States, 1989 to 1998," *Circulation*, Vol. 104, 2001, pp. 2158–2163.

[2] Smith, J. M., et al., "Electrical Alternans and Cardiac Electrical Instability," *Circulation*, Vol. 77, 1988a, pp. 110–121.

[3] Rosenbaum, D. S., et al., "Electrical Alternans and Vulnerability to Ventricular Arrhythmias," *N. Engl. J. Med.*, Vol. 330, 1994, pp. 235–241.

[4] Narayan, S. M., and J. M. Smith, "Exploiting Rate Hysteresis in Repolarization Alternans to Optimize the Sensitivity and Specificity for Ventricular Tachycardia," *J. Am. Coll. Cardiol.*, Vol. 35, 2000c, pp. 1485–1492.

[5] Kleinfeld, M. J., and J. J. Rozanski, "Alternans of the ST Segment in Prinzmetal's Angina," *Circulation*, Vol. 55, 1977, pp. 574–577.

[6]   Gold, M. R., et al., "A Comparison of T Wave Alternans, Signal Averaged Electrocar-diography and Programmed Ventricular Stimulation for Arrhythmia Risk Stratification," *J. Am. Coll. Cardiol.*, Vol. 36, 2000a, pp. 2247–2253.

[7]   Bloomfield, D. M., et al., "Microvolt T-Wave Alternans Distinguishes Between Patients Likely and Patients Not Likely to Benefit from Implanted Cardiac Defibrillator Therapy: A Solution to the Multicenter Automatic Defibrillator Implantation Trial (MADIT) II Conundrum," *Circulation*, Vol. 110, 2004b, pp. 1885–1889.

[8]   Pastore, J. M., et al., "Mechanism Linking T-Wave Alternans to the Genesis of Cardiac Fibrillation," *Circulation*, Vol. 99, 1999, pp. 1385–1394.

[9]   Pastore, J. M., and D. S. Rosenbaum, "Role of Structural Barriers in the Mechanism of Alternans-Induced Reentry," *Circulation Research*, Vol. 87, 2000, pp. 1157–1163.

[10]   CMS and C. f. M. a. M. Services, "Medicare Announces Its Intention to Expand Coverage of Implantable Cardioverter Defibrillators," Vol. 2005, 2005.

[11]   Nearing, B. D., et al., "Dynamic Tracking of Cardiac Vulnerability by Complex Demod-ulation of the T-Wave," *Science*, Vol. 252, 1991a, pp. 437–440.

[12]   Habbab, M. A., and N. El-Sherif, "TU Alternans, Long QTU, and Torsade de Pointes: Clinical and Experimental Observations," *Pacing & Clinical Electrophysiology*, Vol. 15, 1992, pp. 916–931.

[13]   Narayan, S. M., et al., "Demonstrating the Pro-Arrhythmic Preconditioning of Single Premature Extrastimuli Using the Magnitude, Phase and Temporal Distribution of Repo-larization Alternans," *Circulation*, Vol. 100, 1999d, pp. 1887–1893.

[14]   Hering, H., "Experimentelle Studien an Saugentieren uber das Electrocardiogram," *Z. Exper. Med.*, Vol. 7, 1909, p. 363.

[15]   Lewis, T., "Notes upon Alternation of the Heart," *Q. J. Med.*, Vol. 4, 1910, pp. 141–144.

[16]   Narayan, S. M., "T-Wave Alternans and the Susceptibility to Ventricular Arrhythmias: State of the Art Paper," *J. Am. Coll. Cardiol.*, Vol. 47, 2006a, pp. 269–281.

[17]   Martinez, J. P., and S. Olmos, "Methodological Principles of T-Wave Alternans Analysis: A Unified Framework," *IEEE Trans. Biomed. Eng.*, Vol. 52, 2005, pp. 599–613.

[18]   Chinushi, M., et al.,"Electrophysiological Basis of Arrhythmogenicity of QT/T Alternans in the Long QT Syndrome: Tridimensional Analysis of the Kinetics of Cardiac Repolar-ization," *Circulation Research*, Vol. 83, 1998a, pp. 614–628.

[19]   Smith, J. M., and R. J. Cohen, "Simple Finite-Element Model Accounts for a Wide Range of Cardiac Dysrhythmias," *Proc. Natl. Sci. USA*, Vol. 81, 1984b, pp. 233–237.

[20]   Weiss, J., et al., "Chaos and the Transition to Ventricular Fibrillation: A New Approach to Anti-Arrhythmic Drug Evaluation," *Circulation*, Vol. 99, 1999, pp. 2819–2826.

[21]   Banville, I., and R. A. Gray, "Effect of Action Potential Duration and Conduction Velocity Restitution and Their Spatial Dispersion on Alternans and the Stability of Arrhythmias," *J. Cardiovasc. Electrophysiol.*, Vol. 13, 2002, pp. 1141–1149.

[22]   Cherry, E., and F. Fenton, "Suppression of Alternans and Conduction Blocks Despite Steep APD Restitution: Electrotonic, Memory, and Conduction Velocity Restitution Effects," *Am. J. Physiol. Heart Circ. Physiol.*, Vol. 286, 2004, pp. H2332–H2341.

[23]   Narayan, S. M., et al., "Alternans of Atrial Action Potentials as a Precursor of Atrial Fibrillation," *Circulation*, Vol. 106, 2002b, pp. 1968–1973.

[24]   Franz, M. R., et al., "Cycle Length Dependence of Human Action Potential Duration in Vivo. Effects of Single Extrastimuli, Sudden Sustained Rate Acceleration and Deceleration, and Different Steady-State Frequencies," *J. Clin. Invest.*, Vol. 82, 1988a, pp. 972–979.

[25]   Narayan, S. M., et al., "Alternans in Ventricular Monophasic Action Potentials Precedes the Induction of Ventricular Arrhythmias [abstract]," *Pacing and Clinical Electrophysiol-ogy (PACE)*, Vol. 23 (4 part II), 2000f, p. 738.

[26]   Karma, A., "Spiral Breakup in Model Equations of Action Potential Propagation in Car-diac Tissue," *Phys. Rev. Lett.*, Vol. 71, 1993, pp. 1103–1106.

[27]   Franz, M., "The Electrical Restitution Curve Revisited: Steep or Flat Slope—Which Is Better?" *J. Cardiovasc. Electrophysiol.*, Vol. 14, 2003, pp. S140–S147.

[28]   Spear, J., and E. Moore, "A Comparison of Alternation in Myocardial Action Potentials and Contractility," *Am. J. Physiol.*, Vol. 220, 1971, pp. 1708–1716.

[29]   Hirayama, Y., et al., "Electrical and Mechanical Alternans in Canine Myocardium In Vivo: Dependence on Intracellular Calcium Cycling," *Circulation*, Vol. 88, 1993, pp. 2894–2902.

[30]   Pruvot, E. J., et al., "Role of Calcium Cycling Versus Restitution in the Mechanism of Repolarization Alternans," *Circ. Res.*, Vol. 94, 2004, pp. 1083–1090.

[31]   Rubenstein, D. S., and S. L. Lipsius, "Premature Beats Elicit a Phase Reversal of Mechanoelectrical Alternans in Cat Ventricular Myocytes: A Possible Mechanism for Reentrant Arrhythmias," *Circulation*, Vol. 91, 1995, pp. 201–214.

[32]   Narayan, S. M., and J. M. Smith, "Spectral Analysis of Periodic Fluctuations in ECG Repolarization," *IEEE Trans. Biomed. Eng.*, Vol. 46, 1999b, pp. 203–212.

[33]   Hashimoto, H., et al., "Effects of the Ventricular Premature Beat on the Alternation of the Repolarization Phase in Ischemic Myocardium During Acute Coronary Occlusion in Dogs," *J. Electrocardiology*, Vol. 17, 1984a, pp. 229–238.

[34]   Hashimoto, H., et al., "Alternation in Refractoriness and in Conduction Delay in the Ischemic Myocardium Associated with the Alternation in the ST-T Complex During Acute Coronary Occlusion in Anesthetized Dogs," *J. Electrocardiology*, Vol. 19, 1986, pp. 77–84.

[35]   Green, L. S., et al., "Three-Dimensional Distribution of ST-T Wave Alternans During Acute Ischemia," *J. Cardiovasc. Electrophysiol.*, Vol. 8, 1997, pp. 1413–1419.

[36]   Narayan, S. M., et al., "T-Wave Alternans Phase Following Ventricular Extrasystoles Predicts Arrhythmia-Free Survival," *Heart Rhythm*, Vol. 2, 2005a, pp. 234–241.

[37]   Klingenheben, T., et al., "Quantitative Assessment of Microvolt T-Wave Alternans in Patients with Congestive Heart Failure," *J. Cardiovasc. Electrophysiol.*, Vol. 16, 2005, pp. 620–624.

[38]   Bloomfield, D. M., et al., "Interpretation and Classification of Microvolt T-Wave Alternans Tests," *J. Cardiovasc. Electrophysiol.*, Vol. 13, 2002, pp. 502–512.

[39]   Garfinkel, A., et al., "Preventing Ventricular Fibrillation by Flattening Cardiac Restitution," *Proc. Natl. Acad. Sci. USA*, Vol. 97, 2000, pp. 6061–6066.

[40]   Walker, M. L., et al., "Hysteresis Effect Implicates Calcium Cycling as a Mechanism of Repolarization Alternans," *Circulation*, Vol. 108, 2003, pp. 2704–2709.

[41]   Kaufman, E. S., et al., "Influence of Heart Rate and Sympathetic Stimulation on Arrhythmogenic T Wave Alternans," *Am. J. Physiol. Heart Circ. Physiol.*, Vol. 279, 2000, pp. H1248–H1255.

[42]   Narayan, S. M., and J. M. Smith, "Differing Rate Dependence and Temporal Distribution of Repolarization Alternans in Patients with and Without Ventricular Tachycardia," *J. Cardiovasc. Electrophysiol.*, Vol. 10, 1999a, pp. 61–71.

[43]   Martinez, J. P., et al., "Simulation Study and Performance Evaluation of T-Wave Alternans Detectors," *Proc. 22nd Ann. Int. Conf. IEEE Engineering in Medicine and Biology Society*, Vol. CD-ROM, 2000, 2000.

[44]   Narayan, S. M., et al., "Relation of T-Wave Alternans to Regional Left Ventricular Dysfunction and Eccentric Hypertrophy Secondary to Coronary Artery Disease," *Am. J. Cardiol.*, Vol. 97, No. 6, March 15, 2006, pp. 775–780.

[45]   Verrier, R. L., et al., "Ambulatory Electrocardiogram Based Tracking of T Wave Alternans in Postmyocardial Infarction Patients to Assess Risk of Cardiac Arrest or Arrhythmic Events," *J. Cardiovasc. Electrophysiol.*, Vol. 14, 2003, pp. 705–711.

[46]   Burattini, L., et al., "Optimizing ECG Signal Sampling Frequency for T-Wave Alternans Detection," *Comput. Cardiol.*, Vol. 25, 1998, pp. 721–724.

[47]   Nearing, B. D., et al., "Frequency-Response Characteristics Required for Detection of T-Wave Alternans During Ambulatory ECG Monitoring," *Ann. Noninvasive Electrocardiol.*, Vol. 1, 1996, pp. 103–112.

[48]   Adam, D. R., et al., "Fluctuations in T-Wave Morphology and Susceptibility to Ventricular Fibrillation," *J. Electrocardiol.*, Vol. 17, 1984, pp. 209–218.

[49]   Laguna, P., et al., "Repolarization Alternans Detection Using the KL Transform and the Beatquency Spectrum," *Comput. Cardiol.*, Vol. 22, 1996, pp. 673–676.

[50]   Malik, M., "Problems of Heart Rate Correction in Assessment of Drug-Induced QT Interval Prolongation," *J. Cardiovasc. Electrophysiol.*, Vol. 12, 2001, pp. 411–420.

[51]   Kurz, R. W., et al., "Ischaemia Induced Alternans of Action Potential Duration in the Intact Heart: Dependence on Coronary Flow, Preload and Cycle Length," *Eur. H. J.*, Vol. 14, 1993, pp. 1410–1420.

[52]   Osman, A. F., et al., "Prognostic Value of Voltage Magnitude During T-Wave Alternans (TWA) Assessment with Exercise and Pacing in Patients with Ischemic Cardiomyopathy [Abstract]," *PACE*, Vol. 24, 2001, p. 530.

[53]   Tanno, K., et al., "Microvolt T-Wave Alternans as a Predictor of Ventricular Tachyarrhythmias: A Prospective Study Using Atrial Pacing," *Circulation*, Vol. 109, 2004, pp. 1854–1858.

[54]   Kavesh, N. G., et al., "Effect of Heart Rate on T-Wave Alternans," *J. Cardiovasc. Electrophysiol.*, Vol. 9, 1998, pp. 703–708.

[55]   Verrier, R. L., et al., "T-Wave Alternans Monitoring to Assess Risk for Ventricular Tachycardia and Fibrilation," in E. A. J. Moss, and S. Stern, (eds.), *Noninvasive Electrocardiology: Clinical Aspects of Holter Monitoring*, London, U.K.: Saunders, 1996, pp. 445–464.

[56]   Rosenbaum, D. S., et al., "Predicting Sudden Cardiac Death from T Wave Alternans of the Surface Electrocardiogram: Promise and Pitfalls. (Review)," *J. Cardiovasc. Electrophysiol.*, Vol. 7, 1996a, pp. 1095–1111.

[57]   Srikanth, T., et al., "Presence of T Wave Alternans in the Statistical Context — A New Approach to Low Amplitude Alternans Measurement," *Comput. Cardiol.*, Vol. 29, 2002, pp. 681–684.

[58]   Burattini, L., et al., "Correlation Method for Detection of Transient T-Wave Alternans in Digital Holter ECG Recordings," *Ann. Electrocardiol*, Vol. 4, 1999, pp. 416–426.

[59]   Nearing, B., and R. Verrier, "Tracking Cardiac Electrical Instability by Computing Interlead Heterogeneity of T-Wave Morphology," *J. Appl. Physiol.*, Vol. 95, 2003, pp. 2265–2272.

[60]   Martinez, J. P., and S. Olmos, "A Robust T-Wave Alternans Detector Based on the GLRT for Laplacian Noise Distribution," *Proc. Comput. Cardiol.*, 2002, pp. 677–680.

[61]   Kitamura, H., et al., "Onset Heart Rate of Microvolt-Level T-Wave Alternans Provides Clinical and Prognostic Value in Nonischemic Dilated Cardiomyopathy," *J. Am. Coll. Cardiol.*, Vol. 39, 2002, pp. 295–300.

[62]   Rosenbaum, D. S., et al., "How to Detect ECG T-Wave Alternans in Patients at Risk for Sudden Cardiac Death?" *J. Am. Coll. Cardiol.*, Vol. 25, 1995, p. 409A.

[63]   Bullinga, J., et al., "Resonant Pacing Improves T-Wave Alternans Testing in Patients with Dilated Cardiomyopathy," *Heart Rhythm*, Vol. I, 2004, p. S128.

CHAPTER 8

ECG-Derived Respiratory Frequency Estimation

Raquel Bailón, Leif Sörnmo, and Pablo Laguna

8.1 Introduction

The respiratory signal is usually recorded with techniques like spirometry, pneumography, or plethysmography. These techniques require the use of cumbersome devices that may interfere with natural breathing, and which are unmanageable in certain applications such as ambulatory monitoring, stress testing, and sleep studies. Nonetheless, the joint study of the respiratory and cardiac systems is of great interest in these applications and the use of methods for indirect extraction of respiratory information is particularly attractive to pursue. One example of application would be the analysis of the influence of the respiratory system in heart rate variability (HRV) during stress testing, since it has been observed that the power in the very high frequency band (from 0.4 Hz to half the mean heart rate expressed in Hz) exhibits potential value in coronary artery disease diagnosis [1], and HRV power spectrum is dependent on respiratory frequency. Another field of application would be sleep studies, since the diagnosis of apnea could be based on fewer and simpler measurements, like the ECG, rather than on the polysomnogram, which is expensive to record.

It is well known that the respiratory activity influences electrocardiographic measurements in various ways. During the respiratory cycle, chest movements and changes in the thorax impedance distribution due to filling and emptying of the lungs cause a rotation of the electrical axis of the heart which affects beat morphology. The effect of respiration-induced heart displacement on the ECG was first studied by Einthoven et al. [2] and quantified in further detail in [3, 4]. It has been experimentally shown that "electrical rotation" during the respiratory cycle is mainly caused by the motion of the electrodes relative to the heart, and that thoracic impedance variations contribute to the electrical rotation just as a second-order effect [5].

Furthermore, it is well known that respiration modulates heart rate such that it increases during inspiration and decreases during expiration [6, 7]. It has also been shown that the mechanical action of respiration results in the same kind of frequency content in the ECG spectrum as does HRV [8].

Figure 8.1 displays an ECG lead as well as the related heart rate (HR) and respiratory signals in which the ECG amplitude is modulated with a frequency similar to that of the respiratory signal. It seems that the ECG amplitude modulation is not in phase with the respiratory signal. It can also be seen that the HR and the

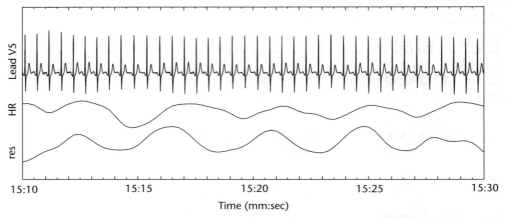

Figure 8.1 Simultaneous ECG lead V5 (top), HR (middle), and respiration (bottom) signals.

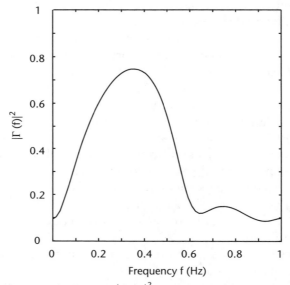

Figure 8.2 Magnitude squared coherence $|\Gamma(f)|^2$ between HR and respiratory signals of Figure 8.1. The largest value of $|\Gamma(f)|^2$ is located around 0.3 Hz.

respiratory signal fluctuate at a similar frequency. Figure 8.2 displays the magnitude squared coherence between HR and respiratory signal. The magnitude squared coherence is defined as being a measure of the correlation between two signals at a given frequency [9]. It can be seen that the largest value is located around 0.3 Hz, meaning that the signals are strongly correlated at this frequency.

Several studies have developed signal processing techniques to extract respiratory information from the ECG, so-called ECG-derived respiratory (EDR) information. Some techniques are based on respiration-induced variations in beat-to-beat morphology [5, 10–24], while others attempt to extract respiratory information from the HR [25–27].

The first EDR method based on morphologic variations dates back to 1974 when Wang and Calvert [10] proposed a model for the mechanics of the heart with respect to respired air volume of the lungs, and a technique for monitoring respiratory rate and depth using the vectorcardiogram (VCG). Later, Pinciroli et al. [11] and Moody et al. [5] proposed algorithms which exploit variations in the direction of the heart's electrical axis. Recently, the respiratory frequency was obtained as the dominant frequency of the estimated rotation angles of the electrical axis [22]; this method was later extended to handle noisy exercise ECGs [28]. Variations in the inertial axes and center of gravity of QRS-VCG loops were also used to estimate the respiratory signal [23]. For single-lead recordings, amplitude modulation of ECG waves has been used to derive a respiratory signal, especially in the context of sleep apnea studies [14, 18, 24]. Yet another approach to the EDR problem has been to apply a bandpass filter to the single-lead ECG, selecting the usual respiratory frequency band from 0.2 to 0.4 Hz [20].

Some methods derive respiratory information solely from the HR series. The respiratory frequency was estimated from the RR interval series using singular value decomposition (SVD) to track the most important instantaneous frequencies of the interval series [25]. Some years later, the respiratory frequency present in the HR series was derived using the S-transform [26]. Respiratory frequency patterns were derived from the RR interval series using autoregressive (AR) model-based methods in stationary [29] and nonstationary situations [27].

There are also some methods which derive the respiratory signal using both beat morphology and HR information. The cross-power spectrum of the EDR signals obtained from morphologic variations and HR was used to enhance the respiratory frequency [22]. Another approach was to use an adaptive filter so as to enhance the respiration-related common component present in the EDR signals derived from beat morphology and HR [30].

In this chapter the estimation of respiratory frequency from the ECG will be addressed. Algorithms deriving a respiratory signal from the ECG, so-called EDR algorithms, are presented, as well as the signal preprocessing needed for their proper performance. Electrocardiogram-derived respiration algorithms may be divided into three categories: Section 8.2 presents EDR algorithms based on beat-to-beat morphologic variations (which can be applied to single- or multilead ECGs), Section 8.3 describes EDR algorithms based on HR information, and Section 8.4 describes EDR algorithms using both beat morphology and HR information. One of the main interests in deriving the EDR signal is the estimation of respiratory frequency. Therefore, spectral analysis of the previously derived EDR signals is described in Section 8.5 and related estimation of the respiratory frequency. The general procedure to estimate the respiratory frequency from the ECG is summarized in Figure 8.3.

In order to evaluate and compare the performance of the EDR algorithms, the derived respiratory information should be compared to respiratory information simultaneously recorded. Performance measurements may vary depending on the particular goal for which the EDR algorithm is applied. For example, the respiratory frequency estimated from the ECG can be compared to that estimated from a simultaneously recorded respiratory signal, considered as gold standard [28]. When simultaneous recordings of ECG and respiratory signal are unavailable, an alternative is the design of a simulation study, where all signal parameters can be controlled and compared to the derived ones. This approach is described in Section 8.6.

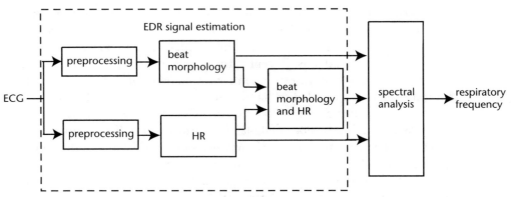

Figure 8.3   Block diagram of the estimation of the respiratory frequency from the ECG.

8.2   EDR Algorithms Based on Beat Morphology

Several methods have been proposed to derive the respiratory signal from the ECG using beat-to-beat morphologic variations. The underlying idea behind these methods is that the electrical axis of the heart changes its direction during the respiratory cycle due to motion of the electrodes relative to the heart and heterogeneous variations in the thorax impedance caused by the filling and emptying of the lungs. Therefore, the EDR signal may be estimated from the fluctuations of the heart's electrical axis. The way to estimate variations in axis direction is what mainly differs from one method to another.

In this section, three different types of EDR algorithms based on beat morphology are described, namely those based on wave amplitudes (Section 8.2.1), the multilead QRS area (Section 8.2.2) and the QRS-VCG loop alignment (Section 8.2.3). Amplitude EDR algorithms can be applied to single-lead ECGs while the multilead QRS area and the QRS-VCG loop alignment methods require at least two orthogonal leads.

Adequate performance of an EDR algorithm requires certain types of preprocessing of the raw ECG. First of all, QRS complexes must be detected and clustered based on their morphology, since only beats with the dominant morphology should be analyzed. The dominant morphology is the one corresponding to the largest class, whose beats typically originate from the sinoatrial node. Baseline wander should be attenuated in order not to introduce a rotation of the electrical axis unrelated to respiration. Certain EDR algorithms, like the QRS-VCG loop alignment, require VCG signals which, if unavailable, may have to be synthesized from the standard 12-lead ECG by means of the inverse Dower transformation [31]; see Appendix 8A for further details.

Additional preprocessing has been proposed to make the EDR algorithm robust when processing noisy ECGs such as those recorded during exercise [28]. Noisy beats can be substituted on a lead-by-lead basis using an exponentially updated average beat. The idea is that excessive noise present in a single lead would mask the rotation information present in the remaining leads. In such cases, the noisy beat is substituted so that the rotation information of the remaining leads is preserved.

Two different kinds of noise are common in ECGs: high-frequency (HF) noise mainly due to muscle activity, and low-frequency (LF) noise due to remaining baseline wander unattenuated by the preprocessing step. Consequently, a high frequency SNR, SNR_{HF}, and a low-frequency SNR, SNR_{LF}, can be defined to determine beats for substitution. The SNR_{HF} is defined as the ratio of the peak-to-peak amplitude in an interval centered around the QRS mark, and the root-mean-square (RMS) value of the HF noise in an HR-dependent interval following the QRS mark to avoid QRS mediated HF components. The SNR_{LF} is defined as the ratio of the peak-to-peak amplitude of the exponentially updated average beat and the RMS value of the residual ECG after average beat substraction and lowpass filtering computed over the whole beat interval. Figure 8.4 displays an example of a noisy beat, the exponentially updated average beat, the HF noise resulting from highpass filtering the noisy beat with a cutoff frequency of 20 Hz, and the residual ECG after average beat substraction and lowpass filtering with a cutoff frequency of 20 Hz. Beats whose SNR_{HF} is below a threshold, η_{HF}, or whose SNR_{LF} is below another threshold, η_{LF}, are substituted by their corresponding averaged beats. Figure 8.5 displays a VCG before and after substitution of noisy beats, as well as the estimated EDR signals and related respiratory signal. The spectra obtained from the EDR signals and the respiratory signal of Figure 8.5 are displayed in Figure 8.6. The substitution of noisy beats improves the estimation of the respiratory frequency since the largest

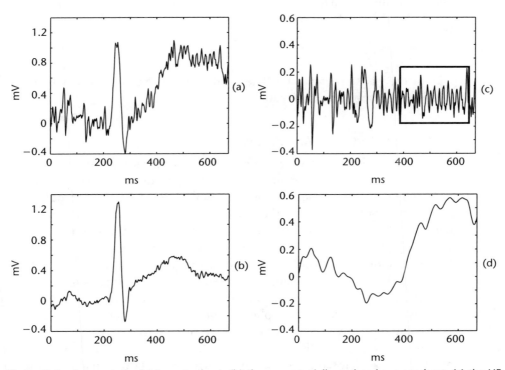

Figure 8.4 An example of (a) a noisy beat, (b) the exponentially updated average beat, (c) the HF noise resulting from highpass filtering the noisy beat with a cutoff frequency of 20 Hz (the interval over which the RMS is computed has been marked with a box), and (d) the residual ECG after average beat substraction and lowpass filtering with a cutoff frequency of 20 Hz.

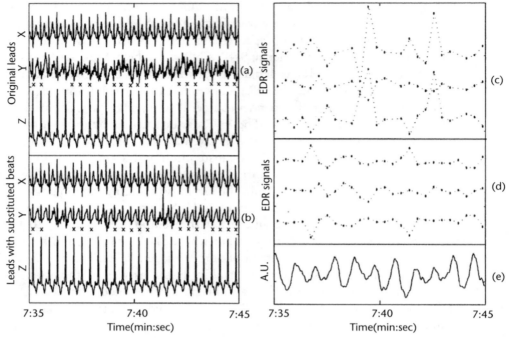

Figure 8.5 The VCG leads (a) before and (b) after substitution of noisy beats. The EDR signals (linear interpolation points have been used) estimated (c) before and (d) after substitution of noisy beats, and (e) the related respiratory signal. Recordings were taken during a stress test. Substituted beats in lead Y have been marked ($\times$). The following parameter values are used: $\eta_{HF} = 20$ and $\eta_{LF} = 3$.

peak of the EDR spectrum has been shifted such that it coincides with the largest peak of the respiratory spectrum.

8.2.1 Amplitude EDR Algorithms

When only single-lead ECGs are available, amplitude modulation of the ECG waves has been used to derive a respiratory signal, especially in the context of sleep apnea studies. For example, the sum of the absolute R and S wave amplitudes is used as a respiratory estimate in the detection of apneic events in infants [14]. Two methods for deriving an EDR signal from single-lead ECG amplitudes have been compared [18]: The amplitude of the R wave is measured either with respect to the baseline or differentially with respect to the amplitude of the S wave for each QRS complex. Both EDR signals are used to detect breaths using a peak detection algorithm; the EDR signal based on the differential measure of the R wave amplitude with respect to the S wave amplitude obtained higher sensitivity (77% compared to 68%) and positive predictivity (56% compared to 49%).

Alternatively, an EDR signal can be obtained from single-lead ECGs by calculating the area enclosed by the baseline-corrected ECG within a fixed interval of the QRS complex. The area measurements have been found to be more stable and less prone to noise than amplitude measurements [5]. Such an EDR signal has been used in the detection of obstructive sleep apnea [21, 32]. The error between respiratory

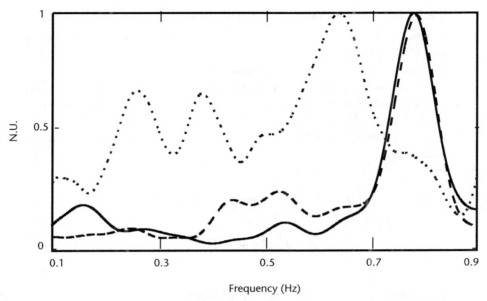

Figure 8.6   Power spectrum of the respiratory signal (solid line), and the EDR signals before (dotted line) and after (dashed line) substitution of noisy beats in normalized units (N.U.).

rate extracted from such an EDR signal and from a simultaneous airflow signal was reported to be −0.3 breaths per minute (−0.005 Hz) [32].

An EDR signal can also be obtained from the T wave rather than from the QRS complex: the signal segment following each QRS complex is linearly detrended and its average absolute value can be used as a sample of an EDR signal [17].

A different approach to the EDR problem is to filter the single-lead ECG with a passband corresponding to the usual respiratory frequency band. For example, the discrete wavelet transform has been applied to the single-lead ECG and the scale corresponding to the frequency band 0.2 to 0.4 Hz can be selected as an EDR signal [20]. Correlation coefficients between respiratory frequency extracted from the EDR signal and from simultaneous airflow signal exceeding 0.9 were reported.

Due to the thorax anisotropy and its intersubject variability together with the intersubject electrical axis variability, respiration may have a different effect on different ECG leads, implying that the lead most influenced by respiration often changes from subject to subject [33]. Single-lead EDR algorithms are reported to work better if the lead axis is significantly different from the mean electrical axis since a relatively larger EDR signal results in such cases. It has been experimentally shown that respiration-related ECG changes are reflected primarily in the direction (affected mainly by motion of the electrodes relative to the heart) and not in the magnitude (affected mainly by thoracic impedance variations) of the mean electrical axis; therefore, a lead perpendicular to the mean electrical axis would produce a larger EDR signal than a parallel lead [5]. Principal component analysis may be applied to the 12-lead ECG in order to obtain a virtual lead, linear combination of the original ones, most influenced by respiration [32].

8.2.2   Multilead QRS Area EDR Algorithm

In this method, the projection of the mean electrical axis on the plane defined by two leads is considered. The variation in angle between this projection and a reference lead is used as an estimate of the EDR signal [5]. The area of the ith QRS complex, occurring at time instant t_i, is computed over a fixed time interval in each lead, thus being proportional to the projection of the mean electrical axis on that lead. Consider the projection of the mean electrical axis on the plane jk, defined by orthogonal leads j and k, at time instant t_i, which is denoted as the vector $\overline{\mathbf{m}}(t_i)$,

$$
\overline{\mathbf{m}}(t_i) = \begin{bmatrix} \dfrac{1}{\delta_2 + \delta_1} \displaystyle\int_{t_i-\delta_1}^{t_i+\delta_2} \|\mathbf{m}(t)\|_2 \cos(\theta_{jk}(t))dt \\[2mm] \dfrac{1}{\delta_2 + \delta_1} \displaystyle\int_{t_i-\delta_1}^{t_i+\delta_2} \|\mathbf{m}(t)\|_2 \sin(\theta_{jk}(t))dt \end{bmatrix} = \dfrac{1}{\delta_2 + \delta_1} \begin{bmatrix} A_j(t_i) \\[2mm] A_k(t_i) \end{bmatrix} \quad (8.1)
$$

where $\mathbf{m}(t)$ is the instantaneous projection of the electrical axis on the plane jk, $\theta_{jk}(t)$ is the angle between $\mathbf{m}(t)$ and lead j, $A_j(t_i)$ represents the QRS area in lead j, δ_1 and δ_2 define the integration interval over which the mean is computed, and the operator $\|.\|_2$ denotes the Euclidean distance. The term $\|\mathbf{m}(t)\|_2 \cos(\theta_{jk}(t))$ represents the projection of $\mathbf{m}(t)$ on lead j, and $\|\mathbf{m}(t)\|_2 \sin(\theta_{jk}(t))$ the projection of $\mathbf{m}(t)$ on lead k. The projection angle of the mean electrical axis on the plane jk with respect to lead j, $\overline{\theta}_{jk}(t_i)$, can be estimated as

$$
\overline{\theta}_{jk}(t_i) = \arctan(A_k(t_i)/A_j(t_i)) \quad (8.2)
$$

See Figure 8.7. Finally, the fluctuations of the $\overline{\theta}_{jk}(t_i)$ series are used as an EDR signal. The values of δ_1 and δ_2 depend on the application; they can be chosen so as to comprise the whole QRS complex, a symmetric window around the QRS fiducial point, or an asymmetric window in order to reduce the QRS morphologic variations unrelated to respiration but related to other conditions such as exercise. Figure 8.8 displays an example of the multilead QRS area EDR algorithm, where the angle series $\overline{\theta}_{YZ}(t_i)$ can be seen as well as the two orthogonal VCG leads Y and Z and the related respiratory signal.

The multilead QRS area EDR algorithm has been further studied [13] and applied in HRV analysis [12], sleep studies [19], and used for ambulatory monitoring [16].

Using a similar principle, the areas of the QRS complexes in eight leads have been used to define an EDR signal [15]. First, an eight-dimensional space is defined by eigenvalue analysis of a learning set; then, each eight-dimensional QRS area vector is projected onto the main direction, which is considered as particularly sensitive to respiratory information, and then used as an EDR signal.

A different approach has been addressed to estimate the direction of the projection of the mean electrical axis on the plane defined by two orthogonal leads. The least-squares (LS) straight line is computed which fits the projection of the VCG

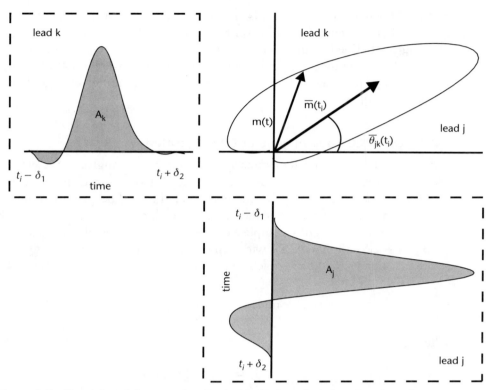

Figure 8.7 Illustration of the mean heart's electrical axis projected on the plane jk.

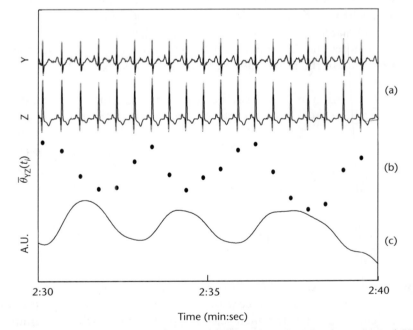

Figure 8.8 Multilead QRS area EDR algorithm: (a) leads Y and Z, (b) the estimated EDR signal $\overline{\theta}_{YZ}(t_i)$, and (c) the related respiratory signal. Recordings were taken during a stress test. The parameter values used are: $\delta_1 = 60$ ms, $\delta_2 = 20$ ms.

on the plane defined by two leads. Then, the variations of the angle that forms the LS fit with a reference direction constitutes the EDR signal [11]. It has been stated that angles obtained from different pairs of orthogonal leads cannot be expected to provide the same range of amplitude variation. Furthermore, the lead configuration yielding the EDR signal with largest amplitude variation often changes from subject to subject [33].

8.2.3   QRS-VCG Loop Alignment EDR Algorithm

This method is based on LS estimation of the rotation angles of the electrical axis around the three-dimensional orthogonal axes between successive VCG loops and a reference loop [22]. At each time instant t_i, the method performs minimization of a normalized distance ε between a reference loop ($N \times 3$ matrix $\mathbf{Y_R}$, where the columns contain the QRS complex of the X, Y, and Z leads) and each observed loop (($N + 2\Delta) \times 3$ matrix $\mathbf{Y}$), with respect to rotation (3×3 matrix $\mathbf{Q}$), amplitude scaling (scalar γ), and time synchronization ($N \times (N + 2\Delta)$ matrix $\mathbf{J}_\tau$) [34, 35]:

$$\varepsilon_{min} = \min_{\gamma, \tau, Q}(\varepsilon) = \min_{\gamma, \tau, Q} \frac{\|\mathbf{Y_R} - \gamma \mathbf{J}_\tau \mathbf{YQ}\|_F^2}{\|\gamma \mathbf{J}_\tau \mathbf{YQ}\|_F^2} \tag{8.3}$$

where

$$\mathbf{J}_\tau = [\, 0_{\Delta - \tau} \ \mathbf{I} \ 0_{\Delta + \tau} \,] \tag{8.4}$$

and N is the number of samples of the QRS complex analysis window. The parameter Δ denotes the number of symmetrically augmented samples which allow for time synchronization with $\tau = -\Delta, \ldots, \Delta$. The dimensions of the $0_{\Delta - \tau}$, $0_{\Delta + \tau}$, and $\mathbf{I}$ (identity) matrices are $N \times (\Delta - \tau)$, $N \times (\Delta + \tau)$, and $N \times N$, respectively. The operator $\| \cdot \|_F^2$ denotes the Frobenius norm. For simplicity, the dependence on time instant t_i is omitted in the notation [i.e., $\varepsilon = \varepsilon(t_i)$, $\mathbf{Y_R} = \mathbf{Y_R}(t_i)$, $\mathbf{Y} = \mathbf{Y}(t_i)$, $\mathbf{Q} = \mathbf{Q}(t_i)$, and $\gamma = \gamma(t_i)$].

The rotation matrix $\mathbf{Q}$ can be viewed as three successive rotations around each axis (lead), defined by the rotation angles ϕ_X, ϕ_Y, and ϕ_Z,

$$
\begin{aligned}
\mathbf{Q} &= \begin{bmatrix} 1 & 0 & 0 \\ 0 & \cos(\phi_X) & \sin(\phi_X) \\ 0 & -\sin(\phi_X) & \cos(\phi_X) \end{bmatrix} \begin{bmatrix} \cos(\phi_Y) & 0 & \sin(\phi_Y) \\ 0 & 1 & 0 \\ -\sin(\phi_Y) & 0 & \cos(\phi_Y) \end{bmatrix} \begin{bmatrix} \cos(\phi_Z) & \sin(\phi_Z) & 0 \\ -\sin(\phi_Z) & \cos(\phi_Z) & 0 \\ 0 & 0 & 1 \end{bmatrix} \\
&= \begin{bmatrix} * & \sin(\phi_Z)\cos(\phi_Y) & \sin(\phi_Y) \\ * & * & \sin(\phi_X)\cos(\phi_Y) \\ * & * & * \end{bmatrix}
\end{aligned} \tag{8.5}
$$

where the asterisk $*$ denotes an omitted matrix entry.

The normalized distance ε is minimized by first finding estimates of γ and $\mathbf{Q}$ for every value of τ and then selecting that τ for which ε is minimum. For a fixed value of τ, the optimal estimator of $\mathbf{Q}$ is given by [34]

$$\hat{\mathbf{Q}}_\tau = \mathbf{V}_\tau \mathbf{U}_\tau^T \tag{8.6}$$

where the matrices $\mathbf{U}_\tau$ and $\mathbf{V}_\tau$ contain the left and right singular vectors from the SVD of $\mathbf{Z}_\tau = \mathbf{Y}_R^T \mathbf{J}_\tau \mathbf{Y}$. The estimate of γ is then obtained by [35]

$$\hat{\gamma}_\tau = \frac{tr(\mathbf{Y_R}^T \mathbf{Y_R})}{tr(\mathbf{Y_R}^T \mathbf{J}_\tau^T \mathbf{Y} \hat{\mathbf{Q}}_\tau)} \tag{8.7}$$

The parameters $\hat{\mathbf{Q}}_\tau$ and $\hat{\gamma}_\tau$ are calculated for all values of τ, with $\hat{\mathbf{Q}}$ resulting from that τ which yields the minimal error ε. Finally, the rotation angles are estimated from $\hat{\mathbf{Q}}$ using the structure in (8.5) [22],

$$\hat{\phi}_Y = \arcsin(\hat{q}_{13}) \tag{8.8}$$

$$\hat{\phi}_X = \arcsin\left(\frac{\hat{q}_{23}}{\cos(\hat{\phi}_Y)}\right) \tag{8.9}$$

$$\hat{\phi}_Z = \arcsin\left(\frac{\hat{q}_{12}}{\cos(\hat{\phi}_Y)}\right) \tag{8.10}$$

where the estimate $\hat{q}_{kl}$ denotes the (k,l) entry of $\hat{\mathbf{Q}}$.

In certain situations, such as during ischemia, QRS morphology exhibits long-term variations unrelated to respiration. This motivates a continuous update of the reference loop in order to avoid the estimation of rotation angles generated by such variations rather than by respiration [28]. The reference loop is exponentially updated as

$$\mathbf{Y_R}(i+1) = \alpha \mathbf{Y_R}(i) + (1-\alpha)\mathbf{Y}(i+1) \tag{8.11}$$

where i denotes the beat index at time instant t_i [i.e., $\mathbf{Y_R}(t_i) = \mathbf{Y_R}(i)$ and $\mathbf{Y}(t_i) = \mathbf{Y}(i)$]. The parameter α is chosen such that long-term morphologic variations are tracked while adaptation to noise and short-term respiratory variations is avoided. The initial reference loop $\mathbf{Y_R}(1)$ can be defined as the average of the first loops in order to obtain a reliable reference. Figure 8.9 displays lead X of $\mathbf{Y_R}$ at the beginning and peak exercise of a stress test, and illustrates the extent by which QRS morphology may change during exercise.

An example of the method's performance is presented in Figure 8.10 where the estimated rotation angle series are displayed as well as the VCG leads and the related respiratory signal.

Unreliable angle estimates may be observed at poor SNRs or in the presence of ectopic beats, calling for an approach which makes the algorithm robust against outlier estimates [28]. Such estimates are detected when the absolute value of the angle estimates exceed a lead-dependent threshold $\eta_j(t_i)$ ($j \in \{X, Y, Z\}$). The threshold $\eta_j(t_i)$ is defined as the running standard deviation (SD) of the N_e most recent angle estimates, multiplied by a factor C. For $i < N_e$, $\eta_j(t_i)$ is computed from the available estimates. Outliers are replaced by the angle estimates obtained by reperforming the minimization in (8.3), but excluding the value of τ which produced the outlier estimate. The new estimates are only accepted if they do not exceed the threshold $\eta_j(t_i)$; if no acceptable value of τ is found, the EDR signal contains a gap and the reference loop $\mathbf{Y_R}$ in (8.11) is not updated. This procedure is illustrated by Figure 8.11.

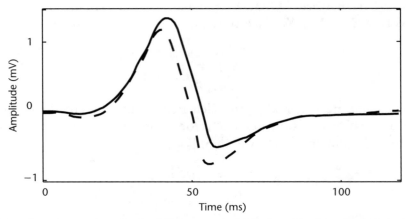

Figure 8.9 The reference loop $\mathbf{Y_R}$ (lead X) at onset (solid line) and peak exercise (dashed line) of a stress test.

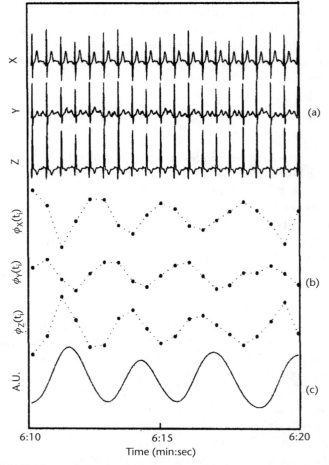

Figure 8.10 QRS-VCG loop alignment EDR algorithm: (a) the VCG leads, (b) the estimated EDR signals (linear interpolation points have been used), and (c) the related respiratory signal. Recordings were taken during a stress test. The following parameter values are used: $N = 120$ ms, $\Delta = 30$ ms in steps of 1 ms, and $\alpha = 0.8$.

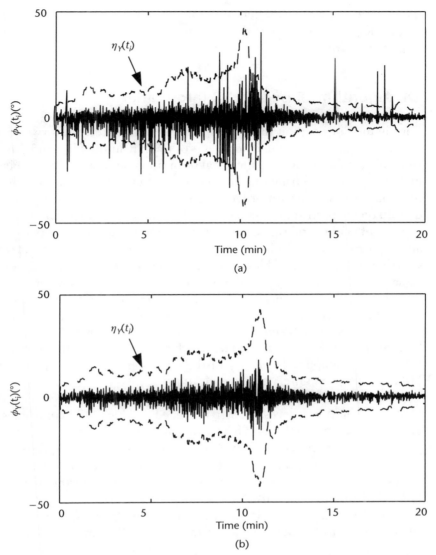

Figure 8.11   The EDR signal $\phi_Y(t_i)$ estimated (a) before and (b) after outlier correction/rejection. Dashed lines denote the running threshold $\eta_Y(t_i)$. The parameter values used are $N_e = 50$ and $C = 5$.

Although the QRS-VCG loop alignment EDR algorithm is developed for recordings with three orthogonal leads, it can still be applied when only two orthogonal leads are available. In this case the rotation matrix $\mathbf{Q}$ would be 2×2 and represent rotation around the lead orthogonal to the plane defined by the two leads.

Another approach to estimate the rotation angles of the electrical axis is by means of its intrinsic components, determined from the last 30 ms of the QR segment for each loop [10]. Using a similar idea, principal component analysis is applied to measurements of gravity center and inertial axes of each loop [23]; for each beat a QRS loop is constructed comprising 120 ms around the R peak and its center of gravity is computed yielding three coordinates referred to the axes of the reference system; the inertial axes in the space are also obtained and characterized by the three angles that each inertial axis forms with the axes of reference; finally, the first principal component of the set of the computed parameters is identified as the respiratory activity.

8.3 EDR Algorithms Based on HR Information

Certain methods exploit the HRV spectrum to derive respiratory information. The underlying idea is that the component of the HR in the HF band (above 0.15 Hz) generally can be ascribed to the vagal respiratory sinus arrhythmia. Figure 8.12 displays the power spectrum of a HR signal during resting conditions and 90° head-up tilt, obtained by a seventh-order AR model. Although the power spectrum patterns depend on the particular interactions between the sympathetic and parasympathetic systems in resting and tilt conditions, two major components are detectable at low and high frequencies in both cases. The LF band (0.04 to 0.15 Hz) is related to short-term regulation of blood pressure whereas the extended HF band (0.15 Hz to half the mean HR expressed in Hz) reflects respiratory influence on HR.

Most EDR algorithms based on HR information estimate the respiratory activity as the HF component in the HRV signal and, therefore, the HRV signal itself can be used as an EDR signal. The HRV signal can be filtered (e.g., from 0.15 Hz to half the mean HR expressed in Hz, which is the highest meaningful frequency since the intrinsic sampling frequency of the HRV signal is given by the HR) to reduce HRV components unrelated to respiration.

The HRV signal is based on the series of beat occurrence times obtained by a QRS detector. A preprocessing step is needed in which QRS complexes are detected and clustered, since only beats from sinus rhythm (i.e., originated from the sinoatrial node) should be analyzed. Several definitions of signals for representing HRV have been suggested, for example, based on the interval tachogram, the interval function, the event series, or the heart timing signal; see [36] for further details on different HRV signal representations.

The presence of ectopic beats, as well as missed or falsely detected beats, results in fictitious frequency components in the HRV signal which must be avoided.

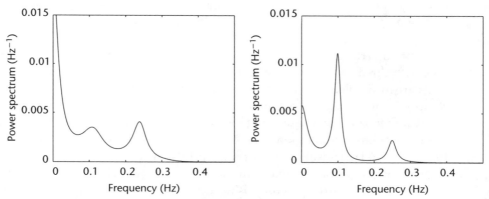

Figure 8.12 Power spectrum of a HR signal during resting conditions (left) and 90° head-up tilt (right).

A method to derive the HRV signal in the presence of ectopic beats based on the heart timing signal has been proposed [37].

8.4   EDR Algorithms Based on Both Beat Morphology and HR

Some methods derive respiratory information from the ECG by exploiting beat morphology and HR [22, 30]. A multichannel EDR signal can be constructed with EDR signals obtained both from the EDR algorithms based on beat morphology (Section 8.2) and from HR (Section 8.3). The power spectra of the EDR signals based on beat morphology can be crosscorrelated with the HR-based spectrum in order to reduce components unrelated to respiration [22].

A different approach is to use an adaptive filter which enhances the common component present in two input signals while attenuating uncorrelated noise. It was mentioned earlier that both ECG wave amplitudes and HR are influenced by respiration, which can be considered the common component. Therefore, the respiratory signal can be estimated by an adaptive filter applied to the series of RR intervals and R wave amplitudes [30]; see Figure 8.13(a). The series $a_r(i)$ denotes the R wave amplitude of the ith beat and is used as the reference input, whereas $rr(i)$ denotes the RR interval series and is the primary input. The filter output $r(i)$ is the estimate of the respiratory activity. The filter structure is not symmetric with respect to its inputs. The effectiveness of the two possible input configurations depends on the application [30]. This filter can be seen as a particular case of a more general adaptive filter whose reference input is the RR interval series $rr(i)$ and whose primary input is any of the EDR signals based on beat morphology, $e_j(i)$ ($j = 1, \ldots, J$), or even a combination of them; see Figure 8.13(b). The interchange of reference and primary inputs could be also considered.

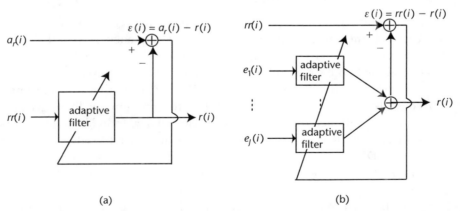

(a)   (b)

Figure 8.13   Adaptive estimation of respiratory signal. (a) The reference input is the R wave amplitude series $a_r(i)$, the primary input is the RR interval series $rr(i)$, and the filter output is the estimate of the respiratory signal $r(i)$. (b) The reference input is the RR interval series $rr(i)$ and the primary input is a combination of different EDR signals based on beat morphology $e_j(i)$, $j = 1,\ldots,J$, J denotes the number of EDR signals; the filter output is the estimate of the respiratory signal $r(i)$.

8.5   Estimation of the Respiratory Frequency

In this section the estimation of the respiratory frequency from the EDR signal, obtained by any of the methods previously described in Sections 8.2, 8.3, and 8.4, is presented. It may comprise spectral analysis of the EDR signal and estimation of the respiratory frequency from the EDR spectrum.

Let us define a multichannel EDR signal $e_j(t_i)$, where $j = 1, \ldots, J, i = 1, \ldots, L$, J denotes the number of EDR signals, and L the number of samples of the EDR signals. For single-lead EDR algorithms based on wave amplitudes (Section 8.2.1) and for EDR algorithms based on HR (Section 8.3), $J = 1$. For EDR algorithms based on multilead QRS area (Section 8.2.2) or on QRS-VCG loop alignment (Section 8.2.3), the value of J depends on the number of available leads. The value of J for EDR algorithms based on both beat morphology and HR depends on the particular choice of method.

Each EDR signal can be unevenly sampled, $e_j(t_i)$, as before, or evenly sampled, $e_j(n)$, coming either from interpolating and resampling of $e_j(t_i)$ or from an EDR signal which is intrinsically evenly sampled. The EDR signals coming from any source related to beats could be evenly sampled if represented as a function of beat order or unevenly sampled if represented as function of beat occurrence time t_i, but which could become evenly sampled when interpolated. An EDR signal based on direct filtering of the ECG is evenly sampled.

The spectral analysis of an evenly sampled EDR signal can be performed using either nonparametric methods based on the Fourier transform or parametric methods such as AR modeling. An unevenly sampled EDR signal may be interpolated and resampled at evenly spaced times, and then processed with the same methods as for an evenly sampled EDR signal. Alternatively, an unevenly sampled signal may be analyzed by spectral techniques designed to directly handle unevenly sampled signals such as Lomb's method [38].

8.5.1   Nonparametric Approach

In the nonparametric approach, the respiratory frequency is estimated from the location of the largest peak in the respiratory frequency band of the power spectrum of the multichannel EDR signal, using the Fourier transform if the signal is evenly sampled or Lomb's method if the signal is unevenly sampled.

In order to handle nonstationary EDR signals with a time-varying respiratory frequency, the power spectrum is estimated on running intervals of T_s seconds, where the EDR signal is assumed to be stationary. Individual running power spectra of each EDR signal $e_j(t_i)$ are averaged in order to reduce their variance. For the jth EDR signal and kth running interval of T_s- second length, the power spectrum $S_{j,k}(f)$ results from averaging the power spectra obtained from subintervals of length T_m seconds ($T_m < T_s$) using an overlap of $T_m/2$ seconds. A T_s-second spectrum is estimated every t_s seconds. The variance of $S_{j,k}(f)$ is further reduced by "peak-conditioned" averaging in which selective averaging is performed only on those $S_{j,k}(f)$ which are sufficiently peaked. Here, "peaked" means that a certain percentage (ξ) of the spectral power must be contained in an interval centered around the largest peak $f_p(j,k)$, otherwise the spectrum is omitted from averaging. In mathematical terms, peak-conditioned averaging is defined by

$$\overline{S}_k(f) = \sum_{l=0}^{L_s-1} \sum_{j=1}^{J} \chi_{j,k-l} S_{j,k-l}(f), \quad k = 1, 2, \ldots \tag{8.12}$$

where the parameter L_s denotes the number of T_s-second intervals used for computing the averaged spectrum $\overline{S}_k(f)$. The binary variable $\chi_{j,k}$ indicates if the spectrum $S_{j,k}(f)$ is peaked or not, defined by

$$\chi_{j,k} = \begin{cases} 1 & P_{j,k} \geq \xi \\ 0 & \text{otherwise} \end{cases} \tag{8.13}$$

where the relative spectral power $P_{j,k}$ is given by

$$P_{j,k} = \frac{\displaystyle\int_{(1-\mu) f_p(j,k)}^{(1+\mu) f_p(j,k)} S_{j,k}(f) df}{\displaystyle\int_{0.1}^{f_{max}(k)} S_{j,k}(f) df} \tag{8.14}$$

where the value of $f_{max}(k)$ is given by half the mean HR expressed in Hz in the kth interval and μ determines the width of integration interval.

Figure 8.14 illustrates the estimation of the power spectrum $S_{j,k}(f)$ using different values of T_m. It can be appreciated that larger values of T_m yield spectra with better resolution and, therefore, more accurate estimation of the respiratory frequency. However, the respiratory frequency does not always correspond to a unimodal peak (i.e., showing a single frequency peak), but to a bimodal peak,

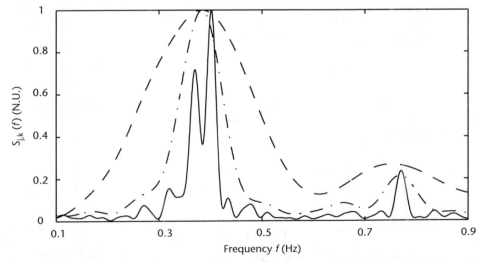

Figure 8.14   The power spectrum $S_{j,k}(f)$ computed for $T_m = 4$ seconds (dashed line), 12 seconds (dashed/dotted line), and 40 seconds (solid line), using $T_s = 40$ seconds.

sometimes observed in ECGs recorded during exercise. In such situations, smaller values of T_m should be used to estimate the gross dominant frequency.

Estimation of the respiratory frequency $\hat{f}_r(k)$ as the largest peak of $\overline{S}_k(f)$ comes with the risk of choosing the location of a spurious peak. This risk is, however, considerably reduced by narrowing down the search interval to only include frequencies in an interval of $2\delta_f$ Hz centered around a reference frequency $f_w(k)$: $[f_w(k) - \delta_f, f_w(k) + \delta_f]$. The reference frequency is obtained as an exponential average of previous estimates, using

$$f_w(k+1) = \beta f_w(k) + (1 - \beta)\hat{f}_r(k) \tag{8.15}$$

where β denotes the forgetting factor. The procedure to estimate the respiratory frequency is summarized in Figure 8.15.

Respiratory frequency during a stress test has been estimated using this procedure in combination with both the multilead QRS area and the QRS-VCG loop alignment EDR algorithms, described in Sections 8.2.2 and 8.2.3, respectively [28]. Results are compared with the respiratory frequency obtained from simultaneous airflow respiratory signals. An estimation error of 0.022±0.016 Hz (5.9±4.0%) is achieved by the QRS-VCG loop alignment EDR algorithm and of 0.076±0.087 Hz (18.8±21.7%) by the multilead QRS area EDR algorithm. Figure 8.16 displays an example of the respiratory frequency estimated from the respiratory signal and from the ECG using the QRS-VCG loop alignment EDR algorithm. Lead X of the observed and reference loop are displayed at different time instants during the stress test.

8.5.2 Parametric Approach

Parametric AR model-based methods have been used to estimate the respiratory frequency in stationary [29] and nonstationary situations [27, 39]. Such methods offer automatic decomposition of the spectral components and, consequently, estimation of the respiratory frequency. Each EDR signal $e_j(n)$ can be seen as the output of an AR model of order P,

$$e_j(n) = -a_{j,1}e_j(n-1) - \cdots - a_{j,P}e_j(n-P) + v(n) \tag{8.16}$$

where n indexes the evenly sampled EDR signal, $a_{j,1}, \ldots, a_{j,P}$ are the AR parameters, and $v(n)$ is white noise with zero mean and variance σ^2. The model transfer function is

$$H_j(z) = \frac{1}{A_j(z)} = \frac{1}{\sum_{l=0}^{P} a_{j,l}z^{-l}} = \frac{1}{\prod_{p=1}^{P}(1 - z_{j,p}z^{-1})} \tag{8.17}$$

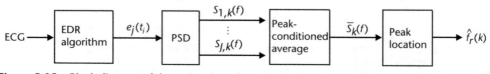

Figure 8.15 Block diagram of the estimation of respiratory frequency. PSD: power spectral density.

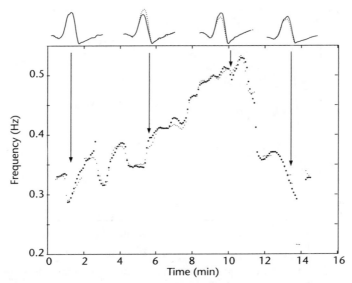

Figure 8.16   The respiratory frequency estimated from the respiratory signal (f_r, small dots) and from the ECG ($\hat{f}_r$, big dots) during a stress test using QRS-VCG loop alignment EDR algorithm. Lead X of the observed (solid line) and reference (dotted line) loop are displayed above the figure at different time instants. Parameter values: $T_s = 40$ seconds, $t_s = 5$ seconds, $T_m = 12$ seconds, $L_s = 5$, $\mu = 0.5$, $\xi = 0.35$, $\beta = 0.7$, $\delta_f = 0.2$ Hz, and $f_w(1) = \arg\max_{0.15 \leq f \leq 0.4} (\bar{S}_1(f))$.

where $a_{j,0} = 1$ and the poles $z_{j,p}$ appear in complex-conjugate pairs since the EDR signal is real. The corresponding AR spectrum can be obtained by evaluating the following expression for $z = e^{j\omega}$,

$$S_j(z) = \frac{\sigma^2}{A_j(z)\, A_j(z^{-1})} = \frac{\sigma^2}{\prod_{p=1}^{P}(1 - z_{j,p}z^{-1})(1 - z_{j,p}^* z)} \tag{8.18}$$

It can be seen from (8.18) that the roots of the polynomial $A_j(z)$ and the spectral peaks are related. A simple way to estimate peak frequencies is by the phase angle of the poles $z_{j,p}$,

$$\hat{f}_{j,p} = \frac{1}{2\pi} \arctan\left(\frac{\Im(z_{j,p})}{\Re(z_{j,p})}\right) \cdot f_s \tag{8.19}$$

where f_s is the sampling frequency of $e_j(n)$. A detailed description on peak frequency estimation from AR spectrum can be found in [36]. The selection of the respiratory frequency $\hat{f}_r$ from the peak frequency estimates $\hat{f}_{j,p}$ depends on the chosen EDR signal and the AR model order P. An AR model of order 12 has been fitted to a HRV signal and the respiratory frequency estimated as the peak frequency estimate with the highest power lying in the expected frequency range [27]. Another approach has been to determine the AR model order by means of the Akaike criterion and then to select the central frequency of the HF band as the respiratory frequency [29]. Results have been compared to those extracted from simultaneous strain gauge respiratory signal and a mean error of 0.41±0.48 breaths per minute (0.007±0.008 Hz) has been reported.

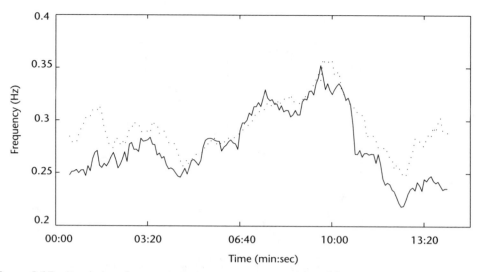

Figure 8.17 Respiratory frequency during a stress test, estimated from the respiratory signal (f_r, dotted) and from the HRV signal ($\hat{f}_r$, solid) using seventh-order AR modeling. The parameter values used are: $P = 7$, $T_s = 60$ seconds, and $t_s = 5$ seconds.

Figure 8.17 displays an example of the respiratory frequency during a stress test, estimated both from an airflow signal and from the ECG using parametric AR modeling. The nonstationarity nature of the signals during a stress test is handled by estimating the AR parameters on running intervals of T_s seconds, shifted by t_s seconds, where the EDR signal is supposed to be stationary, as in the nonparametric approach of Section 8.5.1. The EDR signal in this case is made to be the HRV signal which has been filtered in each interval of T_s second duration using a FIR filter with passband from 0.15 Hz to the minimum between 0.9 Hz (respiratory frequency is not supposed to exceed 0.9 Hz even in the peak of exercise) and half the mean HR expressed in Hz in the corresponding interval. The AR model order has been set to $P = 7$, as in Figure 8.12. The peak frequency estimate $\hat{f}_{j,p}$ with the highest power is selected as the respiratory frequency $\hat{f}_r$ in each interval.

The parametric approach can be applied to the multichannel EDR signal in a way similar to the nonparametric approach of Section 8.5.1. Selective averaging can be applied to the AR spectra $S_j(z)$ of each EDR signal $e_j(n)$, and the respiratory frequency can be estimated from the averaged spectrum in a restricted frequency interval. Another approach is the use of multivariate AR modeling [9] in which the cross-spectra of the different EDR signals are exploited for identification of the respiratory frequency.

8.5.3 Signal Modeling Approach

In Sections 8.5.1 and 8.5.2, nonparametric and parametric approaches have been applied to estimate the respiratory frequency from the power spectrum of the EDR signal. In this section, a different approach based on signal modeling is considered for identifying and quantifying the spectral component related to respiration.

The evenly sampled EDR signal $e_j(n)$ is assumed to be the sum of K complex undamped exponentials, according to the model

$$e_j(n) = \sum_{k=1}^{K} h_k e^{j\omega_k n} \tag{8.20}$$

where h_k denotes the amplitude and ω_k denotes the angular frequency. Since $e_j(n)$ is a real-valued signal, it is necessary that the complex exponentials in (8.20) occur in complex-conjugate pairs (i.e., K must be even). The problem of interest is to determine the frequencies of the exponentials given the observations $e_j(n)$, and to identify the respiratory frequency, f_r.

A direct approach would be to set up a nonlinear LS minimization problem in which the signal parameters h_k and ω_k would be chosen so as to minimize

$$\left\| e_j(n) - \sum_{k=1}^{K} h_k e^{j\omega_k n} \right\|_F^2 \tag{8.21}$$

However, since nonlinear minimization is computationally intensive and cumbersome, indirect approaches are often used. These are based on the fact that, in the absence of noise and for the model in (8.20), $e_j(n)$ is exactly predictable as a linear combination of its K past samples,

$$e_j(n) = -a_{j,1} e_j(n-1) - \cdots - a_{j,K} e_j(n-K), \quad n = K, \ldots, 2K-1 \tag{8.22}$$

which can be seen as an AR model of order K.

One such approach is due to Prony [40], developed to estimate the parameters of a sum of complex damped exponentials. Our problem can be seen as a particular case in which the damping factors are zero; further details on the derivation of Prony's method for undamped exponentials are found in [9].

A major drawback of Prony-based methods is the requirement of a priori knowledge of the model order K (i.e., the number of complex exponentials). When it is unknown, it must be estimated from the observed signal, for example, using techniques similar to AR model order estimation.

Another approach to estimate the frequencies of a sum of complex exponentials is by means of state space methods [41]. The EDR signal $e_j(n)$ is assumed to be generated by the following state space model:

$$\mathbf{e}_j(n+1) = \mathbf{F}\mathbf{e}_j(n)$$
$$e_j(n) = \mathbf{h}^T \mathbf{e}_j(n) \tag{8.23}$$

where

$$\mathbf{e}_j(n) = \begin{bmatrix} e_j(n-1) \\ e_j(n-2) \\ \vdots \\ e_j(n-K) \end{bmatrix}, \quad \mathbf{F} = \begin{bmatrix} a_1 & a_2 & \ldots & a_{K-1} & a_K \\ 1 & 0 & \ldots & 0 & 0 \\ 0 & 1 & \ldots & 0 & 0 \\ \vdots & \vdots & & \vdots & \\ 0 & 0 & \ldots & 1 & 0 \end{bmatrix}, \quad \mathbf{h} = \begin{bmatrix} a_1 \\ a_2 \\ \ldots \\ a_K \end{bmatrix} \tag{8.24}$$

It can be shown that the eigenvalues of the $K \times K$ matrix $\mathbf{F}$ are equal to $e^{j\omega_k}$, $k = 1, \ldots, K$, and thus the frequencies can be obtained once $\mathbf{F}$ is estimated from data [41]. Then, respiratory frequency has to be identified from the frequency estimates.

Such an approach has been applied to HR series to estimate the respiratory frequency, considered as the third lowest frequency estimate [25]. Respiratory frequency estimated is compared to that extracted from simultaneous respiratory recordings. A mean absolute error lower than 0.03 Hz is reported during rest and tilt-test. However, the method fails to track the respiratory frequency during exercise due to the very low SNR.

8.6 Evaluation

In order to evaluate the performance of EDR algorithms, the derived respiratory information should be compared to the respiratory information simultaneously recorded. However, simultaneous recording of ECG and respiratory signals is difficult to perform in certain situations, such as sleep studies, ambulatory monitoring, and stress testing. In such situations, an interesting alternative is the design of a simulation study where all signal parameters can be controlled.

A dynamical model for generating simulated ECGs has been presented [42]. The model generates a trajectory in a three-dimensional state space with coordinates (x, y, z), which moves around an attracting limit cycle of unit radius in the (x, y) plane; each cycle corresponds to one RR interval. The ECG waves are generated by attractors/repellors in the z direction. Baseline wander is introduced by coupling the baseline value in the z direction to the respiratory frequency. The z variable of the three-dimensional trajectory yields a simulated ECG with realistic PQRST morphology. The HRV is incorporated in the model by varying the angular velocity of the trajectory as it moves around the limit cycle according to variations in the length of RR intervals. A bimodal power spectrum consisting of the sum of two Gaussian distributions is generated to simulate a peak in the LF band, related to short-term regulation of blood pressure, and another peak in the HF band, related to respiratory sinus arrhythmia. An RR interval series with the former power spectrum is generated and the angular velocity of the trajectory around the limit cycle is defined from it. Time-varying power spectra can be used to simulate respiratory signals with varying frequency. Observational uncertainty is incorporated by adding zero-mean Gaussian noise. Simulated ECGs generated by this model can be used to evaluate EDR algorithms based on HR information (Section 8.3) and single-lead EDR algorithms based on the modulation of wave amplitudes (Section 8.2.1). However, it is not useful to evaluate multilead EDR algorithms based on estimating the rotation of the heart's electrical axis.

A simulation study to evaluate multilead EDR algorithms based on beat morphology (Sections 8.2.2 and 8.2.3) on exercise ECGs has been presented [28]. The study consists of a set of computer-generated reference exercise ECGs to which noise and respiratory influence have been added.

First, a noise-free 12-lead ECG is simulated from a set of 15 beats (templates) extracted from rest, exercise, and recovery of a stress test using weighted averaging. The HR and ST depression of each template is modified to follow a predefined ST/HR pattern. The simulated signals result from concatenation of templates such that HR and ST depression evolve linearly with time. Then, the VCG signal is synthesized from the simulated 12-lead ECG.

In order to account for respiratory influence, the simulated VCG is transformed on a sample-by-sample basis with a three-dimensional rotation matrix defined by time-varying angles. The angular variation around each axis is modeled by the product of two sigmoidal functions reflecting inhalation and exhalation [43], such that for lead X,

$$\phi_X(n) = \sum_{p=0}^{\infty} \zeta_X \frac{1}{1 + e^{-\lambda_i(p)(n-\kappa_i(p))}} \frac{1}{1 + e^{\lambda_e(p)(n-\kappa_e(p))}} \tag{8.25}$$

$$\lambda_i(p) = 20\frac{f_r(p)}{f_s}, \kappa_i(p) = \kappa_i(p-1) + \frac{f_s}{f_r(p-1)}, \kappa_i(0) = 0.35 f_s,$$

$$\lambda_e(p) = 15\frac{f_r(p)}{f_s}, \kappa_e(p) = \kappa_e(p-1) + \frac{f_s}{f_r(p-1)}, \kappa_e(0) = 0.6 f_s$$

where n denotes sample index, p denotes each respiratory cycle index, $\frac{1}{\lambda_i(p)}$ and $\frac{1}{\lambda_e(p)}$ are the duration of inhalation and exhalation, respectively, $\kappa_i(p)$ and $\kappa_e(p)$ are the time delays of the sigmoidal functions, f_s is the sampling rate, $f_r(p)$ is the respiratory frequency, and ζ_X is the maximum angular variation around lead X, which has been set to $5°$. The same procedure is applied to leads Y and Z, with $\zeta_Y = \zeta_Z = \zeta_X$. To account for the dynamic nature of the respiratory frequency during a stress test, the simulated respiratory frequency $f_r(p)$ follows a pattern varying from 0.2 to 0.7 Hz, see Figure 8.18. A similar respiratory pattern has been observed in several actual stress tests.

Finally, noise is added to the concatenated ECG signals, obtained as the residual between raw exercise ECGs and a running average of the heartbeats [1]. The noise contribution to the VCG is synthesized from the 12-lead noise records. In Figure 8.19 lead X of a simulated VCG is displayed during different stages of a stress test. The simulation procedure is summarized in Figure 8.20.

This simulation study has been used to evaluate the performance of the methods based on the multilead QRS area and the QRS-VCG loop alignment in estimating the respiratory frequency from the ECG [28]. An estimation error of 0.002±0.001 Hz (0.5±0.2%) is achieved by QRS-VCG loop alignment while an error of 0.005±0.004 Hz (1.0±0.7%) is achieved by multilead QRS area. The mean and the standard deviation of the estimated respiratory frequency by both approaches are displayed in Figure 8.21.

This simulation study is not useful for evaluating EDR algorithms based on HR information (Section 8.3) since respiratory influence only affects beat morphology but not beat occurrence time. However, it can be easily upgraded to include respiration effect on HR. For example, HR trends can be generated by an AR model like those in Figure 8.12 whose HF peak is driven by respiratory frequency.

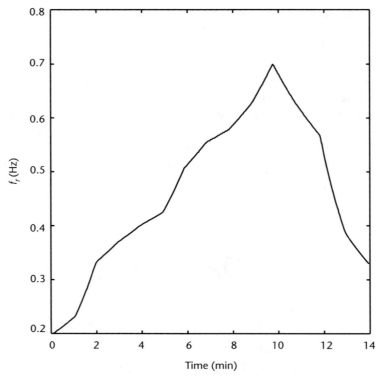

Figure 8.18   Simulated respiratory frequency pattern.

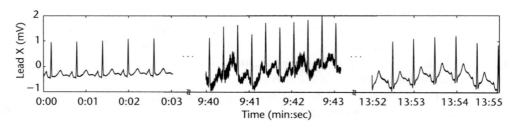

Figure 8.19   Simulated ECG signal at onset, peak exercise, and end of a stress test.

The above simulation designs can be seen as particular cases of a generalized simulation used to evaluate EDR algorithms based on beat morphology (single- or multilead) and EDR algorithms based on HR. First, beat templates are generated, either from a model [42] or from real ECGs [28]. The simulated ECG signals result from concatenation of beat templates following RR interval series with power spectrum such that the HF peak is driven by respiratory frequency. Long-term variations of QRS morphology unrelated to respiration and due to physiological conditions such as ischemia can be added to the simulated ECG signals. The respiratory influence on beat morphology is introduced by simulating the rotation of the heart's electrical axis induced by respiration. Finally, noise is generated either from a model [42] or from real ECGs [28] and added to the simulated ECGs. The generalized simulation design is summarized in Figure 8.22.

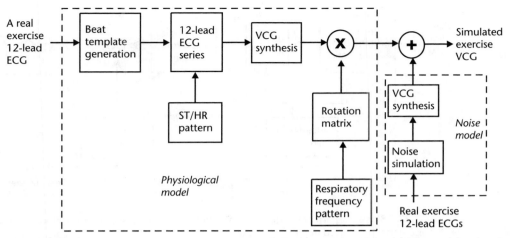

Figure 8.20 Block diagram of the simulation design. Note that the 12-lead ECGs used for signal and noise generation are different.

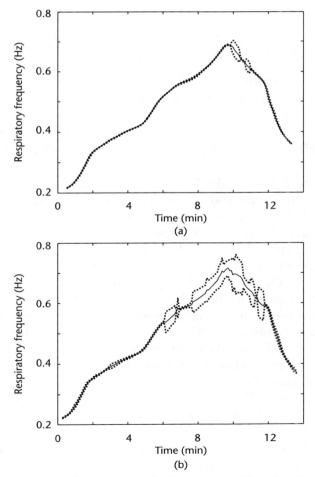

Figure 8.21 The mean respiratory frequency (solid line) ± the SD (dotted line) estimated in the simulation study using (a) QRS-VCG loop alignment and (b) multilead QRS area approaches.

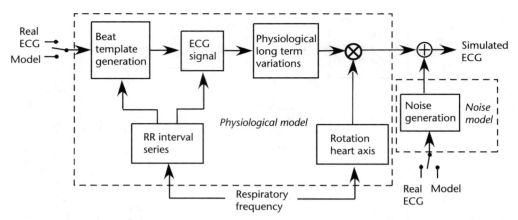

Figure 8.22 Block diagram of the generalized simulation design. Note that the ECGs used for signal and noise generation are different.

8.7 Conclusions

In this chapter, several EDR algorithms have been presented which estimate a respiratory signal from the ECG. They have been divided into three categories:

1. EDR algorithms based on beat morphology, namely, those based on ECG wave amplitude, on multilead QRS area, and on QRS-VCG loop alignment (Section 8.2);
2. EDR algorithms based on HR information (Section 8.3);
3. EDR algorithms based on both beat morphology and HR (Section 8.4).

The choice of a particular EDR algorithm depends on the application. In general, EDR algorithms based on beat morphology are more accurate than EDR algorithms based on HR information, since the modulation of HRV by respiration is sometimes lost or embedded in other parasympathetic interactions.

Amplitude EDR algorithms have been reported to perform satisfactorily when only single-lead ECGs are available, as is usually the case in sleep apnea monitoring [14, 17, 18, 20, 21, 32]. When multilead ECGs are available, EDR algorithms based on either multilead QRS area or QRS-VCG loop alignment are preferable. The reason is that due to thorax anisotropy and its intersubject variability together with the intersubject electrical axis variability, respiration influences ECG leads in different ways; the direction of the electrical axis, containing multilead information, is likely to better reflect the effect of respiration than wave amplitudes of a single lead. In stationary situations, both multilead QRS area or QRS-VCG loop alignment EDR algorithms estimate a reliable respiratory signal from the ECG [5, 22]. However, in nonstationary situations, such as in stress testing, the QRS-VCG loop alignment approach is preferred over the multilead QRS area [28]. Electrocardiogram-derived respiration algorithms based on both beat morphology and HR may be appropriate when only a single-lead ECG is available and the respiration effect on that lead is not pronounced [30]. The power spectra of the EDR signals based on morphology and HR can be cross-correlated to reduce spurious peaks and enhance the respiratory frequency. However, the likelihood of having an EDR signal with pronounced respiration modulation is better when the signal is derived from multilead ECGs; cross-correlation with the HR power spectrum may in those situations worsen the results due to poor respiratory HR modulation [22].

There are still certain topics in the EDR field which deserve further study. One is the robustness of the EDR algorithms in different physiological conditions. In this chapter, robustness to long-term QRS morphologic variations due to, for example, ischemia, has been addressed. The study of nonunimodal respiratory patterns should be considered when estimating the respiratory frequency from the ECG by techniques like, for example, spectral coherence. Finally, one of the motivations and future challenges in the EDR field is the study of the cardio-respiratory coupling and its potential value in the evaluation of the autonomic nervous system activity.

References

[1]   Bailón, R., et al., "Coronary Artery Disease Diagnosis Based on Exercise Electrocardiogram Indexes from Repolarisation, Depolarisation and Heart Rate Variability," *Med. Biol. Eng. Comput.*, Vol. 41, 2003, pp. 561–571.

[2]   Einthoven, W., G. Fahr, and A. Waart, "On the Direction and Manifest Size of the Variations of Potential in the Human Heart and on the Influence of the Position of the Heart on the Form of the Electrocardiogram," *Am. Heart J.*, Vol. 40, 1950, pp. 163–193.

[3]   Flaherty, J., et al., "Influence of Respiration on Recording Cardiac Potentials," *Am. J. Cardiol.*, Vol. 20, 1967, pp. 21–28.

[4]   Riekkinen, H., and P., Rautaharju, "Body Position, Electrode Level and Respiration Effects on the Frank Lead Electrocardiogram," *Circ.*, Vol. 53, 1976, pp. 40–45.

[5]   ...rivation of Respiratory Signals from Multi-Lead ECGs," *Proc.* ..., IEEE Computer Society Press, 1986, pp. 113–116.

[6]   ...ntjes, "Respiratory Sinus Arrhythmia and Parasympathetic Car... Issues Concerning Quantification, Applications and Implica... Janssen, and D. Vaitl, (eds.), *Cardiorespiratory and Cardioso...* w York: Plenum Press, 1986, pp. 117–138.

[7]   ... Response Curve Analysis of Heart Rate Variability," *IEEE* ... 1997, pp. 321–325.

[8]   ...Balagué, and F. Rosell, "The Effect of Respiration-Induced ...G," *IEEE Trans. Biomed. Eng.*, Vol. 36, No. 6, 1989,

[9]   ...nalysis with Applications*, Englewood Cliffs, NJ: Prentice-Hall ...

[10] ...A Model to Estimate Respiration from Vectorcardiogram ...d. Eng.*, Vol. 2, 1974, pp. 47–57.

[11] ... Vergani, "Detection of Electrical Axis Variation for the ...ormation," *Proc. Computers in Cardiology*, IEEE Computer ...-502.

[12] Zhao, L., S. Reisman, ... Findley, "Derivation of Respiration from Electrocardiogram During Heart Rate Variability Studies," *Proc. Computers in Cardiology*, IEEE Computer Society Press, 1994, pp. 53–56.

[13]   Caggiano, D., and S. Reisman, "Respiration Derived from the Electrocardiogram: A Quantitative Comparison of Three Different Methods," *Proc. of the IEEE 22nd Ann. Northeast Bioengineering Conf.*, IEEE Press, 1996, pp. 103–104.

[14]   Dobrev, D., and I. Daskalov, "Two-Electrode Telemetric Instrument for Infant Heart Rate and Apnea Monitoring," *Med. Eng. Phys.*, Vol. 20, 1998, pp. 729–734.

[15]   Travaglini, A., et al., "Respiratory Signal Derived from Eight-Lead ECG," *Proc. Computers in Cardiology*, Vol. 25, IEEE Press, 1998, pp. 65–68.

[16]   Nazeran, H., et al., "Reconstruction of Respiratory Patterns from Electrocardiographic Signals," *Proc. 2nd Int. Conf. Bioelectromagnetism*, IEEE Press, 1998, pp. 183–184.

[17]   Raymond, B., et al., "Screening for Obstructive Sleep Apnoea Based on the Electrocardiogram—The Computers in Cardiology Challenge," *Proc. Computers in Cardiology*, Vol. 27, IEEE Press, 2000, pp. 267–270.

[18]   Mason, C., and L. Tarassenko, "Quantitative Assessment of Respiratory Derivation Algorithms," *Proc. 23rd Ann. IEEE EMBS Int. Conf.*, Istanbul, Turkey, 2001, pp. 1998–2001.

[19]   Behbehani, K., et al., "An Investigation of the Mean Electrical Axis Angle and Respiration During Sleep," *Proc. 2nd Joint EMBS/BMES Conf.*, Houston, TX, 2002, pp. 1550–1551.

[20]   Yi, W., and K. Park, "Derivation of Respiration from ECG Measured Without Subject's Awareness Using Wavelet Transform," *Proc. 2nd Joint EMBS/BMES Conf.*, Houston, TX, 2002, pp. 130–131.

[21]   Chazal, P., et al., "Automated Processing of Single-Lead Electrocardiogram for the Detection of Obstructive Sleep Apnoea," *IEEE Trans. Biomed. Eng.*, Vol. 50, No. 6, 2003, pp. 686–696.

[22]   Leanderson, S., P. Laguna, and L. Sörnmo, "Estimation of the Respiratory Frequency Using Spatial Information in the VCG," *Med. Eng. Phys.*, Vol. 25, 2003, pp. 501–507.

[23]   Bianchi, A., et al., "Estimation of the Respiratory Activity from Orthogonal ECG Leads," *Proc. Computers in Cardiology*, Vol. 30, IEEE Press, 2003, pp. 85–88.

[24]   Yoshimura, T., et al., "An ECG Electrode-Mounted Heart Rate, Respiratory Rhythm, Posture and Behavior Recording System," *Proc. 26th Ann. IEEE EMBS Int. Conf.*, Vol. 4, IEEE Press, 2004, pp. 2373–2374.

[25]   Pilgram, B., and M. Renzo, "Estimating Respiratory Rate from Instantaneous Frequencies of Long Term Heart Rate Tracings," *Proc. Computers in Cardiology*, IEEE Computer Society Press, 1993, pp. 859–862.

[26]   Varanini, M., et al., "Spectral Analysis of Cardiovascular Time Series by the S-Transform," *Proc. Computers in Cardiology*, Vol. 24, IEEE Press, 1997, pp. 383–386.

[27]   Meste, O., G. Blain, and S. Bermon, "Analysis of the Respiratory and Cardiac Systems Coupling in Pyramidal Exercise Using a Time-Varying Model," *Proc. Computers in Cardiology*, Vol. 29, IEEE Press, 2002, pp. 429–432.

[28]   Bailón, R., L. Sörnmo, and P. Laguna, "A Robust Method for ECG-Based Estimation of the Respiratory Frequency During Stress Testing," *IEEE Trans. Biomed. Eng.*, Vol. 53, No. 7, 2006, pp. 1273–1285.

[29]   Thayer, J., et al., "Estimating Respiratory Frequency from Autoregressive Spectral Analysis of Heart Period," *IEEE Eng. Med. Biol.*, Vol. 21, No. 4, 2002, pp. 41–45.

[30]   Varanini, M., et al., "Adaptive Filtering of ECG Signal for Deriving Respiratory Activity," *Proc. Computers in Cardiology*, IEEE Computer Society Press, 1990, pp. 621–624.

[31]   Edenbrandt, L., and O. Pahlm, "Vectorcardiogram Synthesized from a 12-Lead ECG: Superiority of the Inverse Dower Matrix," *J. Electrocardiol.*, Vol. 21, No. 4, 1988, pp. 361–367.

[32] Mazzanti, B., C. Lamberti, and J. de Bie, "Validation of an ECG-Derived Respiration Monitoring Method," *Proc. Computers in Cardiology*, Vol. 30, IEEE Press, 2003, pp. 613–616.

[33] Pinciroli, F., et al., "Remarks and Experiments on the Construction of Respiratory Waveforms from Electrocardiographic Tracings," *Comput. Biomed. Res.*, Vol. 19, 1986, pp. 391–409.

[34] Sörnmo, L., "Vectorcardiographic Loop Alignment and Morphologic Beat-to-Beat Variability," *IEEE Trans. Biomed. Eng.*, Vol. 45, No. 12, 1998, pp. 1401–1413.

[35] Åström, M., et al., "Detection of Body Position Changes Using the Surface ECG," *Med. Biol. Eng. Comput.*, Vol. 41, No. 2, 2003, pp. 164–171.

[36] Sörnmo, L., and P. Laguna, *Bioelectrical Signal Processing in Cardiac and Neurological Applications*, Amsterdam: Elsevier (Academic Press), 2005.

[37] Mateo, J., and P. Laguna, "Analysis of Heart Rate Variability in the Presence of Ectopic Beats Using the Heart Timing Signal," *IEEE Trans. Biomed. Eng.*, Vol. 50, 2003, pp. 334–343.

[38] Lomb, N. R., "Least-Squares Frequency Analysis of Unequally Spaced Data," *Astrophys. Space Sci.*, Vol. 39, 1976, pp. 447–462.

[39] Mainardi, L., et al., "Pole-Tracking Algorithms for the Extraction of Time-Variant Heart Rate Variability Spectral Parameters," *IEEE Trans. Biomed. Eng.*, Vol. 42, No. 3, 1995, pp. 250–258.

[40] de Prony, G., "Essai expérimental et analytique: sur les lois de la dilatabilité de fluides élastiques et sur celles de la force expansive de la vapeur de l'eau et de la vapeur de l'alkool, à différentes températures," *J. E. Polytech.*, Vol. 1, No. 2, 1795, pp. 24–76.

[41] Rao, B., and K. Arun, "Model Based Processing of Signals: A State Space Approach," *Proc. IEEE*, Vol. 80, No. 2, 1992, pp. 283–306.

[42] McSharry, P., et al., "A Dynamical Model for Generating Synthetic Electrocardiogram Signals," *IEEE Trans. Biomed. Eng.*, Vol. 50, No. 3, 2003, pp. 289–294.

[43] Åström, M., et al., "Vectorcardiographic Loop Alignment and the Measurement of Morphologic Beat-to-Beat Variability in Noisy Signals," *IEEE Trans. Biomed. Eng.*, Vol. 47, No. 4, 2000, pp. 497–506.

[44] Dower, G., H. Machado, and J. Osborne, "On Deriving the Electrocardiogram from Vectorcardiographic Leads," *Clin. Cardiol.*, Vol. 3, 1980, pp. 87–95.

[45] Frank, E., "The Image Surface of a Homogeneous Torso," *Am. Heart J.*, Vol. 47, 1954, pp. 757–768.

Appendix 8A Vectorcardiogram Synthesis from the 12-Lead ECG

Although several methods have been proposed for synthesizing the VCG from the 12-lead ECG, the inverse transformation matrix of Dower is the most commonly used [31]. Dower et al. presented a method for deriving the 12-lead ECG from Frank lead VCG [44]. Each ECG lead is calculated as a weighted sum of the VCG leads X, Y, and Z using lead-specific coefficients based on the image surface data from the original torso studies by Frank [45]. The transformation operation used to derive the eight independent leads (V1 to V6, I and II) of the 12-lead ECG from the VCG leads is given by

$$s(n) = Dv(n), \quad D = \begin{bmatrix} -0.515 & 0.157 & -0.917 \\ 0.044 & 0.164 & -1.387 \\ 0.882 & 0.098 & -1.277 \\ 1.213 & 0.127 & -0.601 \\ 1.125 & 0.127 & -0.086 \\ 0.831 & 0.076 & 0.230 \\ 0.632 & -0.235 & 0.059 \\ 0.235 & 1.066 & -0.132 \end{bmatrix} \tag{8A.1}$$

where $s(n) = [V_1(n) \ V_2(n) \ V_3(n) \ V_4(n) \ V_5(n) \ V_6(n) \ I(n) \ II(n)]^T$ and $v(n) = [X(n) \ Y(n) \ Z(n)]^T$ contain the voltages of the corresponding leads, n denotes the sample index, and D is called the Dower transformation matrix. From (8A.1) it follows that the VCG leads can be synthesized from the 12-lead ECG by

$$v(n) = Ts(n) \tag{8A.2}$$

where $T = (D^T D)^{-1} D^T$ is called the inverse Dower transformation matrix and given by

$$T = \begin{bmatrix} -0.172 & -0.074 & 0.122 & 0.231 & 0.239 & 0.194 & 0.156 & -0.010 \\ 0.057 & -0.019 & -0.106 & -0.022 & 0.041 & 0.048 & -0.227 & 0.887 \\ -0.229 & -0.310 & -0.246 & -0.063 & 0.055 & 0.108 & 0.022 & 0.102 \end{bmatrix} \tag{8A.3}$$

CHAPTER 9

Introduction to Feature Extraction

Franc Jager

In this chapter we describe general signal processing techniques that robustly generate diagnostic and morphologic feature-vector time series of ECG. These techniques allow efficient, accurate, and robust extraction, representation, monitoring, examination, and characterization of ECG diagnostic and morphologic features. In particular, an emphasis is made on the efficient and accurate automated analysis of transient ST segment changes. Traditional time-domain approaches and an orthonormal function model approach using principal components are explored.

9.1 Overview of Feature Extraction Phases

Figure 9.1 shows typical ECG data from an ambulatory ECG (AECG) record. A transient ST segment episode compatible with ischemia (ischemic ST episode) begins in the second part of the third data segment shown. Two abnormal beats can be observed in the final strip. In the field of arrhythmia detection, we are mostly interested in the global beat morphology (i.e., normal or abnormal morphology). However, in the field of ST segment change analysis, wave measurements and robust construction of ECG diagnostic and morphologic feature time series are of direct interest. Due to enormous amount of data in long-term AECG records, standard visual analysis of raw ECG waveforms does not readily permit assessment of the features that allow one to detect and classify QRS complexes, to analyze many types of transient ECG events, to distinguish ischemic from nonischemic ST changes, nor possibly to distinguish among ischemic and heart rate related ST change episodes. Questions concerning representation, characterization, monitoring, automatic analysis of ECG waveforms, and detection and differentiation of different types of transient ST segment events require the development of automated techniques. The major problems facing automated AECG record analysis include the nonstationary nature of diagnostic and morphologic feature time series and their unknown a priori distributions. Due to the frequent occurrence of severe noise contamination, random shifts, and other noisy outliers, robust automated techniques to estimate heartbeat diagnostic and morphologic features are necessary.

The representation of M-dimensional ECG *pattern vectors*, x (e.g., QRS complexes, ST segments, or any other set of consecutive original ECG signal samples), in terms of a set of a few features or numerical parameters, is a critical step in automated ECG analysis. The aim of such a feature (or parameter) extraction technique is to properly modify data according to the context of the specific problem at hand for the purposes of automated analysis. Since the information content of a set of

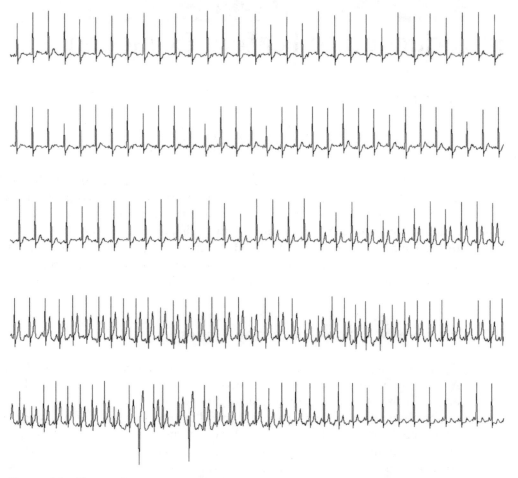

Figure 9.1 Five contiguous segments of a single lead of an ambulatory ECG record. A transient ischemic ST segment episode begins in the second part of the third data segment, notable by the sudden increase in T-wave amplitude. Two abnormal heartbeats can also be observed in the final segment.

signal samples that constitutes a pattern vector usually far exceeds what is necessary for the analysis, the feature extraction techniques reduce the data dimensionality yielding an N-dimensional, $N < M$, *feature vector*, $\mathbf{y}$, whose components are termed *features*. Feature vectors of a reduced dimension allow efficient implementation of techniques to detect and classify QRS complexes, and to distinguish transient ischemic from nonischemic ST changes. A commonly used approach for the task of feature extraction involves heuristic descriptors such as the QRS wave amplitude, duration, and area, or the ST segment level, slope, and area. However, classification techniques based on heuristic features are known to be more vulnerable to noise. Since proper selection of the features is of key importance when reducing the dimensionality of the feature space, without discarding significant information, suitable feature extraction techniques that derive formal features are required. An example of such a method is the orthonormal function model (OFM) [1]. Due to the orthogonality of the basis functions of the OFM, each feature contains independent information (in a second-order sense) and the ECG pattern vectors can be represented with low dimensional feature vectors.

In this chapter, we focus on efficient techniques to extract ECG diagnostic and morphologic features that allow one to detect transient ST segment episodes and to differentiate them from nonischemic ST segment changes. Traditional time-domain metrics are presented that permit quantitative measurement of ECG pattern vectors in conventional terms and have proved to be useful to represent, characterize, and detect transient ST segment changes of automatically derived conventional time-domain ECG variables plotted in high temporal trend format, which allows retrospective identification of beginnings and ends of transient ST episodes [2], proved to be superior (sensitivity of 100%, positive predictivity of 100%) to conventional visual scrutiny of raw ECG signals (sensitivity of 82.5%, positive predictivity of 95.7%), and proved to be suitable for quantification of transient ST segment episodes. However, ST segment morphology changes may not be apparent on the basis of these conventional differential (level or slope) measurements. The OFM approach using principal components, or the Karhunen-Loève

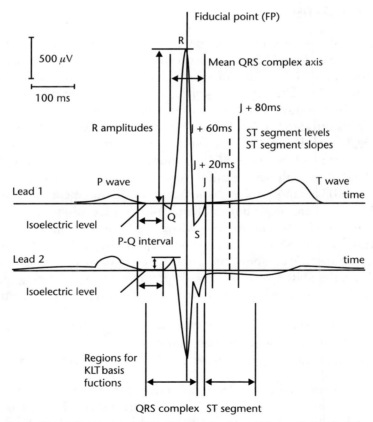

Figure 9.2 A heartbeat of a two-lead ECG with amplitudes and intervals required to estimate ECG diagnostic and morphologic features.

transform (KLT) representation is an alternative approach and is also presented in this chapter.

Figure 9.2 illustrates a normal heartbeat of ECG with important ECG diagnostic and morphologic features relevant to the analysis of transient ST segment changes. While time-domain ST segment feature vectors provide direct and easy measurement of raw ST segment pattern vectors, the KLT-based QRS complex and ST segment morphology feature vectors provide efficient feature extraction, high representational power of subtle morphology features, differentiation between nonnoisy and noisy events, and differentiation between transient ischemic and nonischemic ST segment events.

A general system for robust estimation of transient heartbeat diagnostic and morphologic feature-vector time series in long-term ECGs for the purpose of ST segment analysis may involve following phases:

1. Preprocessing;
2. Derivation of time-domain and OFM transform-based diagnostic and morphologic feature vectors;
3. Shape representation in terms of feature-vector time series.

9.2 Preprocessing

In general, the aim of the preprocessing steps is to improve the signal-to-noise ratio (SNR) of the ECG for more accurate analysis and measurement. Noises may disturb the ECG to such an extent that measurements from the original signals are unreliable. The main categories of noise are: low-frequency baseline wander caused by respiration and body movements, high-frequency random noises caused by mains interference (50 Hz, 60 Hz) and muscular activity, and random shifts of the ECG signal amplitude caused by poor electrode contact and body movements. The spectrum of the noise can be randomly spread over the entire ECG spectrum. In the field of arrhythmia detection, we are mostly interested in the global (normal or abnormal) beat morphology, whereas wave measurements are not of direct interest. Robust classical deterministic digital filtering techniques are mostly used. In the domain of ST segment analysis where accurate wave measurements are the main features of interest, filtering must not disturb the fine structure of the useful signal. Since the spectral components of noise overlap those of the ECG, it is not possible to improve the SNR solely by using deterministic digital filtering techniques, and advanced nonlinear techniques are required. The preprocessing comprises three steps:

1. QRS complex detection and beat classification;
2. Removal of high-frequency noise;
3. Removal of baseline wander (elimination of very low frequencies).

The main tasks of a QRS complex detector include detecting QRS complexes of heartbeats in single or multilead ECG signal and generating a stable fiducial point for each individual heartbeat, $FP(i, j)$, where i denotes the ECG lead number and j denotes the heartbeat number. The fiducial point of jth heartbeat is desired to be unique for all ECG leads, $FP(j)$, and its placement should be robust and insensitive to subtle morphological variability in the QRS complex. In the literature, there are some excellent QRS complex detectors presented [3–7]. The characteristic of a robust fiducial point is its placement in the QRS's "center of mass." In the case of biphasic QRS complex, it should be placed close to the more significant deflection, while in the case of monophasic QRS complex, it should be placed close to a peak of the QRS complex. A stable fiducial point in each heartbeat is a prerequisite for the automatic identification of the isoelectric levels, calculation of QRS complex and ST segment diagnostic and morphologic feature vectors, and time averaging of pattern vectors. Accurate beat classification which distinguishes between normal and abnormal heartbeats is necessary. Furthermore, erroneous QRS complex waveforms and atypical ST-T waves of abnormal beats may result in erroneous wave measurements. Therefore, abnormal beats have to be accurately detected and rejected.

Butterworth 4-pole or 6-pole lowpass digital filters [8] with a cutoff frequency from 45 to 55 Hz appear to be acceptable for rejecting high-frequency noises in the ECG. A smooth frequency characteristic of the filter in the passband and in the cutoff region is desirable. The distortion of output signal due to nonlinear phase of the filter at higher frequencies is not significant, and does not affect ST level measurements.

Baseline wander results in erroneous measurements of the ST segment level (which is measured relative to isoelectric level estimated in the PQ segment). It has been shown [9] that baseline wander can be filtered using a highpass linear phase digital filter with a cutoff frequency up to 0.8 Hz. A cutoff frequency above 0.8 Hz would distort any relatively long interval between the PQ interval and the ST segment. Nonlinear phase-response digital filters with similar frequency characteristics require far fewer coefficients but do lead to ST segment distortion. The large number of coefficients in a linear phase digital filter required to achieve an acceptable frequency response, together with the fact that the spectral components of baseline wander often extend above 0.8 Hz, suggest the use of a nonlinear cubic spline approximation (polynomial fit) and subtraction technique [10, 11] that does not significantly distort P-QRS-ST cycle. A third-order polynomial fit and subtraction technique to correct the baseline requires three reference points: baseline estimates (nodes) of two subsequent heartbeats in addition to the baseline estimate of the current heartbeat. Nodes are chosen typically from the PQ segment, which is also used for an estimate of the isoelectric level and is close to the fiducial point of each beat. The establishing of such stable reference points one beat-by-beat basis in the PQ segment must be reliable and accurate. This procedure is crucial since further procedures of baseline wander removal, ST segment level measurement and the derivation of the KLT-based QRS complex and ST segment morphology feature vectors depend on the accurate estimation of the isoelectric level.

Next, a reliable and accurate example of such a procedure (developed in [12]) to locate the PQ segment and to estimate the isoelectric level is described. This method was successfully used in a KLT-based system to detect transient ST change episodes [13] and during the development of the long-term ST database (LTST DB) [14], a standard reference for assessing the quality of AECG analyzers. The procedure appears to be reliable and accurate and is illustrated in Figure 9.3. The procedure uses a priori knowledge of the form of the ECG heartbeat morphology.

Constants:

f_{samp}:   Sampling frequency
ΔT $=$ $1/f_{samp}$; Time step
T_Q: Interval to search for Q peak (60 ms)
QS $=$ $T_Q / \Delta T$; Samples to search for Q peak
T_{PQ}:   Interval to search for PQ segment (80 ms)
PQS $=$ $T_{PQ} / \Delta T$;Samples to search for PQ
T_f: Flatness interval (20 ms)
L $=$ $T_f / \Delta T$; Samples for flatness interval

Input:

i :   Lead number
j :   Heart-beat number
$FP(j)$:   Fiducial point [ms]
$x(i,.)$:   ECG signal samples [μV]

Output:

$I(i,j)$:   Position of the isoelectric point [ms]
$z(i,j)$:   Estimated isoelectric level [μV]

procedure pq_segment($I(i,j)$, $z(i,j)$);

k $=$ $FP(j) / \Delta T$;
sp $=$ sign $(x(i, k - 2) - x(i, k))$;
k $=$ $k - 2$;
s $=$ sign $(x(i, k - 1) - x(i, k))$;
while $(s \neq 0) \wedge (s = sp) \wedge (FP(j)/\Delta T - k < QS)$ **do**

  sp $=$ s ;
  k $=$ $k - 1$;
  s $=$ sign $(x(i, k - 1) - x(i, k))$;

enddo

k $=$ $k - 2$;
$z(i,j)$ $=$ $\frac{1}{L} \sum_{l=-L/2}^{L/2} x(i, k + l)$;
$I(i,j)$ $=$ $k \cdot \Delta T$;
$minabsdev$ $=$ $\sum_{l=-L/2}^{L/2} | x(i, k + l) - z(i,j) |$;

for $m = k - 1$ **downto** $k - PQS + 2$ **do**

  $mean$ $=$ $\frac{1}{L} \sum_{l=-L/2}^{L/2} x(i, m + l)$
  $absdev$ $=$ $\sum_{l=-L/2}^{L/2} | x(i, m + l) - mean |$;
  if $absdev < minabsdev$ **then**

    $z(i,j)$ $=$ $mean$;
    $I(i,j)$ $=$ $m \, \Delta T$;
    $minabsdev$ $=$ $absdev$;

  endif

enddo

end_procedure

Figure 9.3   Procedure to locate PQ segment and to estimate the isoelectric level. $FP(j)$ is the fiducial point for jth heartbeat and $x(i, k)$ denote the sequence of original signal samples in ith ECG lead. $I(i, j)$ is the position of the isoelectric reference point found in the PQ segment, and $z(i, j)$ is the estimated isoelectric level.

The procedure first searches backwards from fiducial point $FP(j)$ located by a QRS detector, for up to $T_Q = 60$ ms, for a sample in which the slope of the waveform equals zero or changes sign. The endpoint of the search may be the R peak, the Q peak, or the end of the PQ segment, depending on the type of the QRS complex (monophasic or biphasic) and on the position of the fiducial point. If such a sample is not found, searching ends at the last sample. From this point, the procedure searches backwards for the "flattest" $T_f = 20$ ms segment within the $T_{PQ} = 80$ ms. For this purpose, the mean absolute deviation of each segment from its own mean is determined, and the segment for which this value is minimum is judged the flattest or the PQ interval. The middle sample of this flattest waveform segment found in each ECG lead defines the position of the isoelectric reference point, $I(i, j)$, while the mean amplitude of this flattest segment is taken as an estimate of the isoelectric level, $z(i, j)$.

9.3 Derivation of Diagnostic and Morphologic Feature Vectors

In this section we will explore methods for the derivation of diagnostic and morphologic features that are necessary to represent, characterize, detect, and differentiate transient ischemic and nonischemic ST segment changes.

9.3.1 Derivation of Orthonormal Function Model Transform–Based Morphology Feature Vectors

The OFM is an attractive and powerful general approach to the feature extraction and shape-representation process if the probability densities of population of pattern vectors of a problem domain are unknown. Among the classes of orthonormal transforms, the principal component transform (i.e., the KLT) is theoretically optimal (in a least-square sense) in terms of separating signal from noise. Consider an ECG pattern vector (e.g., QRS complex or ST segment pattern vector of a given dimension). It is desirable to reduce data dimensionality to effect a noise filter while retaining the information related to the useful signal. Representing ECG morphology by coefficients of the KLT results in robust estimates of a few descriptive signal parameters, accurate representation of normal and deviating ECG pattern vectors by exposing subtle features of pattern vectors, good approximation properties that facilitate distinguishing between noisy and clean events, and good discrimination of waveforms with different morphology. The use of principal component analysis in ECG signal analysis has included compression, filtering and QRS complex classification [15], visual identification of acute ischemic episodes [16], shape representation of the ECG morphology [15, 17], automated detection of transient ST segment episodes during AECG monitoring [13], and analysis of the cardiac repolarization period (ST-T complex) [18, 19].

9.3.1.1 The Karhunen-Loève Transform

The KLT is an operation through which a nonperiodic random process can be expanded over a series of orthonormal functions with uncorrelated features. Theoretical basis of the KLT may be found in [1, 20, 21]. A short description of KLT is given in Appendix 9A. The KLT is optimal in the sense that the expected least mean squared error (MSE) obtained by approximating a given pattern of a random process using any given number of the first few coefficients is minimal in comparison to other suboptimal transforms.

The residual error of a truncated KLT is an optimal estimate of noise content. Note that this property holds only in the sense of expected MSE. The actual error of the approximation for a given sample pattern vector $\mathbf{x} = (x_1, x_2, \ldots, x_M)^T$ where M is dimension of pattern vectors, is not necessarily minimal, but can be greater.

This is particularly true for those pattern vectors that were poorly represented in the sample population from which the covariance matrix, $\mathbf{R}$, of pattern vectors $\{\mathbf{x}\}$ was calculated when performing a KLT. Let us assume the existence of a few pattern classes. Intervals of ECG signals containing nonischemic or ischemic ST segment episodes, or intervals of ECG signals containing no significant ST deviations, can be considered as intervals containing pattern vectors (QRS complexes and ST segments of heartbeats) that belong to different pattern classes. Therefore, our random patterns $\{\mathbf{x}\}$ may originate from more than one source. The origin of the "incoming" pattern vectors $\mathbf{x}_l$, where l denotes the lth pattern class, is not known (except during the "training" phase), so the condition for the KLT expansion to yield optimal results [i.e., the expected mean of centralized observations, $E(\mathbf{x}_l - \boldsymbol{\mu}_l) = 0$, where $\boldsymbol{\mu}_l$ is the lth class mean] cannot be satisfied. This condition is satisfied if the various pattern classes are characterized by zero means. If this condition is not satisfied, only suboptimal results may be expected. It seems that this problem may be overcome by centralizing the patterns of each class with regard to their means, but the origin of the patterns is unknown (except during the training phase). Besides, centralizing the patterns of the training set with regard to their means would imply altering the characteristics of the pattern classes under consideration. The special case, in which all pattern classes possess identical means, regardless of their origin, does not in any way guarantee optimal results either, but does utilize information on the class means and class variances [21].

Modeling of the distribution of pattern vectors $\{\mathbf{x}\}$ and estimating of eigenvectors is also complicated by the presence of noisy patterns. Derived eigenvectors would be sensitive to noisy pattern vectors, if such noisy outliers were members of a distribution modeled by a covariance matrix. Furthermore, other feature vectors may be confined closely together in the feature space and their correlation coefficient would be undesirably high.

To avoid the problem of suboptimal approximation of sample pattern vectors, and to avoid the problem of noisy patterns, it is appropriate to use kernel-approximation method [22, 23] by which we replace pattern classes by their means, and to exclude noisy outliers. Using these two approaches, the covariance matrix can be written in the following form:

$$\mathbf{R} = E\left\{(\mathbf{x} - \boldsymbol{\mu}_0)(\mathbf{x} - \boldsymbol{\mu}_0)^T\right\} = \sum_{l=1}^{L} p(\omega_l) E\left\{(\overline{\mathbf{x}}_l - \boldsymbol{\mu}_0)(\overline{\mathbf{x}}_l - \boldsymbol{\mu}_0)^T\right\} \qquad (9.1)$$

where $\overline{\mathbf{x}}_l$ is the lth class mean, $p(\omega_l)$ is a priori probability of the occurrence of the lth class, and the mean vector $\boldsymbol{\mu}_0$ is defined as

$$\boldsymbol{\mu}_0 = E\{\mathbf{x}\} \qquad \forall \mathbf{x} \qquad (9.2)$$

Input pattern classes are thus replaced by their means, and centralized over all classes by subtracting the mean vector obtained over all classes. The eigenvalues of the covariance matrix $\mathbf{R}$ are functions of the means of each class. Such a single mean multiclass approach retains means and therefore utilizes the spatial distribution of individual classes, while exclusion of noisy outliers yields a robust covariance matrix.

If the KLT is applied to the pattern vector $\mathbf{x}$ with means included, then a new feature vector $\mathbf{y}$ is obtained

$$\mathbf{y} = \Phi^T \mathbf{x} \tag{9.3}$$

where Φ is the matrix of KLT basis functions (i.e., the matrix of eigenvectors of the covariance matrix $\mathbf{R}$). Components of such a feature vector $\mathbf{y}$ are termed KLT coefficients. The eigenvalues ψ_m of the covariance matrix of the new feature vectors $\{\mathbf{y}\}$ are then the variances σ_m^2 of these new features,

$$\psi_m = \sigma_m^2 = \sum_{l=1}^{L} p(\omega_l) E \left\{ (y_{lm} - (v_{lm} + v_{0m}))^2 \right\} \tag{9.4}$$

where v_{lm} is the transformed mean of the feature y_{lm} [i.e., the mth component of the transformed mean $\mu_l = E(\mathbf{x}_l - \mu_0)$ of the pattern vectors $\mathbf{x}_l$ from the lth class relative to the overall mean μ_0], and v_{0m} is the mth component of the transformed mean μ_0 of the overall set of pattern vectors $\{\mathbf{x}\}$.

9.3.1.2   Feature Selection

Since transient nonischemic ST segment changes can be efficiently differentiated from real ischemic ST changes by tracking the QRS complex morphology changes independently from the ST segment morphology changes, it is appropriate to derive two sets of KLT basis functions, one from the data window covering the PQ segment and QRS complex, and the other from the data window covering the ST segment and the initial portion of the T wave (see Figure 9.2). QRS complex and ST segment pattern vectors typically show interrecord and intrarecord variability due to the presence of noise. To avoid problems with the distribution of means of pattern classes and noisy outliers, it is appropriate during the training phase to derive robust covariance matrices according to (9.1) with noisy outliers excluded.

We now describe the derivation of such KLT basis functions [12] that were used in [13, 14]. The KLT basis functions were derived using all the records of the European Society of Cardiology ST-T Database (ESC DB) [24], the first standard reference database for assessing the quality of ST segment and T wave change analyzers. To obtain the correct representative pattern vectors, $\{\mathbf{x}\}$, for covariance matrices, an accurately placed fiducial point and accurately estimated isoelectric level for each heartbeat were necessary. Approximately 800,000 heartbeats of the ESC DB were detected and classified using the Aristotle arrhythmia detector [4] of which fiducial point placement is robust and insensitive to subtle morphological variability of QRS complexes. To locate the PQ segment in each individual heartbeat and to estimate the isoelectric level, the procedure [12], described in Section 9.2, was used. For exclusion of noisy beats, time-domain noise detection procedures from [25] were used, and abnormal beats and their neighbors were discarded. The remaining heartbeats (744, 840) were used for computation of both covariance matrices. Then, all intervals of the records of the database containing nonischemic or ischemic ST episodes and corresponding intervals with no significant ST deviation were considered as separate classes of pattern vectors, $\mathbf{x}_l$, and their means, μ_l, and the a priori probabilities of their occurrence, $p(\omega_l)$, where l denotes the lth pattern class, were calculated. All the patterns, $\{\mathbf{x}\}$, were centralized over all classes by subtracting the mean vector, $\boldsymbol{\mu}_0$, obtained over all classes. The number of pattern classes N was 120 for the QRS complex and 605 for the ST segment covariance matrix with regard to nonischemic and ischemic ST episodes. Each set of KLT basis functions was derived over each of the two ECG leads using standard techniques (see Figure 9.2). The QRS complex basis functions start at the point 96 ms prior to the QRS center of mass, ARISTOTLE'S fiducial point (*FP*), and end at the point *FP*+24 ms. The set of ST segment basis functions covers the interval from *FP*+40 ms to *FP*+160 ms. Figure 9.4 shows the first eight QRS complex and ST segment KLT basis functions thus derived.

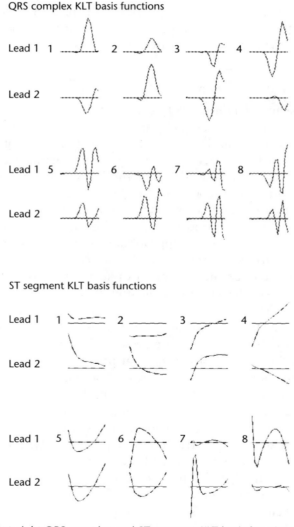

Figure 9.4 The first eight QRS complex and ST segment KLT basis functions plotted as a function of time. Each basis function expands over each of the ECG leads.

9.3.1.3   Estimation of Dimensionality of Feature Vectors

To estimate the necessary dimensionality of the QRS complex and the ST segment feature vectors, a useful approach is the calculation of the expected fractions of the remaining energy $\eta(N)$ (9A.15) when using the first N basis functions for approximation of patterns. The first five coefficients corresponding to the QRS complex and ST segment basis functions derived in Section 9.3.1.2 contribute approximately 93% and 97%, respectively, to the total expected power of approximation for the QRS and the ST basis function sets. To estimate the optimal number of KLT coefficients for distinguishing between noisy and clean patterns, a method originally introduced in [15] can be used. By this method, histograms of normalized residual errors of a truncated KLT for clean and noisy pattern vectors can be used as an estimate of separability between useful signal and noise. The normalized residual error $r_{\mathbf{x}}(N)$ for a given pattern $\mathbf{x}$, given N, is defined as

$$r_{\mathbf{x}}(N) = \frac{\|\widetilde{\mathbf{x}}_N - \mathbf{x}\|}{\|\mathbf{x}\|} \tag{9.5}$$

where $\widetilde{\mathbf{x}}_N$ is an approximated pattern. Table 9.1 summarizes such results as obtained in [13] for the QRS complex and ST segment basis functions derived in the previous subsection. In this study [13], the annotations of noisy heartbeats were taken those as performed by human expert annotators of the ESC DB and those as determined by a time-domain algorithms for noise detection from [25]. The average residual errors for clean, $\bar{r}_c(N)$, and noisy patterns, $\bar{r}_n(N)$, decrease as the dimensionality of approximation, N, increases. Besides, the average residual errors for clean patterns are lower than those for noisy ones. The differences in the average residual errors, $\Delta \bar{r}(N)$, increase for small values of N, but after that decrease beyond $N = 5$. We can conclude that five KLT coefficients for ST segment and five for the QRS complex are sufficient and necessary for separating between noisy and clean patterns and for accurately representing the features. The dimensionality of five for the QRS complex is the same as that estimated in [15].

9.3.1.4   Derivation of Morphology Feature Vectors

Tracking of a specific subset of the heartbeat morphology feature vectors over time may reveal changes corresponding to transient ischemic and nonischemic ST segment changes. An ST segment change analyzer would need to derive an n-dimensional QRS complex feature vector, $\mathbf{y}_{qrs}(j)$, where j is the beat number, and another n-dimensional ST segment feature vector, $\mathbf{y}_{st}(j)$, for each single isoelectric corrected heartbeat. Given the overall feature space, we consider a normal distribution of feature vectors. Recognition procedures of an ST change analyzer may use the Mahalanobis distance measure (normalized Euclidean distance measure) between feature vectors, $d(\mathbf{y}(j), \mathbf{y}(k))$, or squared Mahalanobis distance measure between feature vectors,

$$d^2(\mathbf{y}(j), \mathbf{y}(k)) = (\mathbf{y}(j) - \mathbf{y}(k))^T \mathbf{C}^{-1}(\mathbf{y}(j) - \mathbf{y}(k)) \tag{9.6}$$

where $\mathbf{C}^{-1}$ is the inverse of the covariance matrix of the KLT expansion coefficient vectors obtained during training. $\mathbf{C}^{-1}$ is a diagonal and symmetric matrix. Since the

Table 9.1 The Expected Fractions of the Remaining Energy for QRS Complex, $\eta_{qrs}(N)$, and ST Segment, $\eta_{st}(N)$, Pattern Vectors, Average Normalized Residual Errors for Clean, $\bar{r}_c(N)$, and Noisy, $\bar{r}_n(N)$, QRS Complex and ST Segment Patterns of the ESC DB When Using the First N Basis Functions for Approximation

Dimensionality on Approximation:									
N		1	2	3	4	5 ⇑	6	7	8
Expected Fractions of the Remaining Energy:									
$\eta_{qrs}(N)$	[%]	55	26	16	10	7	4	3	2
$\eta_{st}(N)$	[%]	58	26	13	5	3 ⇑	1	1	0
QRS Complex Patterns, Algorithm Annotator:									
$\bar{r}_c(N)$	[%]	53	22	14	9	6	5	4	3
$\bar{r}_n(N)$	[%]	54	23	16	11	9	7	6	5
$\Delta\bar{r}(N)$	[%]	1	1	2	2	3 ⇑	2	2	2
ST Segment Patterns, Algorithm Annotator:									
$\bar{r}_c(N)$	[%]	74	47	27	14	7	5	4	4
$\bar{r}_n(N)$	[%]	77	54	37	27	21	19	18	16
$\Delta\bar{r}(N)$	[%]	3	7	10	13	14 ⇑	14	14	12
ST Segment Patterns, Human Annotator:									
$\bar{r}_c(N)$	[%]	74	47	27	14	7	5	4	4
$\bar{r}_n(N)$	[%]	74	48	29	21	15	12	11	10
$\Delta\bar{r}(N)$	[%]	0	1	2	7	8 ⇑	7	7	6

coefficients in the KLT expansion vectors are statistically independent, then the off-diagonal elements of $\mathbf{C}^{-1}$ are zero. This means that each feature in $\mathbf{y}$ is normalized with the corresponding standard deviation such that its standard deviation ς is 1. This means that subtle features of pattern vectors corresponding to basis functions with lower standard deviations are emphasized. If $\mathbf{C}^{-1}$ was the identity matrix, d^2 would represent the squared Euclidean distance between the feature vectors and would be more sensitive to fluctuations in features with larger standard deviations. Furthermore, we set an assumption that the features are independent and normally distributed. This assumption yields that d^2 is distributed as χ_n^2 (i.e., a chi-squared random variable with n degrees of freedom). In the case when $n = 5$, the expected mean value, $m_{d^2}(n)$, of d^2 is $n\varsigma = 5$, and the expected standard deviation, $\sigma_{d^2}(n)$, of d^2 is $\sqrt{2n\varsigma} \approx 3.16$. Multiples of these values could be used for feature space boundaries or decision thresholds in recognition algorithms.

9.3.1.5 Removal of Outliers

In ST segment analysis, it is desirable to use only those heartbeats for ST change measurements which are expected not to be disturbed by waves of the previous or following heartbeats. Therefore, abnormal beats like ventricular premature and atrial premature beats that may have atypical ST-T waves, and their neighbors, should be excluded from the beat sequence. The exception to this rule could be right bundle branch block (RBBB) beats, and if RBBB is the dominant heart rhythm, such beats could be left in the sequence.

Even though the signals may have passed the noise detection phase, erroneous waveform morphologies due to noise with spectra in the same frequency band as the useful signal (but differ markedly from clean waveforms of normal heartbeats) are still present in the signals and must be rejected. The KLT representation of such noisy beats may be expected to have relatively large residual errors, and to differ markedly from those of neighboring beats. Precisely, feature vector corresponding to the pattern vector not belonging to the distribution modeled by the covariance matrix (outlier), will result in high residual error. Besides, the QRS complex or ST segment feature vector of a noisy beat is far from the neighboring feature vector trajectory in the feature space. We next describe a technique to reject noisy outliers that exploit these two observations of the feature vector time series and that was successfully used in [13, 14]. The procedure considers the jth heartbeat noisy if the normalized residual error for the QRS complex, $r_{qrs}(j)$, or for the ST segment, $r_{st}(j)$, exceeds a certain percentage,

$$r_{qrs}(j) > K_r \vee r_{st}(j) > K_r \tag{9.7}$$

where K_r is the residual threshold, or if the QRS or ST feature vector differs sufficiently from those of the past few beats such that

$$d^2(\mathbf{y}_{qrs}(j), \bar{\mathbf{y}}_{qrs}(j)) > \Theta \quad \vee d^2(\mathbf{y}_{st}(j), \bar{\mathbf{y}}_{st}(j)) > \Theta \tag{9.8}$$

where $\bar{\mathbf{y}}_{qrs}(j)$ and $\bar{\mathbf{y}}_{st}(j)$ are the mean feature vectors for the last M nonnoisy beats, and Θ is a distance threshold. In [13, 14] the parameters were taken to be: $n = 5$, $M = 15$, $K_r = 25\%$, and $\Theta = m_{d^2} + 1\sigma_{d^2} = 8.16$.

9.3.2 Derivation of Time-Domain Diagnostic and Morphologic Feature Vectors

Instantaneous heart rate is an important diagnostic feature and is defined by consecutive measurements of RR intervals between heartbeats. A sample of heartrate time series may be defined following

$$HR(j) = \frac{1}{FP(j) - FP(j-1)} \cdot 60 \, [\text{beats min}^{-1}] \tag{9.9}$$

9.3.2.1 Estimating Dominant Beat Morphology

It is necessary to estimate the dominant heartbeat morphology in order to obtain as accurate wave measurements as possible. After the preprocessing step, the remaining heartbeat sequence may still include heartbeats containing noise with spectral overlap with the useful ECG signal. A possible noise reduction approach is to operate in blockwise manner, processing intervals of input heartbeat sequence of a predetermined length, T_a, (typically $T_a = 16$ seconds) and producing a single heartbeat morphology estimate during each interval suitable for wave measurements. An alternative approach is recursive in nature, such that the dominant beat morphology is updated for each new heartbeat.

Beat averaging and median filtering are widely used estimators in determining the dominant beat morphology [26]. Beat averaging is expected to provide efficient suppression of muscle noise, while median filtering of beats is known to be less sensitive to outliers, such as sudden baseline shifts, spikes, or abnormal beats. A variant of the recursive beat averaging following the removal of outliers (described in the previous section) is an efficient combinatorial method, suppressing noise and resulting in a high performance. Estimating beat averages is not in itself a robust estimation method. Median filtering provides a better filter [27]. However, in the field of ECG signal analysis, we need a local estimate of the average heartbeat morphology and ST segment level over a given time interval, and not just an estimate based on a single heartbeat morphology. The average value does yield an estimate of local heartbeat morphology while median filtering provides only information of a single heartbeat. The latter estimate is not acceptable due to beat-by-beat measurement jitter. Furthermore, outliers may sequentially appear in longer intervals up to few minutes. In such cases, averaging results in a local estimate of noise while median results in an estimate of the noise in an individual heartbeat. A robust technique that rejects outliers and estimates local heartbeat morphology or ST segment level is therefore needed. Recursive beat averaging with rejection of outliers is known as the *skipped mean robust estimator* [27]. This method (with a time window of $T_a = 16$ seconds) together with the outlier rejection procedure described in the previous section was successfully used for deriving a time series of diagnostic and morphologic feature vectors during development of the LTST DB [14].

In beat averaging, beats are time aligned by the fiducial point of each QRS complex and added together. Assuming that the noise is uncorrelated with the useful ECG signal and it is uncorrelated with itself on a beat-by-beat basis, then the expected SNR of the average beat under consideration is improved for $\sqrt{Q(j)}$ where $Q(j)$ is the number of beats included into the jth average. To ensure that each average comprises a sufficient number of heartbeats and yet produces a frequent enough measurement, averaging over a window of $T_a = 16$ seconds is performed. A heart rate criterion and a procedure to reject outliers determine how many beats are included in each average.

9.3.2.2   Wave Amplitude, Level, and Slope Measurements

Time-domain diagnostic and morphologic features such as wave amplitude, level, and slope (see Figure 9.2) could be estimated using a sequence of individual heartbeats or using a sequence of averaged heartbeats after estimating the dominant beat morphology. The ST segment level is measured with respect to the isoelectric level at the selected point in the ST segment. A sample of the ST segment level time series, $s_l(i, j)$, could be defined as

$$s_l(i, j) = a(i, j) - z(i, j) \tag{9.10}$$

where $a(i, j)$ is the ST segment amplitude of an individual heartbeat and $z(i, j)$ is its isoelectric level, measured at the point $I(i, j)$. The point of measurement,

$ST(j)$, of the ST segment amplitudes, $a(i, j)$, is equal for all ECG leads and should be adaptive with regard to heart rate. The following rule was used in [12] and in [14]:

$$ST(j) = \begin{cases} J(j) + 80 \text{ ms} & : \text{if} \quad HR(j) < 100 \text{ beats min}^{-1} \\ J(j) + 72 \text{ ms} & : \text{if} \quad HR(j) \geq 100 \text{ beats min}^{-1} \wedge \\ & \quad HR(j) < 110 \text{ beats min}^{-1} \\ J(j) + 64 \text{ ms} & : \text{if} \quad HR(j) \geq 110 \text{ beats min}^{-1} \wedge \\ & \quad HR(j) < 120 \text{ beats min}^{-1} \\ J(j) + 60 \text{ ms} & : \text{if} \quad HR(j) \geq 120 \text{ beats min}^{-1} \end{cases} \tag{9.11}$$

where $J(j)$ is the position of the J point and $HR(j)$ is the instantaneous heart rate at the jth heartbeat. The ST segment amplitude, $a(i, j)$, and the isoelectric level, $z(i, j)$, are actually computed as means of signal segments of length $T_f = 20$ ms surrounding the point $ST(j)$ and the points $I(i, j)$ in order to avoid measurement jitter due to amplitude scatter of the original signal samples.

For the position of the J point, $J(j)$, a similar procedure to that for locating the isoelectric reference point using a priori knowledge of the form of the ECG heartbeat morphology could be used. Here we describe a procedure developed that was successfully used in [28]. The procedure searches forwards in each lead from the $FP(j)$ for up to $T_S = 32$ ms for a sample, where the slope of the waveform equals zero or changes sign. This is usually taken to be the R or S peak. From this point, or from the $FP(j)$ if such a sample is not found, the procedure searches forwards in each ECG lead for up to $T_J = 68$ ms for a part of the waveform which "starts to flatten" (i.e., a part of waveform where slope became smaller than a certain threshold). A slope criterion to estimate the morphology change of signal waveform was originally introduced in [29]. The procedure calculates, for each signal sample, the absolute amplitude difference between the mean of three preceding and of three trailing samples. The first of the three consecutive signal samples (assuming a sampling frequency of 250 samples s^{-1}) for which this absolute amplitude difference is less than $K_J = 15$ μV (a slope of 0.75 μV ms^{-1} in 20 ms) is considered as the position of the J point for this lead, $J(i, j)$. Then the unique reference J point for all ECG leads is taken as the latest J point of the leads, $J(j) = \max_{(i)}(J(i, j))$.

The position of the J point is problematic to find in many ECG signals, resulting in errors in ST level measurements due to J-point position misplacement. Therefore, one may simply assume that the average width of the QRS complex is 80 ms and that the J point position, $J(j)$, is at the point $FP(j) + 40$ ms for all heartbeats (or average heartbeats). This approach was successfully used in [13, 14].

The value of the ST segment slope, $s_s(i, j)$, can simply be estimated as amplitude difference:

$$s_s(i, j) = a(i, j) - a_{20}(i, j) \tag{9.12}$$

where $a(i, j)$ is the ST segment amplitude measured at the variable point dependent on the $HR(j)$ and $a_{20}(i, j)$ is the ST segment amplitude measured at the point $J(j) + 20$ ms.

Measurement of the R wave amplitude, $r_a(i, j)$, is defined as the maximum positive deviation in the interval surrounding the fiducial point, $FP(j)$, relative to the isoelectric level:

$$r_a(i, j) = \begin{cases} \max_{(m)} \mathbf{x}_{\text{qrs},m}(i, j) & : \text{if } \mathbf{x}_{\text{qrs},m}(i, j) > z(i, j) \\ 0 & : \text{if } \mathbf{x}_{\text{qrs},m}(i, j) \leq z(i, j) \end{cases} \tag{9.13}$$

where $\mathbf{x}_{\text{qrs},m}(i, j)$ is the mth signal sample of the jth heartbeat (or average heartbeat) in the ith ECG lead, and the surrounding interval is from $FP(j) - 60$ ms to $FP(j) + 60$ ms.

Finally, the projection of the mean electrical axis to the lead axis, $p_q(i, j)$, a morphologic feature, can be defined as

$$p_q(i, j) = \frac{1}{M_{\text{qrs}}} \sum_m \mathbf{x}_{\text{qrs},m}(i, j) \tag{9.14}$$

that is, as the mean of amplitudes of M_{qrs} samples surrounding the heartbeat fiducial point from $FP(j) - 40$ ms to $FP(j) + 40$ ms.

9.4 Shape Representation in Terms of Feature-Vector Time Series

Morphology changes of the ECG as well as transient events such as ischemic and nonischemic ST events are best represented and characterized using heartbeat diagnostic and morphologic feature vectors represented in terms of a time series. However, feature vectors derived on a beat-by-beat basis when ordered along the time axis still contain scatter (i.e., beat-by-beat measurement jitter). This remaining scatter of feature vectors gives unclear temporal trends as well as unclear feature-vector trajectories (the exception being the feature vector time series derived from average heartbeats) and therefore has to be rejected. A suitable technique involves averaging of sequences of feature vectors in a blockwise or recursive manner.

Furthermore, feature vectors are not equidistantly spaced due to heart rate variability. After the removal of outliers, when events are infrequent, wider intervals or even longer gaps may appear. It is desirable to obtain an equidistant series of events which are visually informative and accessible for analysis at any time instant. Therefore, a technique which converts such point event series into a form suitable for standard analysis techniques is needed. A resampling procedure is used that resamples the original feature vector series using linear interpolation to obtain a time series of events uniformly spaced, accurately estimated feature values of the original event series, and is conceptually and computationally simple. A time step of $\Delta T_r = 2$ seconds (resampling frequency, $f_r = 0.5$ Hz) is short enough to accurately represent transient waveforms of interest (ST segment episodes) and to leave enough events (15) within the shortest ST change episode possible (30 seconds) to accurately identify and analyze ST segment changes. A byproduct of resampling is that the values of equidistant events deducted may contain scatter. Therefore, the time series may be further smoothed. Figure 9.5 shows an example of the derivation and representation of diagnostic and morphologic feature-vector time series

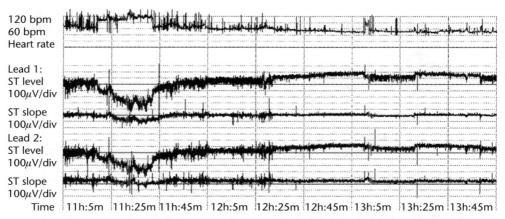

Figure 9.5   Time-domain diagnostic and morphologic feature-vector time series of the record s30661 of the LTST DB after the preprocessing step and prior to removal of outliers. A 3-hour data segment is shown, starting at 11 hours and 5 minutes. The time series contains scatter due to beat-by-beat measurement jitter and outliers. From top to bottom plotted in time scale: heart rate, $HR(j)$, where j is the heartbeat number, and ST segment levels and ST segment slopes, $s_l(i, j)$ and $s_s(i, j)$, $i = 1, 2$, (resolution: 100 μV).

information for a record from the LTST DB. The techniques employed (described in this chapter) were: the ARISTOTLE arrhythmia detector, lowpass filtering using a 6-pole Butterworth filter (with a cutoff frequency of 55 Hz), and a cubic spline approximation and subtraction technique. Figure 9.5 shows in time scale: heart rate, $HR(j)$, where j is the heartbeat number, ST segment levels, $s_l(i, j)$, and ST segment slopes, $s_s(i, j)$. The points of measurement of ST segment levels, $ST(j)$, were determined according to (9.11) with the position of the J point, $J(j)$, assumed to be constant (i.e., 40 ms after ARISTOTLE's fiducial point, $FP(j)$). The time series contains scatter due to beat-by-beat measurement jitter and due to erroneous measurements which manifest as outliers. Figure 9.6 shows the time-domain and KLT-based diagnostic and morphologic feature-vector time series of the same record after preprocessing, removing of outliers in the KLT space, smoothing the time series in a recursive manner (15-point moving average), resampling at a constant rate ($f_r = 0.5$ sample s^{-1}), and further smoothing (9-point moving average). Graphic representation of QRS complex and ST segment KLT coefficient time series on the figure permits robust and accurate display of the information globally in order to have the best opportunity to track changes in these features, and to accurately differentiate between transient ST segment events. Figure 9.6 shows in time scale: heart rate, $HR(k)$, where k is the sample number after resampling, ST segment levels and ST segment slopes, $s_l(i, k)$ and $s_s(i, k)$, R wave amplitudes, $r_a(i, k)$, projections of the mean QRS electrical axis onto both lead axes, $p_q(i, k)$, the first five KLT coefficient representation of ST segments and QRS complexes, $\mathbf{y}_{st}(k)$ and $\mathbf{y}_{qrs}(k)$, and corresponding Mahalanobis distance measures of the first order, $d(\mathbf{y}_{st}(k), \mathbf{y}_{st}(1))$ and $d(\mathbf{y}_{qrs}(k), \mathbf{y}_{qrs}(1))$. A sequence of ST segment KLT feature vectors clearly demonstrates morphology changes in the ST segment. An ST change episode is present. Similarly, a sequence of QRS complex KLT feature vectors contributes information about rapid QRS morphology changes at the beginnings and ends of nonischemic episode-like ST segment events.

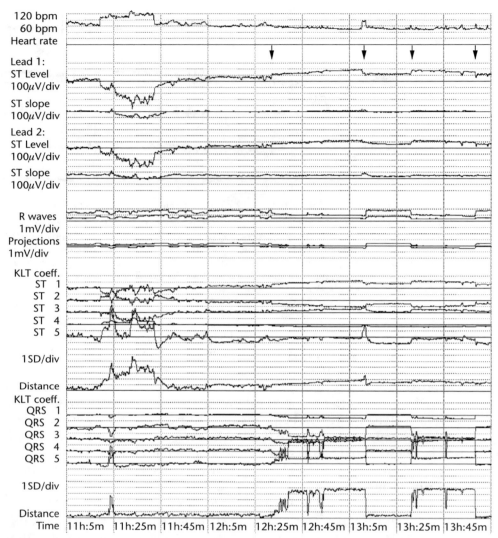

Figure 9.6 Time-domain and KLT-based diagnostic and morphologic feature-vector time series of the record s30661 of the LTST DB after preprocessing, removal of outliers in the KLT space, resampling, and smoothing. A 3-hour data segment is shown. The data segment contains one transient ischemic ST episode (beginning at 11 hours and 19 minutes) and four nonischemic ST segment events due to rapid QRS complex axis shifts (arrows). From top to bottom plotted in time scale: heart rate, $HR(k)$, where k is the sample number after resampling; ST segment levels and slopes, $s_l(i, k)$ and $s_s(i, k)$, $i = 1, 2$, (resolution: 100 μV); R wave amplitudes and projections of the mean QRS electrical axis to both lead axes, $r_a(i, k)$ and $p_q(i, k)$, $i = 1, 2$, (resolution: 1 mV); and the first five ST segment and QRS complex KLT coefficients, $y_{st}(k)$ and $y_{qrs}(k)$, (resolution: 1 SD - eigenvalue λ_m), with the corresponding Mahalanobis distance measures of the first order, $d(y_{st}(k), y_{st}(1))$ and $d(y_{qrs}(k), y_{qrs}(1))$.

The representation of the time series of QRS complex and ST segment KLT coefficients proved to be of key importance during development of the LTST DB [14]. Sample records are available on http://www.physionet.org/physiobank/database/ ltstdb/, the PhysioNet Web site [30]. Expert annotators used an interactive graphical editing tool to annotate transient ischemic and heartrate related nonischemic

ST segment episodes and nonischemic ST segment events [31]. The tool uses the techniques described in this chapter to derive and to represent time series of feature vectors. The next chapter focuses on the practical applications of the techniques described in this chapter on real data and how to assess performance.

References

[1]   Fukunaga, K., *Introduction to Statistical Pattern Recognition*, New York: Academic Press, 1972.

[2]   Gallino, A., et al., "Computer System for Analysis of ST Segment Changes on 24 Hour Holter Monitor Tapes: Comparison with Other Available Systems," *Journal of the American College of Cardiology*, Vol. 4, No. 2, 1984, pp. 245–252.

[3]   Engelse, W. A. H., and C. Zeelenberg, "A Single Scan Algorithm for QRS-Detection and Feature Extraction," *Proc. Computers in Cardiology*, Geneva, Switzerland, September, 1979, pp. 37–42.

[4]   Moody, G. B., and R. G. Mark, "Development and Evaluation of a 2-Lead ECG Analysis Program," *Proc. Computers in Cardiology*, Seattle, WA, October, 1982, pp. 39–44.

[5]   Pahlm, O., and L. Sörnmo, "Software QRS Detection in Ambulatory Monitoring—A Review," *Medical & Biological Engineering & Computing*, Vol. 22, 1984, pp. 289–297.

[6]   Pan, J., and W. J. Tompkins, "A Real-Time QRS Detection Algorithm," *IEEE Trans. Biomed. Eng.*, Vol. 32, No. 3, 1985, pp. 230–236.

[7]   Zong, W., G. B. Moody, and D. Jiang, "A Robust Open-Source Algorithm to Detect Onset and Duration of QRS Complexes," *Proc. Computers in Cardiology*, Thessaloniki, Greece, September 21–24, 2003, pp. 737–740.

[8]   Weaver, C. S., et al., "Digital Filtering with Applications to Electrocardiogram Processing," *IEEE Trans. on Audio and Electroacoustics*, Vol. 16, No. 3, 1968, pp. 350–391.

[9]   Van Alste, J. A., W. Van Eck, and O. E. Herrmann, "ECG Baseline Wander Reduction Using Linear Phase Filters," *Computers and Biomedical Research*, Vol. 19, 1986, pp. 417–427.

[10] Meyer, C., and N. Keiser, "Electrocardiogram Baseline Noise Estimation and Removal Using Cubic Splines and State Computation Techniques," *Computers and Biomedical Research*, Vol. 10, 1977, pp. 459–470.

[11] Talmon, J. L., *Pattern Recognition of the ECG*, Amsterdam: Vrije Universiteit te Amsterdam, 1983.

[12] Jager, F., "Automated Detection of Transient ST-Segment Changes During Ambulatory ECG-Monitoring," Ph.D. dissertation, Ljubljana, Slovenia, University of Ljubljana, Faculty of Electrical and Computer Engineering, 1994.

[13] Jager, F., G. B. Moody, and R. G. Mark, "Detection of Transient ST-Segment Episodes during Ambulatory ECG-Monitoring," *Computers and Biomedical Research*, Vol. 31, 1998, pp. 305–322.

[14] Jager, F., et al., "Long-Term ST Database: A Reference for the Development and Evaluation of Automated Ischaemia Detectors and for the Study of the Dynamics of Myocardial Ischaemia," *Medical & Biological Engineering & Computing*, Vol. 41, No. 2, 2003, pp. 172–182.

[15] Moody, G. B., and R. G. Mark, "QRS Morphology Representation and Noise Estimation Using the Karhunen-Loève Transform," *Proc. Computers in Cardiology*, Chicago, IL, September 23–26, 1990, pp. 269–272.

[16] Buemi, M., et al., "Monitoring Patient Status Through Principal Components Analysis," *Proc. Computers in Cardiology*, Venice, Italy, September 23–26, 1991, pp. 385–388.

[17]   Taddei, A., et al., "An Approach to Cardiorespiratory Activity Monitoring Through Principal Component Analysis," *Journal of Ambulatory Monitoring*, Vol. 5, No. 2–3, 1993, pp. 167–173.

[18]   García, J., et al., "Comparative Study of Local and Karhunen-Loève-Based ST-T Indexes in Recordings from Human Subjects with Induced Myocardial Ischemia," *Computers and Biomedical Research*, Vol. 31, 1998, pp. 271–292.

[19]   Laguna, P., et al., "Analysis of the ST-T Complex of the Electrocardiogram Using the Karhunen-Loève Transform: Adaptive Monitoring and Alternans Detection," *Medical & Biological Engineering & Computing*, Vol. 5, 1999, pp. 175–189.

[20]   Tou, J. T., and R. C. Gonzales, *Pattern Recognition Principles*, Reading, MA: Addison-Wesley, 1974.

[21]   Kittler, J., and P. C. Young, "A New Approach to Feature Selection Based on the Karhunen-Loève Expansion," *Pattern Recognition*, Vol. 5, 1973, pp. 335–352.

[22]   Campbell, N. A. C., "Robust Procedures in Multivariate Analysis I: Robust Covariance Estimation," *Applied Statistics*, Vol. 29, No. 3, 1980, pp. 231–237.

[23]   Devlin, S. J., R. Gnanadesikan, and J. R. Kettenring, "Robust Estimation of Dispersion Matrices and Principal Components," *Journal of the American Statistical Association*, Vol. 76, No. 374, 1981, pp. 354–362.

[24]   Taddei, A., et al., "The European ST-T Database: Standard for Evaluating Systems for the Analysis of ST-T Changes in Ambulatory Electrocardiography," *European Heart Journal*, Vol. 13, 1992, pp. 1164–1172.

[25]   Jager, F., et al., "Analysis of Transient ST Segment Changes During Ambulatory ECG Monitoring," *Proc. Computers in Cardiology*, Venice, Italy, September 23–26, 1991, pp. 453–456.

[26]   Van Alste, J. A., W. Van Eck, and O. E. Herrmann, "Methods for Exercise Electrocardiography in Patients Unable to Perform Leg Exercise: Rowing Ergometry, Robust Averaging and Linear Phase Filtering," *Proc. Computers in Cardiology*, Florence, Italy, September, 1981, pp. 465–468.

[27]   Hampel, F. R., et al., *Robust Statistics*, New York: John Wiley & Sons, 1986.

[28]   Smrdel, A., and F. Jager, "Automated Detection of Transient ST-Segment Episodes in 24h Electrocardiograms," *Medical & Biological Engineering & Computing*, Vol. 42, No. 3, 2004, pp. 303–311.

[29]   Daskalov, I. K., I. A. Dotsinsky, and I. I. Christov, "Development in ECG Acquisition, Preprocessing, Parameter Measurement and Recording," *IEEE Engineering in Medicine and Biology Magazine*, Vol. 17, No. 2, 1998, pp. 50–58.

[30]   Goldberger, A. L., et al., "PhysioBank, PhysioToolkit, and PhysioNet Components of a New Research Resource for Complex Physiologic Signals," *Circulation*, Vol. 101, 2000, pp. e215–e220.

[31]   Dorn, R., and F. Jager, "Semia: Semi-Automatic Interactive Graphic Editing Tool to Annotate Ambulatory ECG Records," *Computer Methods and Programs in Biomedicine*, Vol. 75, 2004, pp. 235–249.

Appendix 9A   Description of the Karhunen-Loève Transform

The KLT expansion [1, 20, 21] is a powerful general approach to feature selection in pattern recognition problems. A pattern vector may be represented as a linear combination of KLT basis functions in a coordinate system in which the coordinate coefficients are mutually uncorrelated.

Consider a set of M-dimensional random vectors, $\{\mathbf{x}\}$, the range of which is part or all of P-dimensional Euclidean space. An efficient eigenbasis to represent $\{\mathbf{x}\}$ requires that the fewest eigenvectors be used to approximate $\{\mathbf{x}\}$ to a desired level of expected MSE. Suppose that any sample pattern vector $\mathbf{x} = (x_1, x_2, ..., x_M)^T$ from this set belongs to L possible pattern classes $\{\omega_l, l = 1, 2, ..., L\}$, where the a priori probability of the occurrence of the lth class is $p(\omega_l)$. Further assume that each class is centralized by subtracting the mean $\boldsymbol{\mu}_l$ of the random pattern vectors $\mathbf{x}_l$ in that class. Denoting the centralized observation from ω_l by $\mathbf{z}_l$, we write

$$\mathbf{z}_l = \mathbf{x}_l - \boldsymbol{\mu}_l \tag{9A.1}$$

The centralized pattern vector $\mathbf{z}_l$ can be represented by a special finite expansion of the following form:

$$\mathbf{z}_l = \sum_{m=1}^{M} c_{lm} \boldsymbol{\Phi}_m \tag{9A.2}$$

where $\boldsymbol{\Phi}_m$ are orthonormal deterministic vectors satisfying the condition

$$\boldsymbol{\Phi}_m \boldsymbol{\Phi}_k = \delta_{mk} \tag{9A.3}$$

and δ_{mk} is the Kronecker delta function,

$$\delta_{mk} = \begin{cases} 1 & m = k \\ 0 & m \neq k \end{cases} \tag{9A.4}$$

while the coefficients c_{lm} satisfy

$$E(c_{lm}) = 0, \qquad (E(\mathbf{c}_l) = 0) \tag{9A.5}$$

and are mutually uncorrelated random coefficients for which

$$\sum_{l=1}^{L} p(\omega_l) E\{c_{lm} c_{lk}\} = \rho_m^2 \delta_{mk} \tag{9A.6}$$

The deterministic vectors $\boldsymbol{\Phi}_m$ in (9A.2) are termed the KLT basis functions. These vectors are the eigenvectors (also known as principal components) of the covariance matrix $\mathbf{R}$ of $\mathbf{z}$,

$$\mathbf{R} = \sum_{l=1}^{L} p(\omega_l) E\{\mathbf{z}_l \mathbf{z}_l^T\} \tag{9A.7}$$

and

$$\lambda_m = \rho_m^2 \tag{9A.8}$$

are their associated eigenvalues, where ρ_m are the standard deviations of the coefficients. Since the basis vectors are the eigenvectors of a real symmetric matrix, they are mutually orthonormal. The eigenvectors $\mathbf{\Phi}_m$ of the covariance matrix $\mathbf{R}$ and their corresponding eigenvalues λ_m are found by solving

$$\mathbf{R}\mathbf{\Phi}_m = \lambda_m \mathbf{\Phi}_m \tag{9A.9}$$

Denoting the KLT basis vectors $(\mathbf{\Phi}_1, \mathbf{\Phi}_2, ..., \mathbf{\Phi}_M)$ in matrix notation Φ, the KLT transformation pair for pattern vector $\mathbf{z}_l$, and the coefficients of the expansion $\mathbf{c}_l$, may be expressed as

$$\mathbf{z}_l = \Phi \mathbf{c}_l \tag{9A.10}$$

$$\mathbf{c}_l = \Phi^T \mathbf{z}_l \tag{9A.11}$$

It is important to arrange the KLT coordinate vectors $\mathbf{\Phi}_m$ in descending order of the magnitude of their corresponding eigenvalues λ_m,

$$\lambda_1 \geq \lambda_2 \geq ... \geq \lambda_N \geq ... \geq \lambda_M \tag{9A.12}$$

By this ordering, the optimal reduced KLT coordinate system is obtained in which the first N coordinate coefficients contain most of the "information" about random patterns $\{\mathbf{x}\}$.

The KLT expansion possesses three optimal properties. If an approximation $\widehat{\mathbf{z}}_l$ of $\mathbf{z}_l$ is constructed as

$$\widehat{\mathbf{z}}_l = \sum_{m=1}^{N} c_{lm} \mathbf{\Phi}_m \tag{9A.13}$$

where $N < M$, the expected MSE,

$$\bar{e}^2(N) = \sum_{l=1}^{L} p(\omega_l) E\{|\mathbf{z}_l - \widehat{\mathbf{z}}_l|^2\} \tag{9A.14}$$

is minimized for all N. Another optimal property of the KLT expansion is that the ratio between the MSE when using N eigenvectors for approximation, $\bar{e}^2(N)$, and the expected total power of $\mathbf{x}$, $E\{\mathbf{z}^T\mathbf{z}\}$, can be calculated as

$$\eta(N) = 1 - \sum_{m=1}^{N} \xi_m \tag{9A.15}$$

where ξ_m defined as:

$$\xi_m = \frac{\lambda_m}{\sum_{k=1}^{M} \lambda_k} \tag{9A.16}$$

represents the expected fraction of the total power of $\mathbf{z}$ associated with the eigenvector $\mathbf{\Phi}_k$. Next, if an approximation $\hat{\mathbf{z}}_l$ of $\mathbf{z}_l$ is constructed according to (9A.13) where $N < M$, the entropy function, given by

$$H(N) = -\sum_{m=N}^{M} \lambda_m \log \lambda_m \qquad (9A.17)$$

is minimized for all N. This property guarantees that the expansion is of minimum entropy and therefore a measure of minimum entropy or dispersion is associated with the coefficients of the expansion.

CHAPTER 10

ST Analysis

Franc Jager

In this chapter, we first review ECG ST segment analysis perspectives/goals and current ST segment analysis approaches. Then, we describe automated detection of transient ST change episodes with special attention to reference databases, the problem of correcting the reference ST segment level, and a procedure to detect transient ST change episodes which strictly models human-expert established criteria. We end the chapter with a description of specific performance measures and an evaluation protocol to assess the performance and robustness of ST change detection algorithms and analyzers. Performance comparisons of a few recently developed ST change analyzers are presented. It is assumed that the reader is familiar with the background presented in Chapter 9.

10.1 ST Segment Analysis: Perspectives and Goals

Typically ambulatory ECG data shows wide and significant ($> 50 \ \mu V$) transient changes in amplitude of the ST segment level which are caused by ischemia, heart rate changes, and a variety of other reasons. The major difficulties in automated ST segment analysis lie in the confounding effects of slow drifts (due to slow diurnal changes), and nonischemic step-shape ST segment shifts which are axis-related (due to shifts of the cardiac electrical axis) or conduction-change related (due to changes in ventricular conduction). These nonischemic changes may be significant, with behavior similar to real transient ischemic or heart rate related ST segment episodes, and complicate manual and automated detection of true ischemic ST episodes. The time-varying ST segment level due to clinically irrelevant nonischemic causes defines the time-varying ST segment reference level. This level must be tracked in order to successfully detect transient ST segment episodes and then to distinguish nonischemic heart rate related ST episodes from clinically significant ischemic ST episodes.

In choosing the ST segment change analysis recognition technique, the following aspects and requirements should be taken into consideration:

1. Accurate QRS complex detection and beat classification is required. The positioning of the fiducial point for each heartbeat should be accurate.
2. Simultaneous analysis of two or more ECG leads offer the improvement of analysis accuracy in comparison to the single channel analysis with regard to noise immunity and ST episode identification.

3. The analysis technique should include robust preprocessing techniques, accurate differentiating between nonnoisy and noisy events, and accurate ST segment level measurements.

4. The representation technique should be able to encode as much information as possible about the subtle structure of ST segment pattern vectors, if possible in terms of uncorrelated features.

5. The distribution of a large collection of ST segment features for normal heartbeats usually form a single cluster. During ST change episodes, significant excursion of ST segment features over the feature space may be observed. The problem of detecting ST change episodes may be formulated as a problem of detecting changes in nonstationary time series.

6. The recognition technique should be able to efficiently and accurately correct the reference ST level by tracking the cluster of normal heartbeats due to the nonischemic slow drift of the ST segment level and due to sudden nonischemic step changes of the ST segment level.

7. Classification between normal and deviating ST segments should take into account interrecord and intrarecord variability of ST segment deviations.

8. The recognition technique should be robust and able to detect transient ST change episodes and to differentiate between ischemic and heart rate related ST episodes.

9. The analysis technique may be required to function online in a single-scan mode with as short a decision delay as possible or in a multiscan mode (or perhaps using retrospective off-line analysis).

10.2 Overview of ST Segment Analysis Approaches

The development and evaluation of automated systems to detect transient ischemic ST episodes has been most prominent since the release of the ESC DB [1], a standardized reference database for development and assessment of transient ST segment and T wave change analyzers. In the recent years, several excellent automated systems were developed based on different approaches and techniques.

Traditional time-domain analysis uses an ST segment function calculated as the magnitude of the ST segment vector determined from two ECG leads [2, 3], or the filtered root mean square series of differences between the heartbeat ST segment (or ST-T complex) and an average pattern segment [4], or ST segment level function determined as ST segment amplitude measured at the heart rate adaptive delays after the heartbeat fiducial point [5]. The Karhunen-Loève transform (KLT) approaches use sequential classification of ST segment KLT coefficients as normal or deviating ones in the KLT feature space [6, 7]. A technique for representing the overall ST-T interval using KLT coefficients was proposed [8, 9] and used to detect ischemia by incorporating a filtered and differentiated KLT-coefficient time series [10]. To improve the SNR of the estimation of the KLT coefficients, an adaptive estimation was proposed [11]. Another study showed that a global representation of the entire ST-T complex appears to be more suitable than local measurements when studying the initial stages of myocardial ischemia [12]. Neural network–based approaches to classify ST segments as normal or ischemic include the use of a counterpropagation algorithm [13], a backpropagation algorithm [14], a three-layer feedforward paradigm [15], a bidirectional associative memory neural network [16], or an adaptive backpropagation algorithm [17]. In these systems, a sequence of ST segments classified as ischemic forms an ischemic ST episode. A variety of neural network architectures to classify ST segments have been implemented, tested, and compared with competing alternatives [18]. Architectures combining principal component analysis techniques and neural networks were investigated as well [18–20]. Further efforts in seeking accurate and reliable neural network architecture to maximize the performance detecting ischemic cardiac heartbeats has resulted in sophisticated architectures like nonlinear principal component analysis neural networks [21] and the network self-organizing map model [22, 23]. The self-organizing map model was successfully used to detect ischemic abnormalities in the ECG without prior knowledge of normal and abnormal ECG morphology [24]. Yet another system successfully detects ischemic ST episodes in long-duration ECG records using a feed-forward neural network and principal component analysis of the input to the network to achieve dimensionality reduction [25]. Other automated systems to detect transient ischemic ST segment and T wave episodes employ fuzzy logic [26–28], wavelet transformation [29], a hidden Markov model approach [30], or a knowledge-based technique [31] implemented in an expert system [32]. Intelligent ischemia monitoring systems employ fuzzy logic [33] or describe ST-T trends as changes in symbolic representations [34].

The detection of transient ST segment episodes is a problem of detecting events that contain a time dimension. There are insufficient distinct classes of ST segments and/or T waves with differing morphologies to allow the use of efficient classification techniques. Some studies on the characterization of ST segment and T wave changes [7, 35] have shown that morphology features of normal heartbeats form a single cluster in the feature space. This cluster of normal heartbeats is moving slowly or in step shape fashion in the feature space due to slow nonischemic changes (drifts) or due to sudden nonischemic changes (axis shifts). Ischemic and heart rate related ST segment episodes are then defined as faster episodic trajectories (or excursions) of morphology features out from and then back to the cluster of normal heartbeats. Therefore, it makes, sense to develop a technique which would efficiently track the cluster of normal heartbeats and would detect faster transient trajectories of morphology features.

The majority of automated systems do not deal adequately (or even at all) with nonischemic events. It was previously thought that the KLT-based systems and in particular neural-network systems (since they extract information of morphology from the entire ST segment), would separate subtle ischemia-related features of the ST segment adequately from nonischemia related features. Unfortunately, the success of these techniques has been limited. The problem of separating ischemic ST episodes from nonischemic ST segment events remains, in part due to the nonstationarity of an ST segment morphology-feature time series, and the lack of a priori knowledge of their distributions. Furthermore, an insufficient number of nonischemic ST segment events present in the ESC DB prevents studying these events at length and only short (biased or unrepresentative) segments of the database records (2 hours) have been used (since they were selected to be sufficiently "clean"). The other reference database for development and assessment of transient ST segment change analyzers, the LTST DB [35], contains long-duration (24-hour) records with a large number of human-annotated ischemic and nonischemic ST segment events.

Only a few automated systems deal explicitly with nonischemic events such as slow drifts and axis shifts. One of the early systems [36] dealt with nonischemic events by discriminating between "stable" and "unstable" ST segment baseline time periods and correcting the ST segment reference level for nonischemic shifts between stable periods. Other systems employ ST segment level trajectory-recognition based on heuristics in time domain [3], in the KLT feature space [7], or a combination of traditional time-domain and KLT-based approaches [37]. These systems are capable (to a certain extent) of detecting transient ST segment episodes and of tracking the time-varying ST segment reference level.

A few other systematic approaches to the problem of detecting body position changes which result in axis shifts have been made. A technique based on a spatial approach by estimating rotation angles of the electrical axis [38] and a technique using a scalar-lead signal representation based on the KLT [39] were investigated. Another study used a measurement of R wave duration to identify changes in body position [40]. In all these investigations, the authors developed their own databases which contain induced axis shifts.

Currently developed ST episode detection systems are capable of detecting transient ST segment episodes which are ischemic or heart rate related ST episodes, but are not able to distinguish between them. Automatic classification of these two types of episodes is an interesting challenge. This task would require additional analysis of heart rate, original raw ST segment patterns, and clinical information concerning the patients. A recognition algorithm would need to distinguish between typical ischemic and nonischemic ST segment morphology changes [35]. These include typical ischemic ST segment morphology changes (horizontal flattening, down sloping, scooping, elevation), which may or may not be accompanied by a change in heart rate, and typical heart rate related ST segment morphology changes (J point depression with positive slope, moving of the T wave into the ST segment, T wave peaking, and parallel shifts of the ST segment compared with the reference or basal ST segment), which are accompanied by an obligatory change in heart rate. The inclusion of clinical information also makes room for the development of sophisticated techniques leading to intelligent ischemia detection systems.

10.3   Detection of Transient ST Change Episodes

Automated detection of transient ST segment changes requires: (1) accurate measurement and tracking of ST segment levels and (2) detection of ST segment change episodes with correct identification of the beginning and end of each episode, and the time and magnitude of the maximum ST deviation. The main features of an ST change detection system may be: (1) the automatic tracking of the time-varying ST segment reference level in the ST segment level time series of each ECG lead, $s_l(i, k)$ (where i denotes the lead number and k denotes the sample number of the ST segment level time series) to construct the ST reference function, $s_r(i, k)$; (2) the ST deviation function, $s_d(i, k)$, in each lead which is constructed by taking the algebraic difference between the ST level and ST reference function; (3) a combination of the ST deviation functions from the leads into the ST detection function, $D(k)$; and (4) the automatic detection of transient ST episode.

10.3.1 Reference Databases

Two freely available international reference databases to develop and evaluate ST segment analyzers are currently in use: the ESC DB [1] and the LTST DB [35], and as such they complement each other in the field of automated analysis of transient ST segment changes.

The ESC DB contains 90 two-channel 2-hour annotated AECG records of varying lead combinations, collected during routine clinical practice. ST segment annotations were made on a beat-by-beat basis by experts. The ischemic ST segment episodes were annotated in each lead separately according to an annotation protocol which incorporates the ST segment deviation defined as a change in the ST segment level from that of the ST segment level of a single reference heartbeat measured at the beginning of a record.

The goal of the LTST DB is to be a representative research resource for development and evaluation of automated systems to detect transient ST segment changes, and for supporting basic research into the mechanisms and dynamics of transient myocardial ischemia. The LTST DB contains 86 two- and three-channel 24-hour annotated AECG records of 80 patients (of varying lead combinations), collected during routine clinical practice. ST segment annotations were made on average heartbeats after considerable preprocessing. A large number of nonischemic ST segment events mixed with transient ischemic ST episodes allows development of reliable and robust ST episode detection systems. The ischemic and heart rate related ST segment episodes were annotated in each lead separately according to an annotation protocol. This protocol incorporates the ST segment deviation defined as the algebraic difference between the ST segment level and the time-varying ST segment reference level (which was annotated throughout the records using local-reference annotations). The annotated events include: transient ischemic ST segment episodes, transient heart rate related nonischemic ST segment episodes, and nonischemic time-varying ST segment reference level trends due to slow drifts and step changes caused by axis shifts and conduction changes.

The expert annotators of the ESC DB and LTST DB annotated transient ST segment episodes which satisfied the following clinically defined criteria:

1. An episode begins when the magnitude of the ST deviation first exceeds a lower annotation detection threshold, $V_{lower} = 50\ \mu V$.
2. The deviation then must reach or exceed an upper annotation detection threshold V_{upper} throughout a continuous interval of at least T_{min} s (the minimum duration of an ST episode).
3. The episode ends when the deviation becomes smaller than $V_{lower} = 50\ \mu V$, provided that it does not exceed V_{lower} in the following $T_{sep} = 30$ seconds (the interval separating consecutive ST episodes).

According to annotation protocol of the ESC DB, the values of the upper annotation detection thresholds and minimum width of ST episodes are $V_{upper} = 100\ \mu V$ and

T_{min} = 30 seconds. The database contains 250 transient lead-independent ischemic ST episodes combined using the logical *OR* function. Episode annotations of the LTST DB are available in three variant annotation protocols:

(A) V_{upper} = 75 μV, T_{min} = 30 seconds;
(B) V_{upper} = 100 μV, T_{min} = 30 seconds, equivalent to the protocol of the ESC DB;
(C) V_{upper} = 100 μV, T_{min} = 60 seconds.

According to the protocol A, the database contains 1,490 transient lead-independent ischemic and heart rate related ST episodes combined using the logical *OR* function. Combining only ischemic ST segment changes yields 1,155 ischemic ST episodes.

10.3.2 Correction of Reference ST Segment Level

Next we describe an efficient technique developed in [37] to correct the reference ST segment level. Using a combination of traditional time-domain and KLT-based approaches, the analyzer derives QRS complex and ST segment morphology features, and by mimicking human examination of the morphology-feature time series and their trends, tracks the time-varying ST segment reference level due to clinically irrelevant nonischemic causes. These include slow drifts, axis shifts, and conduction changes. The analyzer estimates the slowly varying ST segment level trend, identifies step changes in the time series, and subtracts the ST segment reference level thus obtained from the ST segment level to obtain the measured ST segment deviation time series that is suitable for detection of ST segment episodes.

10.3.2.1 Estimation of ST Segment Reference Level Trend

Human experts track the slowly varying trend of ST segment level and skip the more rapid excursions during transient ST segment events. Similarly, the analyzer [37] estimates the time-varying global and local ST segment reference level trend [$s_{rg}(i, k)$ and $s_{rl}(i, k)$, respectively], of the ST level functions, $s_l(i, k)$, by applying two moving-average lowpass filters. The ST level functions were obtained using preprocessing, exclusion of noisy outliers, resampling, and smoothing of the time series (as described in the Chapter 9). The two moving-average lowpass filters are: h_g, over 6 hours and 40 minutes in duration estimating the global nonstationary mean of the ST level function, and h_l, over 5 minutes in duration estimating local excursions of the ST level function. Moving-average lowpass filters posses useful frequency characteristic which are simple to realize and computationally inexpensive. The ST reference function is estimated as follows:

$$s_{r'}(i, k) = \begin{cases} s_{rg}(i, k) & : \text{if } |s_{rg}(i, k) - s_{rl}(i, k)| > K_s \\ s_{rl}(i, k) & : \text{otherwise} \end{cases} \quad (10.1)$$

where K_s = 50 μV is the "significance threshold" (i.e., the threshold to locate significant excursions of the ST level function from its global trend, and is equivalent to a lower annotation detection threshold, V_{lower} = 50 μV). The moving-average filter h_g estimates the global nonstationary trend of the ST level function, $s(i, k)$. The $s_{r'}(i, k)$ is composed from the $s_{rg}(i, k)$ and an excursion of the ST segment level indicates that a transient ST segment episode has occurred at this time.

10.3.2.2 Detection of Sudden Step Changes

A human expert considers each step change of an ST level function (which is accompanied by a step change in the QRS complex morphology, and preceded and followed by a stable interval with no change of the QRS complex and ST segment morphology) as a step-shape path of the ST segment reference level. To detect step changes, the analyzer [37] uses the ST level function, $s_l(i, k)$, and the first-order Mahalanobis distance functions of KLT-coefficient morphology-feature vectors of the QRS complex, $d(\mathbf{y}_{qrs}(k), \mathbf{y}_{qrs}(1))$, and of the ST segment, $d(\mathbf{y}_{st}(k), \mathbf{y}_{st}(1))$. Besides a step change, there has to be a "flat" interval of the three functions before and after the step change. In each of the three functions, the analyzer searches first for a flat interval of 216 seconds in length, which has to have its mean absolute deviation from its own mean value less than $K_f = 20$ μV for the ST level function (and less than $\Sigma = 0.33$ SD for both the QRS and ST Mahalanobis distance functions). Such a flat interval has to be followed by a step change, which is characterized by the moving average value over 72 seconds in length and has to change for more than $K_s = 50$ μV for the ST level function (and for more than $\Lambda_{qrs} = 0.5$ SD and $\Lambda_{st} = 0.4$ SD for QRS and ST Mahalanobis distance functions) within the next 144 seconds in length. This step change has to be followed by another flat interval in each of the functions, defined as for the first flat interval.

The operation used to detect step changes actually computes the derivative of the three functions and therefore behaves like a band-pass filter extracting rapid slopes while rejecting spikes and noises (by attenuating high frequencies) that might be present in the three functions. In the intervals surrounding each step change detected, the ST reference function is updated as follows:

$$s_r(i, k) = \begin{cases} s_{r'}(i, k) & : \text{ if } |s_{rg}(i, k) - s_l(i, k)| < K_s \wedge \\ & \quad |s_{rl}(i, k) - s_l(i, k)| < K_s \\ s_l(i, k) & : \text{ otherwise} \end{cases} \tag{10.2}$$

where the significance threshold, K_s, estimates the significant deviation of the ST level function from its trend. Figure 10.1 shows an example of tracking the reference ST level in the record s30661 of the LTST DB using this technique. In the first 60 minutes of the data segment shown, the ST reference function, $s_r(1, k)$, is estimated by the global ST reference level trend, $s_{rg}(1, k)$, and after that by the ST level function, $s_l(1, k)$, because of detected axis shifts in the region.

10.3.3 Procedure to Detect ST Change Episodes

After estimating the reference ST level, the ST deviation function, $s_d(i, k)$, for each ECG lead can be derived as algebraic difference between the ST level function and ST reference function:

$$s_d(i, k) = s_l(i, k) - s_r(i, k) \tag{10.3}$$

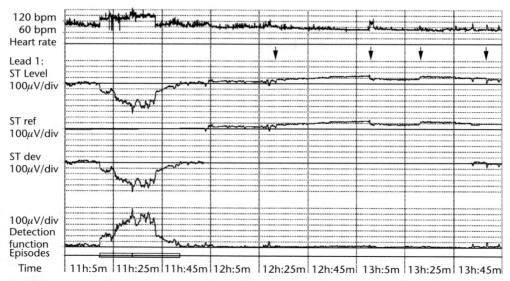

120 bpm
60 bpm
Heart rate

Lead 1:
ST Level
100μV/div

ST ref
100μV/div

ST dev
100μV/div

100μV/div
Detection
function
Episodes

Time   11h:5m   11h:25m 11h:45m 12h:5m   12h:25m 12h:45m 13h:5m   13h:25m 13h:45m

Figure 10.1 Example of tracking the reference ST level, deriving of ST reference, ST deviation, and ST detection function, and of detecting ST change episodes in the record s30661 of the LTST DB using the system in [37]. A 3-hour data segment is shown. During the ischemic ST episode, the ST reference function, $s_r(1, k)$, is estimated by the global ST reference level trend, $s_{rg}(1, k)$, and after that by the ST level function, $s_l(1, k)$, due to detected axis shifts. The arrows mark the axis shifts. From top to bottom plotted in time scale: heart rate; ST level function, $s_l(1, k)$; ST reference function, $s_r(1, k)$; ST deviation function, $s_d(1, k)$; ST detection function, $D(k)$, (resolution: 100 μV); and lead-independent combined ischemic ST episode annotation stream derived by expert annotators (lower line) and ST episodes detected by the analyzer (upper line).

Finally, the ST detection function, $D(k)$, is derived as a combination of ST deviation functions from the ECG leads:

$$D(k) = f(s_d(i, k)) \tag{10.4}$$

An important part of each ST segment analyzer is an algorithm to automatically detect and annotate significant transient ST segment episodes. The algorithm has to classify sequentially samples of the ST detection function, $D(k)$, to normal and deviating ones, has to model human-defined timing criteria for the identification of ST episodes, and must annotate the beginnings, extrema, and ends of transient ST segment episodes. Figure 10.2 symbolically summarizes such an algorithm which strictly follows the human-expert timing criteria of the annotation protocols of the ESC DB and LTST DB with two arbitrary amplitude thresholds. Samples of the detection function, $D(k)$, of the algorithm may be, for example: a time-domain feature [e.g., the ST segment deviation, $s_d(i, k)$]; a combination of features (e.g., the Euclidean distance of ST segment deviations from the leads); or the Mahalanobis distance function d or d^2 of the ST segment KLT-coefficient morphology-feature vectors. (The detection algorithm assumes positive values of the detection function.) Consecutive samples of the detection function, $D(k)$, are classified according to lower and upper feature space boundaries, U_{lower} and U_{upper}, which correspond to human-expert reference annotation thresholds V_{lower} and V_{upper}. Different annotation protocols can be assumed by selecting two thresholds, U_{lower} and U_{upper}, and

Constants:

f_r: Resampling frequency [samples s^{-1}]
$\Delta T_r = 1/f_r$:   Time step between samples [s]
T_{sep}:   Interval separating ST episodes (30 s)

Input:

U_{lower}, U_{upper}:   Lower and upper detection thresholds
T_{min}:   Minimum width of ST episodes [s]
$D(i, 1..K)$:   Detection function

Output:

N_{epis}:   Number of detected ST episodes
$T_{beg}(1..V), T_{ext}(1..V)$:   ST episode beginnings, extrema
$T_{end}(1..V)$:   and ends [s]

Method:

$S = T_{sep}/\Delta T_r$;   /* Samples to separate ST episodes */
$W = T_{min}/\Delta T_r$;   /* Minimum width of ST episodes */
$v = 0$;   /* ST episode counter */
for $k = 1$ **to** K **do   ST_episode_detect**(k);
$N_{epis} = v$;   /* Number of detected ST episodes */
end

procedure ST_episode_detect(k)

/* Segment containing tentative beginning of ST episode */
if $(k \geq S) \wedge (\neg episode) \wedge (D(k) \geq U_{lower}) \wedge$
            $((\forall l \in [1, ..., S]) \, D(k - l) < U_{lower})$ **then**
        $onset = $ TRUE; $Tbeg = k.\Delta T_r$;
/* Segment which is a part of ST episode */
elseif $onset \wedge (\neg episode) \wedge (D(k) \geq U_{upper}) \wedge$
            $((\forall l \in [1, ..., W]) \, D(k - l) \geq U_{upper})$ **then**
        $episode = $ TRUE;
/* Segment separating ST episodes */
elseif $(k \geq S) \wedge (D(k) < U_{lower}) \wedge$
            $((\forall l \in [1, ..., S]) \, D(k - l) < U_{lower})$ **then**
        $onset = $ FALSE;
        if $episode$ **then**   /* End of ST episode */
            $episode = $ FALSE;
            $v = v + 1$;   /* Count ST episode */
            $T_{beg}(v) = Tbeg$; $T_{ext}(v) = Text$;
            $T_{end}(v) = (k - S) \, \Delta T_r$;
        endif
endif
/* Search for extrema */
if $onset \wedge (D(k) > max)$ **then**
        $max = D(k)$; $Text = k \, \Delta T_r$;
endif
end_procedure

Figure 10.2 Algorithm for detecting transient ischemic and heart rate related ST episodes in the ST segment detection function, $D(k)$. On input the algorithm accepts feature space boundaries, U_{lower} and U_{upper}, and minimum width of ST episodes, T_{min}, according to selected criteria for significant ST episodes. On output the algorithm returns the number of detected transient ST episodes, N_{epis}, and arrays of times of beginnings, $T_{beg}(N_{epis})$, extrema, $T_{ext}(N_{epis})$, and ends $T_{end}(N_{epis})$, of detected episodes.

a proper minimum width of ST episodes, T_{min}. A segmentation logic of the algorithm uses segmentation rules which follow human-expert defined criteria for identifying transient ST segment episodes. The logic operates in a sequential manner and identifies segments of the $D(k)$ belonging to normal segments and separating ST episodes, transition segments containing the exact beginning of the ST episode, segments which are a part of ST episodes, and transition segments containing the exact end of the ST episode. Each ST segment episode is then defined between the exact beginning and the exact end of the episode.

Besides tracking the reference ST level using the analyzer [37], Figure 10.1 also shows an example of detecting ST change episodes when using the detection algorithm from Figure 10.2. The detection function in the example uses the Euclidean distance of the $s_d(i, k)$ from the ECG leads. The algorithm correctly detected the ischemic ST episode present in the first part of the data segment shown.

10.4 Performance Evaluation of ST Analyzers

The evaluation of an ST detection algorithm or analyzer should answer the following questions:

- How well are ST episodes detected?
- How well are ischemic and nonischemic heart rate related ST episodes differentiated?
- How reliably are ST episode or ischemic ST episode duration measured?
- How accurately are ST deviations measured?
- How well will the ST analyzer perform in the real world?

In this section we describe performance measures and an evaluation protocol for assessing the performance of ST algorithms and analyzers according to these evaluation questions.

10.4.1 Performance Measures

Three performance measures are commonly used to assess an analyzer performance: sensitivity, specificity, and positive predictive accuracy. Sensitivity, Se, the ratio of the number of correctly detected events, TP (true positives), to the total number of events is given by

$$Se = \frac{TP}{TP + FN} \qquad (10.5)$$

where FN (false negatives) is the number of missed events. The specificity, Sp, the ratio of the number of correctly rejected nonevents, TN (true negatives), to the total number of nonevents is given by

$$Sp = \frac{TN}{TN + FP} \qquad (10.6)$$

where FP (false positives) is the number of falsely detected events. Positive predictive accuracy, $+P$, (or just positive predictivity) is the ratio of the number of correctly detected events, TP, to the total number of events detected by the analyzer and is given by

$$+P = \frac{TP}{TP + FP} \qquad (10.7)$$

These performance measures actually are frequencies in a statistical sense and approximate conditional probabilities [41]. Sensitivity approximates the conditional probability of true positives:

$$p(EVENT|event) \approx \frac{TP}{TP + FN} \tag{10.8}$$

that is, the conditional probability of the decision of $EVENT$ given that the *event* occurred. Specificity approximates the conditional probability of true negatives:

$$p(NONEVENT|nonevent) \approx \frac{TN}{TP + FP} \tag{10.9}$$

that is, the conditional probability of the decision of $NONEVENT$ given that the *nonevent* occurred. Positive predictivity approximates the posterior probability of true positives [i.e., the posterior probability that *event* occurred given the decision (evidence) of $EVENT$]:

$$p(event|EVENT) = \frac{p(EVENT|event)\,p(event)}{p(EVENT)} \approx \frac{TP}{TP + FP} \tag{10.10}$$

In many detection problems, nonevents cannot be counted, so that the number of true negatives, TN, is undefined. In such problems, the commonly used detector-performance measures are sensitivity, Se, the proportion of events which were detected, and positive predictivity, $+P$, the proportion of detections which were events, or the accuracy of classifying detected events.

To evaluate an analyzer's ability to detect significant ($> 50\ \mu V$) ischemic ST episodes (characterized by the beginning, the extrema, and by the end), it is necessary to match reference ST episodes with analyzer-annotated ST episodes. With a matching criteria, the concept of sensitivity (the fraction of correctly detected events) and positive predictivity (the fraction of detections which are events) are applicable, while specificity (the fraction of rejections which are correct) is not applicable, since the number of nonevents, TN, is undefined. We describe next particular sensitivity and positive predictivity metrics which are helpful in quantifying performance. The performance measures to assess the accuracy of detecting ischemic ST episodes and total ischemic time are based on the concepts of matching and overlap between reference and analyzer-annotated episodes.

10.4.1.1   Detection of ST Episode

Transient ST segment episodes (the events of interest) are characterized by: (1) number, (2) length, and (3) extrema deviation. When evaluating multichannel ST-analyzer performance, the ST annotation stream for all leads must be combined into one reference stream using a logical OR function. The fact that at any given time there is either an ST episode or an interval with no ST deviation implies the use of two-by-two performance evaluation matrices. We further assume that all ST episodes are equally important. Evaluation of ST episode detection analyzers consists of comparing analyzer-annotated episodes with reference-annotated episodes. There is not a one-to-one correspondence between analyzer- and reference-annotated episodes; the episodes from the two groups may differ considerably in length. Furthermore, nonevents cannot be counted.

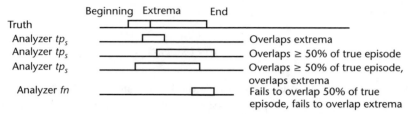

Figure 10.3 Matching criteria defined for a correctly detected ST episode, tp_s, and a missed ST episode, fn.

The performance measures to assess ability to detect ST episodes depend on the concept of matching [42–44]. A match of a reference or analyzer-annotated episode occurs when the period of mutual overlap includes at least a certain portion of the length of the episode according to the defining annotations. In measuring sensitivity (see Figure 10.3), matching of a reference ST episode occurs when the period of overlap includes at least one of the extrema of the reference ST episode, or at least one-half of the length of the reference ST episode. In measuring positive predictivity (see Figure 10.4), the matching of analyzer-annotated ST episodes occurs when the period of overlap includes the extrema of the analyzer-annotated ST episode, or at least one-half of the length of the analyzer-annotated ST episode.

The sensitivity matrix (see Figure 10.5, left) summarizes how the reference ST episodes were labeled by the analyzer (i.e., how many of the reference ST episodes were detected, TP_S, and how many were missed, FN). The positive predictivity matrix (Figure 10.5, right) summarizes how many of the analyzer-annotated ST episodes were actually ST episodes, TP_P, and how many were falsely detected, FP.

ST episode detection sensitivity, $SESe$, an estimate of the likelihood of detecting an ST episode, is defined as

$$SESe = \frac{TP_S}{TP_S + FN} \tag{10.11}$$

The denominator quantifies the number of reference ST episodes, TP_S is the number of matching episodes, and FN is the number of nonmatching episodes where the defining annotations are the reference annotations.

ST episode detection positive predictivity, $SE + P$, an estimate of the likelihood that a detection is a true ST episode, is defined as

$$SE + P = \frac{TP_P}{TP_P + FP} \tag{10.12}$$

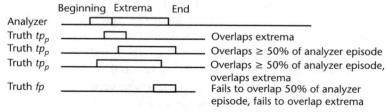

Figure 10.4 Matching criteria defined for an analyzer-annotated ST episode, which is actually an ST episode, tp_p, and a falsely detected ST episode, fp.

Se matrix		Analyzer	
		ST episode	Not epis
Refe-rence	ST episode	TP_S	FN
	Not epis	–	–

+P matrix		Analyzer	
		ST episode	Not epis
Refe-rence	ST episode	TP_P	–
	Not epis	FP	–

Figure 10.5 ST episode sensitivity matrix (left) and ST episode positive predictivity matrix (right). *Not epis* indicates the absence of an ST episode.

The denominator quantifies the number of ST episodes annotated by the analyzer, TP_P is the number of matching episodes, and *FP* is the number of nonmatching episodes, where the defining annotations are the analyzer annotations.

10.4.1.2 Differentiation Between Ischemic and Heart Rate Related ST Episodes

In differentiating ischemic and nonischemic heart rate related ST episodes, we assumed that at any given time there is only one type of episode: either ischemic, nonischemic heart rate related, or an interval without significant ST deviation. This implies three-by-three performance evaluation matrices (see Figure 10.6). Each reference- and analyzer-annotated episode is submitted to the extended matching test [45]. The test is the same as defined previously for ST episodes, but extended in the sense that matching of an episode (ischemic or heart rate related) occurs when the episode is sufficiently and uniquely overlapped by ischemic or by heart rate related ST episodes. The criteria of extended matching test to determine the status of *u*th reference (truth) ST episode (ischemic or heart rate related), $S_R(u)$, are summarized in the following:

> **if** *match with ischemic analyzer-annotated ST episodes* **then**
> $S_R(u) = ischemic$;
> **else if** *match with heart rate related analyzer-annotated ST episodes* **then**
> $S_R(u) = heart\ rate\ related$;
> **else**
> $S_R(u) = missed$;
> **endif**

Se matrix		Analyzer		
		Isch	HR rel	Not epis
	Isch	A	B	C
Ref	HR rel	D	E	F
	Not epis	–	–	–

+P matrix		Analyzer		
		Isch	HR rel	Not epis
	Isch	G	H	–
Ref	HR rel	I	J	–
	Not epis	K	L	–

Figure 10.6 Performance matrices assessing the ability of an ST episode detection analyzer to differentiate ischemic (*Isch*) and nonischemic heart rate related (*HR rel*) ST episodes.

Similarly, the criteria of extended matching test to determine the status of vth analyzer-annotated (analyzer) ST episode (ischemic or heart rate related), $S_A(v)$, are summarized in the following:

> **if** *match with ischemic reference-annotated ST episodes* **then**
> $\quad S_A(v) = ischemic;$
> **else if** *match with heart rate related reference-annotated ST episodes* **then**
> $\quad S_A(v) = heart\ rate\ related;$
> **else**
> $\quad S_A(v) = falsely\ detected;$
> **endif**

The sensitivity matrix (Figure 10.6, left) describes how many reference ischemic, A, and heart rate related, E, ST episodes were correctly detected. B is the number of reference ischemic episodes detected as heart rate related, and D is the number of reference heart rate related episodes detected as ischemic. C and F are the numbers of missed ischemic and heart rate related episodes, respectively. The positive predictivity matrix (Figure 10.6, right) describes how many of the analyzer's ischemic, G, and heart rate related, J, ST episode detections were actually ischemic and heart rate related episodes. H is the number of the analyzer's heart rate related episode detections which actually are reference ischemic episodes, and I is the number of the analyzer's ischemic episode detections which actually are reference heart rate related episodes. K and L are the numbers of falsely detected ischemic and heart rate related episodes, respectively.

Furthermore, if we consider both ischemic and heart rate related ST changes together as ST change episodes of unique type, then the performance matrices can easily be reduced back to two-by-two, with: $TP_S = A + B + D + E$, $TP_P = G + H + I + J$, $FN = C + F$, and $FP = K + L$, yielding the performance matrices in Figure 10.5. Since the events of clinical interest are the ischemic ST episodes, we can further consider all nonischemic heart rate related ST episodes as episodes of no deviation. This consideration yields: $TP_S = A$, $TP_P = G$, $FN = B + C$, and $FP = I + K$, and leads to the ischemic ST episode detection sensitivity, $IESe$, and ischemic ST episode detection positive predictivity, $IE+P$, which are defined in the same manner as the $SESe$ and $SE+P$ in (10.11) and (10.12).

10.4.1.3   Measurement of ST Episode Durations

ST episode duration detection sensitivity, $SD\ Se$, is the estimate of the accuracy with which an analyzer can measure the duration of ST episodes within the observation period. $SD\ Se$ is defined as the fraction of true ST episode durations detected and is given by

$$SD\ Se = \frac{SD_{R\wedge A}}{SD_R} \tag{10.13}$$

ST episode duration detection positive predictivity, $SD+P$, is defined as the fraction of analyzer-annotated ST episode durations which are true ST episodes and is given by

$$SD + P = \frac{SD_{R \wedge A}}{SD_A} \qquad (10.14)$$

where $SD_{R \wedge A}$ is the total duration of analyzer-annotated ST episodes which overlaps reference ST episodes, and SD_R and SD_A are the total durations of reference- and analyzer-annotated ST episodes, respectively [42–44]. Similarly, ischemia duration detection sensitivity, $ID\ Se$, and ischemia duration detection positive predictivity, $ID + P$, can be defined using total duration of analyzer-annotated ischemia, ID_A, which overlaps reference ischemia, ID_R, and their overlap, $ID_{R \wedge A}$.

10.4.1.4   Measurement of ST Segment Deviations

Accuracy of ST-deviation measurement of the extrema of ST episodes is usually summarized by a scatter plot of reference versus test measurements. Such a scatter plot permits rapid visual assessment of any systematic measurement bias, nonlinearity, or unreliable performance of the ST deviation measurement analyzer. Other useful summary statistics are: mean error between the analyzer and reference measurements, standard deviation of errors, correlation coefficient, and linear regression. These statistics do not distinguish between errors resulting from bias or nonlinearity and errors resulting from poor noise tolerance or unreliable measurement techniques. Other more robust and informative statistics in the presence of outliers are: the value of error, which 95% of the measurements do not exceed, and the percentage of measurements for which the absolute difference between the analyzer and reference measurement is greater than 100 μV [42–44].

10.4.1.5   Predicting Real-World Performance

In predicting the analyzer's performance in the real world, it is important to use a test database, which was not used for development. In addition, a second-order aggregate gross statistic which weights each event equally by pooling all the events over all records together and models how the analyzer behaves on a large number of events, and a second-order aggregate average statistic which weights each record equally and models how the analyzer behaves on randomly chosen records, are applicable.

If the database is so small that it could not be divided into development and test subsets, or if additional data is not available, the bootstrap technique [46, 47] is useful for predicting the analyzer's performance in the real world. The method assumes that the database is a well-chosen representative subset of examples for a problem domain and does not require any assumption about the distribution of the data. By this technique, many new databases are chosen at random (with replacement; that is, a newly chosen record put back) from the original database, and performance statistics are derived for each new database. The mean, standard deviation and median of expected performance, as well as the minimum expected performance (5% confidence limits), can be estimated from the distributions of the performance statistics. Due to relative complexity of the performance measures and of the evaluation protocol, an automated tool to objectively evaluate and compare the performance and robustness of transient ST episode detection analyzers is desirable.

The open-source tool EVAL_ST [45] provides first (record-by-record) and second-order (aggregate gross and average) performance statistics for evaluation and comparison of transient ST episode detection analyzers. Inputs to the tool are ST segment annotation streams of a reference database (e.g., the ESC DB or the LTST DB) and ST segment annotation streams of the evaluated analyzers. The tool allows assessing the accuracy of: (1) detecting transient ST episodes, (2) distinguishing between ischemic and nonischemic heart rate related ST episodes, (3) measuring ST episode durations and ischemic ST episode durations, and (4) measuring ST segment deviations. The tool also generates performance distributions using a bootstrap statistical technique for predicting real-world clinical performance and robustness. A graphic user interface module of the tool provides display of all evaluation results. The tool has been made freely available on http://www.physionet.org/physiotools/eval_st/, the PhysioNet Web site [48].

10.4.2 Comparison of Performance of ST Analyzers

Table 10.1 comparatively summarizes the performances of transient ST episode detection systems developed and tested on the the ESC DB and the LTST DB. Only those systems are compared which were developed and tested using the original ESC DB and original LTST DB annotations. These systems incorporate time-domain analysis [3–5], the KLT approach [7], a combination of time-domain analysis and KLT approach [37], a neural network approach [17], and a combination of the KLT transform and a neural network approach [18]. These systems were evaluated using commonly accepted performance measures [42, 49, 50]. (A slightly modified matching test between analyzer's and reference ST episodes were used in [17].) The

Table 10.1 Comparison of Performance of Transient ST Episode Detection Systems Developed and Tested on the ESC DB and LTST DB

System, Technique		ESC DB SE [%] Se	+P	SD [%] Se	+P		LTST DB (Protocol B) SE [%] Se	+P	SD [%] Se	+P
[3], Time domain	[g]	81	76	–	–		–	–	–	–
	[a]	84	81	–	–		–	–	–	–
[4], RMS method	[g]	–	–	–	–		–	–	–	–
	[a]	84.7	86.1	75.3	68.2		–	–	–	–
[5], Time domain	[g]	79.2	81.4	–	–		–	–	–	–
	[a]	81.5	82.5	–	–		–	–	–	–
[7], KLT approach	[g]	85.2	86.2	75.8	78.0	–>	77.0	58.8	48.5	47.8
	[a]	87.1	87.7	78.2	74.1	–>	74.0	61.4	54.8	58.4
[37], Time domain, KLT	[g]	77.2	86.3	67.5	69.2	<–	79.6	78.3	68.4	67.3
	[a]	81.3	89.2	77.6	68.9	<–	78.9	80.7	73.1	74.9
[17], Neural net	[g]	85.0	68.7	73.0	69.5		–	–	–	–
	[a]	88.6	78.4	72.2	67.5		–	–	–	–
[18], Neural net, KLT	[g]	–	–	–	–		–	–	–	–
	[a]	77	86	–	–		–	–	–	–

The system from [7] (the KLT approach) was tested using the LTST DB after its development on the ESC DB, while the system from [37] (time domain, KLT) was developed using the LTST DB and then tested using the ESC DB. SE = ST episode; SD = ST episode duration; Se = sensitivity; $+P$ = positive predictivity; [g] = gross; [a] = average.

published sensitivity and positive predictivity in detecting transient ischemic ST episodes of these systems are about 85%. The KLT-based system [7] was developed using the ESC DB and tested using the LTST DB. A reason for the significant drop of the performance during testing could be too much tuning of the system during its development using the ESC DB. The system that combines time-domain and KLT transform approaches [37] was developed using the LTST DB and tested using the ESC DB. Generally higher average gross performance statistics of this system using the test database suggest that the time domain/KLT system performs well on a randomly chosen record and in the real world. Furthermore, higher performance when using the ESC DB as the test database may suggests that the LTST DB is suitable as a learning set. Only four systems [4, 7, 17, 37] were also evaluated in terms of detecting the total ischemic time. Some of the systems from Table 10.1 were also evaluated using the revised ESC DB annotations [3–5]. Other ischemia detection systems were evaluated using only the revised ESC DB annotations [25, 31]. Yet another group of systems were validated using only a subset of records of the ESC DB [14, 16, 21–23, 27, 30, 33, 34]. It is not possible to make a valid comparison of the performance of these systems nor of those being validated using only revised annotations since each of the development groups made their own choice about a set of records for evaluation, or their own revision of the annotations.

The problem of classification between ischemic and nonischemic events in long-term AECG records was approached in the research challenge conducted by the administrators of the PhysioNet Web site during the international Computers in Cardiology Conference in 2003 [51]. Reference annotated events of the LTST DB were correctly classified as ischemic or nonischemic with sensitivity of 99.0% and specificity of 92.3% [52]. It should be noted that these result are significantly higher than a real analyzer would be able to achieve in any real situation since human annotations were known a priori and hence the problem of detecting the episodes and their precise beginnings were ignored.

Future improvements of transient ST episode detection systems are possible. Incorporating raw signals (i.e., QRS complex and ST segment pattern vectors, and other time series diagnostic parameters such as heart rate) could lead to improved and sophisticated systems for the detection of axis shifts and conduction changes and for the detection of transient ST episodes. Tracking the time-varying ST segment reference level due to nonischemic causes is crucial for reliable detection. Those systems dealing with time-varying ST segment reference level resulted in the highest performance. The next generation of transient ST episode detection systems will have to deal accurately with a time-varying ST segment reference level.

The LTST DB proved to be an important research resource for development and evaluation of ST episode detection systems. It contains records of long duration and adequately models the real-world conditions by a rich collection of transient ST segment events and noises. A large number of nonischemic ST segment events mixed with transient ischemic ST episodes allows the development of new reliable, robust and sophisticated ST episode detection systems, and testing and improving of existing ones. Besides, the database allows development of systems that are capable of distinguishing between transient ischemic and heart rate related ST episodes.

10.4.3   Assessing Robustness of ST Analyzers

Performance assessment using standard inputs [42, 44, 49, 50] can provide much useful information about an ST analyzer's behavior and its expected performance in the real-world, but these tests do not include methods for assessing robustness, which is another important issue when evaluating a given ST analyzer. In this section we present principles and methods for assessing the robustness of ST segment algorithms and analyzers. Evaluation protocol, procedures, and performance measures suitable for assessing the robustness are discussed. While performance measurements typically characterize how the standard inputs are analyzed, it is important to understand to what extent performance depends critically on the variation and choice of inputs. It is often the case that robustness is achieved at the cost of absolute performance in low noise circumstances, such as those of the ESC DB and LTST DB. Robust methods are generally preferred, because they are less likely to fail catastrophically than are nonrobust methods. Assessing the robustness of ST analyzers should answer the following questions:

1. To what extent performance depends critically on the variation of the noise content of input signals, or, is an ST analyzer robust with respect to the variation of input signals?
2. To what extent performance depends critically on the choice of the database used for testing, or, is an ST analyzer robust with respect to distribution of input signals?
3. To what extent the analysis parameters are critically tuned to the database used for testing, or, is an ST analyzer robust with respect to variation of its architecture parameters?

To answer these questions, protocols to assess the robustness of ST analyzers should include the following procedures [53]:

1. Noise stress tests, to determine the critical (minimum) SNR at which performance remains acceptable;
2. Bootstrap estimation of performance distributions, to determine if performance is critically dependent on the choice of the database used for testing;
3. Sensitivity analysis, to determine if analysis parameters are critically tuned to the test database.

An ST analyzer is considered to be robust if the performance measurements obtained during these procedures remain above predefined critical performance boundaries. An analyzer with a performance that is not critically dependent on the variation of the noise content of input signals is said to be robust with respect to the variation of input signals. An analyzer with a performance that is not critically dependent on the choice of the database used for testing is said to be robust with respect to the distribution of input signals. Similarly, if the analysis parameters do not critically affect performance as they are adjusted within some sensible range, an analyzer is robust with respect to variation of its architecture parameters.

Assessing the robustness offers the authors the facility to reveal how fragile their ST analyzer might be. The only ST analysis system [7] that was evaluated with respect to its robustness [53] showed not only robustness of the KLT-based techniques implemented with respect to variation and distribution of input signals, and with respect to variation its architecture parameters, but also confirmed that a dimensionality of five is also the optimal choice for feature representation and pattern recognition part of the analyzer when using orthogonal KLT basis functions. Noise stress test and bootstrap estimation of performance distributions of the robustness protocol are important to understand to what extent performance depends critically on the variation and choice of inputs. Sensitivity analysis of the robustness protocol allows the developer to make objective comparisons of ST analyzers. Knowing what architecture parameters of a given ST analyzer are relevant to be modified in order to "force" the analyzer's sensitivity to have the same sensitivity as other ST analyzers, and then comparing their positive predictivities, allows direct comparison of the performance of the analyzers.

References

[1]   Taddei, A., et al., "The European ST-T Database: Standard for Evaluating Systems for the Analysis of ST-T Changes in Ambulatory Electrocardiography," *European Heart Journal*, Vol. 13, 1992, pp. 1164–1172.

[2]   Jager, F., et al., "Analysis of Transient ST Segment Changes During Ambulatory ECG Monitoring," *Proc. Computers in Cardiology*, Venice, Italy, September 23–26, 1991, pp. 453–456.

[3]   Taddei, A., et al., "A System for the Detection of Ischemic Episodes in Ambulatory ECG," *Proc. Computers in Cardiology*, Vienna, Austria, September 10–13, 1995, pp. 705–708.

[4]   García, J., et al., "Automatic Detection of ST-T Complex Changes on the ECG Using Filtered RMS Difference Series: Application to Ambulatory Ischemia Monitoring," *IEEE Trans. Biomed. Eng.*, Vol. 47, No. 9, 2000, pp. 1195–1201.

[5]   Stadler, R. W., et al., "A Real-Time ST-Segment Monitoring Algorithm for Implantable Devices," *Journal of Electrocardiology*, Vol. 34, No. 4:2, 2001, pp. 119–126.

[6]   Jager, F., et al., "Analysis of Transient ST Segment Changes During Ambulatory ECG Monitoring Using the Karhunen-Loève Transform," *Proc. Computers in Cardiology*, Durham, NC, October 11–14, 1992, pp. 691–694.

[7]   Jager, F., G. B. Moody, and R. G. Mark, "Detection of Transient ST-Segment Episodes During Ambulatory ECG-Monitoring," *Computers and Biomedical Research*, Vol. 31, 1998, pp. 305–322.

[8]   Laguna, P., G. B. Moody, and R. G. Mark, "Analysis of the Cardiac Repolarization Period Using the KL Transform: Applications on the ST-T Database," *Proc. Computers in Cardiology*, Vienna, Austria, September 10–13, 1995, pp. 233–236.

[9]   Laguna, P., et al., "Analysis of the ST-T Complex of the Electrocardiogram Using the Karhunen-Loève Transform: Adaptive Monitoring and Alternans Detection," *Medical & Biological Engineering & Computing*, Vol. 37, 1999, pp. 175–189.

[10] Laguna, P., et al., "Model-Based Estimation of Cardiovascular Repolarization Features: Ischaemia Detection and PTCA Monitoring," *Journal of Medical Engineering & Technology*, Vol. 22, No. 2, 1998, pp. 64–72.

[11] García, J., et al., "Adaptive Estimation of Karhunen-Loève Series Applied to the Study of Ischemic ECG Records," *Proc. Computers in Cardiology*, Indianapolis, IN, September 8–11, 1996, pp. 249–252.

[12] García, J., et al., "Comparative Study of Local and Karhunen-Loève-Based ST-T Indexes in Recordings from Human Subjects with Induced Myocardial Ischemia," *Computers and Biomedical Research*, Vol. 31, 1998, pp. 271–292.

[13] Strintzis, M.G., et al., "Use of Neural Networks for Electrocardiogram (ECG) Feature Extraction and Classification," *Neural Network World*, Vol. 3–4, 1992, pp. 313–327.

[14] Stamkopoulos, T., et al., "One-Lead Ischemia Detection Using a New Backpropagation Algorithm and the European ST-T Database," *Proc. Computers in Cardiology*, Durham, NC, October 11–14, 1992, pp. 663–666.

[15] Silipo, R., and C., Marchesi, "Neural Techniques for ST-T Change Detection," *Proc. Computers in Cardiology*, Indianapolis, IN, September 8–11, 1996, pp. 677–680.

[16] Maglaveras, N., et al., "ECG Processing Techniques Based on Neural Networks and Bidirectional Associative Memories," *Journal of Medical Engineering & Technology*, Vol. 22, No. 3, 1998, pp. 106–111.

[17] Maglaveras, N., et al., "An Adaptive Backpropagation Neural Network for Real-Time Ischemia Episodes Detection: Development and Performance Analysis Using the European ST-T Database," *IEEE Trans. Biomed. Eng.*, Vol. 45, No. 7, 1998, pp. 805–813.

[18] Silipo, R., and C., Marchesi, "Artificial Neural Networks for Automatic ECG Analysis," *IEEE Trans. on Signal Processing*, Vol. 46, No. 5, 1998, pp. 1417–1425.

[19] Silipo, R., et al., "ST-T Change Recognition Using Artificial Neural Networks and Principal Component Analysis," *Proc. Computers in Cardiology*, Vienna, Austria, September 10–13, 1995, pp. 213–216.

[20] Maglaveras, N., et al., "ECG Pattern Recognition and Classification Using Non-Linear Transformations and Neural Networks: A Review," *International Journal of Medical Informatics*, Vol. 52, 1998, pp. 191–208.

[21] Stamkopoulos, T., et al., "ECG Analysis Using Nonlinear PCA Neural Networks for Ischemia Detection," *IEEE Trans. on Signal Processing*, Vol. 46, No. 11, 1998, pp. 3058–3067.

[22] Bezerianos, A., L. Vladutu, and S. Papadimitriou, "Hierarchical State Space Partitioning with a Network Self-Organising Map for the Recognition of ST-T Segment Changes," *Medical & Biological Engineering & Computing*, Vol. 38, 2000, pp. 406–415.

[23] Papadimitriou, S., et al., "Ischemia Detection with Self-Organizing Map Supplemented by Supervised Learning," *IEEE Trans. on Neural Networks*, Vol. 12, No. 3, 2001, pp. 503–515.

[24] Fernandez, E.A., et al., "Detection of Abnormality in the Electrocardiogram Without Prior Knowledge by Using the Quantisation Error of a Self-Organising Map, Tested on the European Ischaemia Database," *Medical & Biological Engineering & Computing*, Vol. 39, 2001, pp. 330–337.

[25] Papaloukas, C., et al., "An Ischemia Detection Method Based on Artificial Neural Networks," *Artificial Intelligence in Medicine*, Vol. 24, 2002, pp. 167–178.

[26] Presedo, J., et al., "Cycles of ECG Parameter Evolution During Ischemic Episodes," *Proc. Computers in Cardiology*, Indianapolis, IN, September 8–11, 1996, pp. 489–492.

[27] Presedo, J., et al., "Fuzzy Modelling of the Expert's Knowledge in ECG-Based Ischaemia Detection," *Fuzzy Sets and Systems*, Vol. 77, 1996, pp. 63–75.

[28] Zahan, S., "A Fuzzy Approach to Computer-Assisted Myocardial Ischemia Diagnosis," *Artificial Intelligence in Medicine*, Vol. 21, 2001, pp. 271–275.

[29] Sahambi, J. S., S. N., Tandon, and R. K. P., Bhatt, "Wavelet Based ST-Segment Analysis," *Medical & Biological Engineering & Computing*, Vol. 36, 1998, pp. 568–572.

[30] Andreao, R.V., et al., "ST-Segment Analysis Using Hidden Markov Model Beat Segmentation: Application to Ischemia Detection," *Proc. Computers in Cardiology*, Chicago, IL, September 19–22, 2004, pp. 381–384.

[31] Papaloukas, C., et al., "A Knowledge-Based Technique for Automated Detection of Ischemic Episodes in Long Duration Electrocardiograms," *Medical & Biological Engineering & Computing*, Vol. 38, 2001, pp. 105–112.

[32] Papaloukas, C., et al., "Use of a Novel Rule-Based Expert System in the Detection of Changes in the ST Segment and the T Wave in Long Duration ECGs," *Journal of Electrocardiology*, Vol. 35, No. 1, 2002, pp. 27–34.

[33] Vila, J., et al., "SUTIL: Intelligent Ischemia Monitoring System," *International Journal of Medical Informatics*, Vol. 47, 1997, pp. 193–214.

[34] Bosnjak, A., et al., "An Approach to Intelligent Ischaemia Monitoring," *Medical & Biological Engineering & Computing*, Vol. 33, 1995, pp. 749–756.

[35] Jager, F., et al., "Long-Term ST Database: A Reference for the Development and Evaluation of Automated Ischaemia Detectors and for the Study of the Dynamics of Myocardial Ischaemia," *Medical & Biological Engineering & Computing*, Vol. 41, No. 2, 2003, pp. 172–182.

[36] Shook, T. L., et al., "Validation of a New Algorithm for Detection and Quantification of Ischemic ST Segment Changes During Ambulatory Electrocardiography," *Proc. Computers in Cardiology*, Leuven, Belgium, September 12–15, 1987, pp. 57–62.

[37] Smrdel, A., and F. Jager, "Automated Detection of Transient ST-Segment Episodes in 24h Electrocardiograms," *Medical & Biological Engineering & Computing*, Vol. 42, No. 3, 2004, pp. 303–311.

[38] García, J., et al., "ECG-Based Detection of Body Position Changes in Ischemia Monitoring," *IEEE Trans. Biomed. Eng.*, Vol. 50, No. 6, 2003, pp. 677–685.

[39] Åström, M., et al., "Detection of Body Position Changes Using the Surface Electrocardiogram," *Medical & Biological Engineering & Computing*, Vol. 41, 2003, pp. 164–171.

[40] Shinar, Z., A. Baharav, and S. Akselrod, "Detection of Different Recumbent Body Positions from the Electrocardiogram," *Medical & Biological Engineering & Computing*, Vol. 41, 2003, pp. 206–210.

[41] Egan, J. P., *Signal Detection Theory and ROC Analysis*, New York: Academic Press, 1975.

[42] Jager, F., et al., "Performance Measures for Algorithms to Detect Transient Ischemic ST Segment Changes," *Proc. Computers in Cardiology*, Venice, Italy, September 23–26, 1991, pp. 369–372.

[43] Jager, F., "Automated Detection of Transient ST-Segment Changes During Ambulatory ECG-Monitoring," Ph.D. dissertation, Ljubljana, Slovenia, University of Ljubljana, Faculty of Electrical and Computer Engineering, 1994.

[44] Jager, F., "Guidelines for Assessing Performance of ST Analyzers," *Journal of Medical Engineering and Technology*, Vol. 22, 1998, pp. 25–30.

[45] Jager, F., A. Smrdel, and R. G. Mark, "An Open-Source Tool to Evaluate Performance of Transient ST Segment Episode Detection Algorithms," *Proc. Computers in Cardiology*, Chicago, IL, September 19–22, 2004, pp. 585–588.

[46] Efron, B., "Bootstrap Methods: Another Look at the Jackknife," *Annals of Statistics*, Vol. 7, 1979, pp. 1–26.

[47] Albrecht, P., G. B. Moody, and R. G. Mark, "Use of the 'Bootstrap' to Assess the Robustness of the Performance Statistics of the Arrhythmia Detector," *Journal of Ambulatory Monitoring*, Vol. 1, No. 2, 1988, pp. 171–176.

[48] Goldberger A. L., et al., "PhysioBank, PhysioToolkit, and PhysioNet Components of a New Research Resource for Complex Physiologic Signals," *Circulation*, Vol. 101, 2000, pp. e215–e220.

[49] ANSI/AAMI EC38:1998, "Ambulatory Electrocardiographs," *American National Standard Institute / Association for the Advancement of Medical Instrumentation*, Arlington, VA, 1999.

[50] ANSI/AAMI EC57:1998, "Testing and Reporting Performance Results of Cardiac Rhythm and ST Segment Measurement Algorithms," *American National Standard Institute / Association for the Advancement of Medical Instrumentation*, Arlington, VA, 1999.

[51]   Moody, G. B., and F. Jager, "Distinguishing Ischemic from Non-Ischemic ST Changes: The Physionet/Computers in Cardiology Challenge 2003," *Proc. Computers in Cardiology*, Thessaloniki, Greece, September 21–24, 2003, pp. 235–237.

[52]   Langley, P., et al., "An Algorithm to Distinguish Ischaemic and Non-Ischaemic ST Changes in the Holter ECG," *Proc. Computers in Cardiology*, Thessaloniki, Greece, September 21–24, 2003, pp. 239–242.

[53]   Jager, F., R. G. Mark, and G. B. Moody, "Protocol to Assess Robustness of ST Analyzers: A Case Study," *Physiologic Measurements*, Vol. 25, 2004, pp. 629–643.

CHAPTER 11

Probabilistic Approaches to ECG Segmentation and Feature Extraction

Nicholas P. Hughes

11.1 Introduction

The development of new drugs by the pharmaceutical industry is a costly and lengthy process, with the time from concept to final product typically lasting 10 years. Perhaps the most critical stage of this process is the phase one study, where the drug is administered to humans for the first time. During this stage each subject is carefully monitored for any unexpected adverse effects which may be brought about by the drug. Of particular interest is the ECG of the patient, which provides detailed information about the state of the patient's heart.

By examining the ECG signal in detail, it is possible to derive a number of informative measurements from the characteristic ECG waveform. These can then be used to assess the medical well-being of the patient, and more importantly, detect any potential side effects of the drug on the cardiac rhythm. The most important of these measurements is the QT interval. In particular, drug-induced prolongation of the QT interval (so called Long QT Syndrome) can result in a very fast, abnormal heart rhythm known as *torsade de pointes*. This rhythm can degenerate into ventricular fibrillation and hence lead to sudden cardiac death.

In practice, QT interval measurements are carried out manually by specially trained ECG analysts. This is an expensive and time-consuming process, which is susceptible to mistakes by the analysts and provides no associated degree of confidence (or accuracy) in the measurements. This problem was recently highlighted in the case of the antihistamine terfenadine, which had the side effect of significantly prolonging the QT interval in a number of patients. Unfortunately this side effect was not detected in the clinical trials and only came to light after a large number of people had unexpectedly died while taking the drug [1].

In this chapter we consider the problem of automated ECG interval analysis from a probabilistic modeling perspective. In particular, we examine the use of hidden Markov models for automatically segmenting an ECG signal into its constituent waveform features. An undecimated wavelet transform is used to provide an informative representation which is both robust to noise and tuned to the morphological characteristics of the waveform features. Finally we investigate the use of duration constraints for improving the robustness of the model segmentations.

11.2　The Electrocardiogram

11.2.1　The ECG Waveform

Each individual heartbeat is comprised of a number of distinct cardiological stages, which in turn give rise to a set of distinct features in the ECG waveform. These features represent either *depolarization* (electrical discharging) or *repolarization* (electrical recharging) of the muscle cells in particular regions of the heart. Figure 11.1 shows a human ECG waveform and the associated features. The standard features of the ECG waveform are the P wave, the QRS complex, and the T wave. Additionally a small U wave (following the T wave) is occasionally present.

The cardiac cycle begins with the P wave (the start and end points of which are referred to as P_{on} and P_{off}), which corresponds to the period of *atrial depolarization* in the heart. This is followed by the QRS complex, which is generally the most recognizable feature of an ECG waveform, and corresponds to the period of *ventricular depolarization*. The start and end points of the QRS complex are referred to as the Q and J points. The T wave follows the QRS complex and corresponds to the period of *ventricular repolarization*. The end point of the T wave is referred to as T_{off} and represents the end of the cardiac cycle (presuming the absence of a U wave).

11.2.2　ECG Interval Analysis

The timing between the onset and offset of particular features of the ECG (referred to as an *interval*) is of great importance since it provides a measure of the state of the heart and can indicate the presence of certain cardiological conditions. Two of

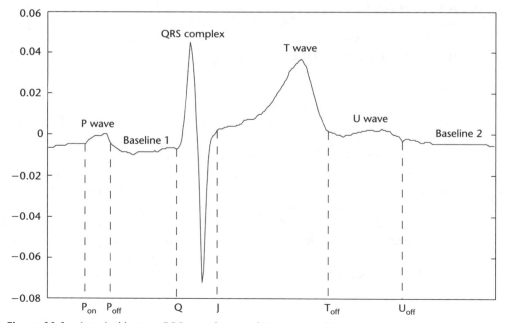

Figure 11.1　A typical human ECG waveform and its associated feature boundaries.

the most important intervals in the ECG waveform are the QT interval and the PR interval. The QT interval is defined as the time from the start of the QRS complex to the end of the T wave (i.e., $T_{off}-Q$) and corresponds to the total duration of electrical activity (both depolarization and repolarization) in the ventricles. Similarly, the PR interval is defined as the time from the start of the P wave to the start of the QRS complex (i.e., $Q-P_{on}$) and corresponds to the time from the onset of atrial depolarization to the onset of ventricular depolarization.

Changes in the QT interval are currently the gold standard for evaluating the effects of drugs on ventricular repolarization. In addition, changes in the PR interval can indicate the presence of specific cardiological conditions such as *atrioventricular block* [2]. Thus, the accurate measurement and assessment of the QT and PR intervals is of paramount importance in clinical drug trials.

11.2.3   Manual ECG Interval Analysis

Manual ECG interval analysis is typically performed by specialist ECG analysis companies known as *centralized ECG core laboratories*. The expert analysts (or "readers") employed by these labs are generally a mixture of professional cardiologists and highly trained cardiac technicians.

The accurate measurement of the QT interval is made difficult by the need to locate the *end* of the T wave to a high level of precision. In theory, the end of the T wave is defined as the point at which the ECG signal (for the T wave) returns to the isoelectric baseline. In practice, however, determining this point precisely is challenging due to the variation in the baseline amplitude, unusual or abnormal T wave morphologies (such as T-U fusions or flat T waves), and the presence of noise or artifact in the signal.

As a result, T wave offset measurements by expert analysts are inherently subjective and the associated QT interval measurements often suffer from a high degree of interanalyst and intra-analyst variability. There has therefore been much focus on the problem of developing an automated ECG interval analysis system, which could provide robust and consistent measurements, together with an associated degree of confidence in each measurement [3].

11.3   Automated ECG Interval Analysis

Standard approaches to ECG segmentation attempt to find the ECG waveform feature boundaries from a given ECG signal in a number of successive stages [4]. In the first stage, a standard QRS detection algorithm (such as the Pan and Tompkins algorithm [5]) is used to locate the R peaks in the ECG signal. Given the location of the R peak in each ECG beat, the next stage in the process is to search forwards and backwards from this point to estimate the locations of the onset and offset boundaries for the various ECG features [4].

In common with manual analysis, the accurate determination of the end of the T wave with automated methods is a challenging problem. The standard approach to this problem is based on the *tangent method*, which is illustrated in Figure 11.2. This technique, which was first introduced in 1952, locates the end of the T wave as the

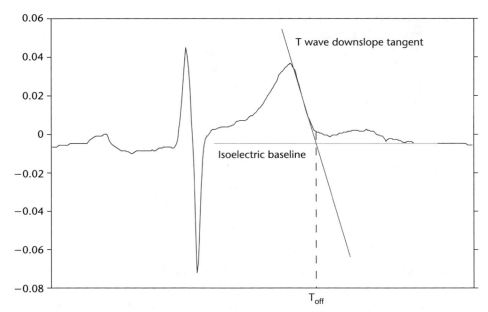

Figure 11.2   An example of the tangent method for determining the end of the T wave. A tangent to the T wave is computed at the point of maximum (absolute) gradient following the T wave peak, and the intersection of this tangent with the estimated isoelectric baseline gives the T wave offset location.

point of intersection between the (estimated) isoelectric baseline and the tangent to the downslope of the T wave (or the upslope for inverted T waves) [6]. The tangent itself is computed at the point of maximum (absolute) gradient following the peak of the T wave.

A significant disadvantage of the tangent method is that it is sensitive to the amplitude of the T wave. In particular, large amplitude T waves can cause the tangent to intersect the isoelectric baseline well before the actual end of the T wave. As a result, the automated QT intervals from the tangent method can significantly underestimate the actual QT interval value. To overcome this problem, Xu and Reddy applied a "nonlinear correction" factor (based on the T wave amplitude) to the T wave offset determined by the tangent method [7].

In practice, automated QT interval measurements continue to be unreliable in the presence of noisy waveforms or unusual T wave morphologies. In addition, it is still the case that automated systems can produce highly unreliable measurements for relatively clean ECGs with regular waveform morphologies [8]. As a result, ECG interval measurements for clinical drug trials are generally performed manually by human experts.

11.4   The Probabilistic Modeling Approach

The *probabilistic modeling* approach to automated ECG interval analysis offers a number of significant advantages compared with traditional approaches. In particular, probabilistic models provide the following benefits:

- The ability to learn from ECG data sets annotated by human experts;
- The ability to incorporate prior knowledge about the statistical characteristics of the ECG waveform features in a principled manner;
- The ability to produce confidence measures in the automated ECG interval measurements.

One of the most powerful features of the probabilistic modeling approach is the ability to learn a model for ECG segmentation from expert annotated ECG data. Such *data-driven* learning allows us to sidestep neatly the problem of having to specify an explicit rule for determining the end of the T wave in the electrocardiogram (e.g., the tangent method). Since rule-based approaches are inherently unreliable for this particular problem (given the wide range of ECG morphologies which can occur in practice), it is much more appropriate to learn the statistical characteristics which define the ECG waveform feature boundaries using measurements from expert analysts. Furthermore, this learning approach enables us to build models from ECG data sets which exhibit specific types of waveform morphologies, or from those corresponding to specific patient cohorts [9].

The most appropriate form of probabilistic model to apply to the task of automated ECG interval analysis is a *hidden Markov model* (HMM). These models can be viewed as a form of *state space model*. Specifically, HMMs make use of a discrete state space to capture the sequential characteristics of the data. This particular formulation offers an attractive framework for ECG signal modeling, since it allows each of the ECG waveform features (i.e., P wave, QRS complex, T wave, and so forth) to be uniquely associated with a particular state in the model. Thus, the model is able to take advantage of the sequence ordering which exists between the different waveform features of normal ECGs.

An additional advantage of utilizing hidden Markov models when considering probabilistic approaches to ECG segmentation is that there are efficient algorithms for HMM training and testing. Specifically, the parameters of an HMM can be estimated straightforwardly in a *supervised* manner using a data set of ECG waveforms together with the corresponding expert measurements of the waveform feature boundaries. Alternatively, if the data set contains only the ECG waveforms (i.e., the associated expert measurements are unavailable), then the EM algorithm can be used to train the model in an *unsupervised* manner [10]. Once the model has been trained, the Viterbi algorithm can be used to segment test ECG signals.

A disadvantage of the probabilistic modeling approach is that the segmentation of ECGs typically requires more computing power (for the same level of processing performance) compared with standard algorithms. For the analysis of 10-second 12-lead ECG signals, this is rarely an issue. However, when very large amounts of ECG data must be processed rapidly (e.g., for the analysis of continuous 12-lead digital Holter recordings), it may be necessary to combine both standard (nonprobabilistic) and probabilistic algorithms to achieve an appropriate rate of segmentation.

Although the use of hidden Markov models for ECG analysis has been considered previously in the literature [11, 12], many of the issues involved in achieving a high level of segmentation accuracy with these models have not previously been discussed in detail. In this chapter, we focus on the core issues which must be addressed when using probabilistic models for automated ECG interval analysis. Specifically, we consider the choice of representation for the ECG signal, and the choice of model architecture for the segmentation.

In the following sections, we describe how wavelet methods (and in particular, the undecimated wavelet transform) can be used to provide an encoding of the ECG which is more appropriate for subsequent modeling with HMMs. In addition, we describe how "duration constraints" can be incorporated into the HMM framework such that the resulting model provides a more appropriate statistical description of the normal ECG waveform, and hence a greater degree of robustness in the waveform segmentations.

11.5 Data Collection

In order to develop an automated system for ECG interval analysis, we collected a data set of over 100 ECG waveforms (sampled at 500 Hz), together with the corresponding waveform feature boundaries as determined by a group of expert ECG analysts. Due to time constraints it was not possible for each expert analyst to label every ECG waveform in the data set. Therefore, we chose to distribute the waveforms at random among the different experts (such that each waveform was measured by one expert only).

For each ECG waveform, the following points were annotated: P_{on}, P_{off}, Q, J, and T_{off} (if a U wave was present, the U_{off} point was also annotated). In addition, the point corresponding to the start of the next P wave (i.e., the P wave of the following heartbeat), NP_{on}, was also annotated. During the data collection exercise, we found that it was not possible to obtain reliable estimates for the T_{on} and U_{on} points, and therefore these were taken to be the J and T_{off} points, respectively.

11.6 Introduction to Hidden Markov Modeling

11.6.1 Overview

Since their development in the late 1960s and early 1970s, hidden Markov models have proved to be a powerful and flexible class of statistical model for describing many different kinds of *sequential* data. The term "sequential" here refers to the fact that there exists a natural ordering inherent in the data itself. This property is particularly true of time-series data, where the individual data samples are ordered according to the particular time point at which they were measured. By incorporating this sequence information into the structure of our model, we can ensure that the model provides a good description of the data and its associated statistical properties.

The utility of hidden Markov models stems from the fact that they offer an effective balance between the core data modeling issues of complexity and tractability. In particular, hidden Markov models are "rich" enough to provide a good statistical description of many different kinds of sequence data, yet they are also sufficiently simple as to admit efficient algorithms for inference and learning. This trade-off between descriptive modeling power and practical ease of use is perhaps the main reason for the success of hidden Markov models in practice.

This section presents a thorough review of hidden Markov models and their associated algorithms for inference and learning. We begin with a brief description of Markov models in the context of stochastic processes, and then proceed to cover the topic of hidden Markov models in more depth.

11.6.2 Stochastic Processes and Markov Models

A natural way to describe a stochastic process is in terms of the probability distribution of the random variable under consideration. In particular, for processes that evolve through time, it is often useful to consider a conditional probability distribution of the form

$$p(x_t \mid x_{t_1}, x_{t_2}, x_{t_3}, \ldots) \tag{11.1}$$

which defines the probability of obtaining a sample value x at time t given a history of previous values. If this distribution is *time-invariant*, such that it is only dependent on the time differences (or "lags") and not the absolute time values, then the process is said to be *strictly stationary*.[1] In this case, (11.1) can be written in the form:

$$p(x_t \mid x_{t-\tau_1}, x_{t-\tau_2}, x_{t-\tau_3}, \ldots) \tag{11.2}$$

A special case of interest occurs when this conditional distribution is dependent on only a *finite* history of previous values, such that:

$$p(x_t \mid x_{t-\tau_1}, x_{t-\tau_2}, \ldots, x_{t-\tau_N}) \tag{11.3}$$

which defines an Nth-order *Markov process*. If we now make the further simplifying assumption that the process depends soley on the previous value, then the conditional distribution becomes

$$p(x_t \mid x_{t-\tau}) \tag{11.4}$$

This equation defines a *first-order Markov process*, which is often referred to simply as a "Markov process" [13]. When dealing with a discrete-time discrete-valued random variable s_t, this Markov process becomes a Markov chain, with the corresponding conditional distribution:

$$P(s_t \mid s_{t-1}) \tag{11.5}$$

A Markov *model* can be used to represent any random variable s_t which can occupy one of K possible discrete "states" at each time step and which satisfies the Markov property

$$P(s_{t+1} \mid s_t, s_{t-1}, s_{t-2}, \ldots) = P(s_{t+1} \mid s_t) \tag{11.6}$$

Equation (11.6) captures the notion that "the *future* is conditionally independent of the *past* given the *present*." Thus when evaluating the probability of the

---

1. A more relaxed definition of stationarity requires that only the first and second moments of the distribution are time-invariant, in which case the process is said to be *weakly stationary*.

system state at a particular time step, we need only consider the state at the previous time step. Statistical models which exploit this Markov property often admit efficient algorithms for computing many practical quantities of interest.

In practice, a Markov model is governed by two distinct parameters: an *initial state distribution* and a *state transition matrix*. The initial state distribution π defines the probabilities of the random variable being in each of the K possible states at the *first* time step (i.e., $t = 1$). Thus, this parameter is simply a K-dimensional vector, where each element π_k gives the corresponding probability $P(s_1 = k)$. The state transition matrix $\mathbf{A}$ defines the probability of the model "transitioning" to a particular state at the next time step, given its state at the current time step. Thus, this parameter is a $K \times K$ matrix, where each element a_{ij} gives the corresponding probability $P(s_{t+1} = j \mid s_t = i)$. If it is possible to transition from any state to any other state (i.e., $a_{ij} \neq 0 \ \forall i, j$), then the model is said to be *ergodic* [7].

11.6.3   Hidden Markov Models

A hidden Markov model is a probabilistic model which describes the statistical relationship between an *observable* sequence O and an *unobservable* or "hidden" state sequence S. The hidden state itself is discrete and governed by an underlying Markov model. The observation values however may be either continuous or discrete in nature.

The key aspect of an HMM is that each observation value is considered to be the result of an additional stochastic process associated with one of the hidden states. Thus, a hidden Markov model can be viewed as a "doubly embedded stochastic process with an underlying stochastic process that is not observable (it is hidden), but can only be observed through another set of stochastic processes that produce the sequence of observations" [10].

More formally, an HMM (with K hidden states) is defined by the following three parameters [10]:

- An initial state distribution π;
- A state transition matrix A;
- An observation probability distribution b_k for each state k.

The first two parameters govern the underlying Markov model which describes the statistical properties of the hidden states. It is the observation probability distributions[2] however which differentiate a hidden Markov model from a standard Markov model. More precisely, the observation probability distribution for a given state models the probability of a particular observation value when the model occupies that particular state.

It is often useful to consider a hidden Markov model from a *generative* perspective. That is, we can consider the HMM as providing a bottom-up description of how the observed sequence O is produced or generated. Viewed as a generative model, the operation of an HMM is as follows:

---

2.   The observation probability distributions are also known as *emission* probability distributions.

1. Select the initial state k by sampling from the initial state distribution π.
2. Generate a observation value from this state by sampling from the associated observation distribution b_k.
3. Select the state at the next time step based upon the transition matrix $\mathbf{A}$.
4. Return to step 2.

In the standard formulation of a hidden Markov model, the observation values "within" a given state are considered to be *independent and identically distributed* (i.i.d.). Hence, when an observation value is generated by a particular state at a given time step, it is generated independently of any previous samples which may have been generated from that same state in previous time steps. Thus, conditioned on the state sequence, we can express the likelihood of a sequence of observations as

$$p(O_{1:T} \mid S_{1:T}, \lambda) = \prod_{t=1}^{T} p(O_t \mid S_t, \lambda) \tag{11.7}$$

where λ represents the set of model parameters for the HMM. It is important to recognize that the factorization shown in (11.7) holds only when the observations are conditioned on the state sequence. Thus, without knowledge of the underlying state sequence, we cannot make any independence assumptions about the probability distribution of the observations [i.e., $p(O_{1:T} \mid \lambda)$].

The assumption of statistical independence between successive observations (within a state) is perhaps the greatest weakness of the standard hidden Markov model. The validity of this assumption in the context of ECG signal modeling is considered in greater detail in Section 11.7.4.

Figure 11.3 shows two different graphical representations of a simple two-state hidden Markov model. The first representation, illustrated in Figure 11.3(a), shows the "architectural" view of an HMM. This form of the model highlights the overall HMM topology together with the role of the individual model parameters. In particular, the two clear nodes correspond to the two individual hidden states

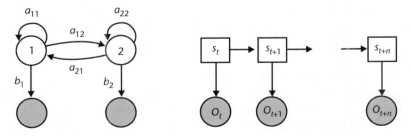

(a) Standard HMM topology   (b) Dynamic Bayesian network

Figure 11.3 Two different graphical representations of a hidden Markov model. (a) In the standard representation the clear nodes corresponds to specific hidden states in the model, and the shaded nodes correspond to the observations which are generated by those hidden states. (b) In the DBN representation each clear node corresponds to the particular state which the model occupies at a given time step, and each shaded node corresponds to the associated observation generated by that state.

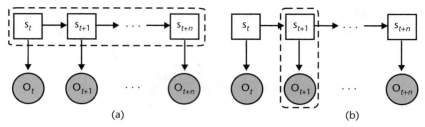

Figure 11.4 Alternative "views" of a hidden Markov model. (a) The HMM as a simple Markov model in which the states are stochastically related to the observations. (b) The HMM as a form of temporal mixture model in which the individual mixture components obey a sequence ordering (governed by the transition matrix).

in the model, and the two shaded nodes correspond to the observations that are generated by those hidden states.

The second representation, illustrated in Figure 11.3(b), shows the HMM as a *dynamic Bayesian network* (DBN) [14]. Here the HMM is shown "unrolled" over a number of time steps. Each clear node[3] now corresponds to the particular state which the model occupies at a given time step, and each shaded node corresponds to the associated observation generated by that state. Both graphical representations serve to illustrate the role of an HMM as a statistical model for sequential data.

Hidden Markov models can also be seen as generalizations of various statistical models [15, 16]. Figure 11.4 shows two such possible "views" of an HMM. The first, shown in Figure 11.4(a), denotes the HMM as a simple Markov model with stochastic observations. This is the view outlined previously in this section. An alternative perspective, however, can be gained by considering the HMM as a form of temporal mixture model, as illustrated in Figure 11.4(b). With a standard (static) mixture model, each data point is considered to have been "generated" by one of the K mixture components independently of the other data points [17]. If we now relax the strong assumption of statistical independence between data points and allow the individual mixture components to possess Markovian "dynamics," the result is a hidden Markov model (where the hidden state at each time step corresponds to the particular mixture component which is active at that time step).

More generally, hidden Markov models can be viewed under the general framework of *probabilistic graphical models* [18]. Such models include standard "state-space" models such as hidden Markov models and Kalman filters as special cases, as well as more advanced models such as coupled HMMs [19] and factorial HMMs [20].

From a purely statistical perspective, an HMM defines a *joint* probability distribution over observation sequences O and hidden state sequences S [i.e., $p(O, S \mid \lambda)$]. Given this joint distribution, it is often of interest to find the particular state sequence which maximizes the conditional distribution $P(S \mid O, \lambda)$. This corresponds to

---

3. In the "language" of Bayesian networks, a *square* node represents a discrete value and a *circular* node represents a continuous value. Similarly a *clear* node represents a hidden (or latent) variable and a *shaded* node represents an observed variable. Hence in Figure 11.3(b), the hidden states are shown as clear square nodes, and the observations (which are assumed to be continuous in this example) are shows as shaded circular nodes.

the state sequence which is most likely to have "generated" the given observation sequence, and thus provides an effective means to segment the observation sequence into its characteristic features. However, before we can use an HMM for such purposes, we must first learn the "optimal" parameters of the model from a given data set (such that the HMM provides a useful statistical model of the data). We now consider the solution to each of these problems in greater detail.

11.6.4 Inference in HMMs

The inference problem for hidden Markov models is typically cast as the problem of determining the single most probable state sequence given the observation data, that is,

$$S^* = \underset{S}{\text{argmax}} \ \{P(S \mid O, \lambda)\} \tag{11.8}$$

This can be reexpressed using Bayes' rule as

$$
\begin{aligned}
S^* &= \underset{S}{\text{argmax}} \ \{P(S \mid O, \lambda)\} \\
&= \underset{S}{\text{argmax}} \ \left\{ \frac{p(S, O \mid \lambda)}{p(O \mid \lambda)} \right\} \\
&= \underset{S}{\text{argmax}} \ \{p(S, O \mid \lambda)\}
\end{aligned}
\tag{11.9}
$$

Hence it suffices to find the state sequence S^* which maximizes the joint distribution $p(S, O \mid \lambda)$. The solution to this problem is known as the *Viterbi algorithm* [21, 22]. More precisely, the Viterbi algorithm is a dynamic programming procedure which takes advantage of the Markov property of the HMM state sequence.

To apply dynamic programming to the HMM inference problem, we must first define the variable $\delta_t(i)$:

$$\delta_t(i) = \max_{s_1 s_2 \cdots s_{t-1}} \{ p(s_1 s_2 \cdots s_t = i, O_1 O_2 \cdots O_t \mid \lambda) \} \tag{11.10}$$

This is the likelihood of the most probable state sequence that accounts for the first t observations and ends in state i at time t. Now consider computing the value of the delta variable at the next time step $t + 1$. We can express this computation as

$$
\begin{aligned}
\delta_{t+1}(i) &= \max_{s_1 s_2 \cdots s_t} \big\{ p(s_1 s_2 \cdots s_{t+1} = i, O_1 O_2 \cdots O_{t+1} \mid \lambda) \big\} \\
&= \max_{j} \Big\{ \max_{s_1 s_2 \cdots s_{t-1}} \{ p(s_1 s_2 \cdots s_t = j, O_1 O_2 \cdots O_t \mid \lambda) \} \\
&\quad \times P(s_{t+1} = i \mid s_t = j) \Big\} \ p(O_{t+1} \mid s_{t+1} = i) \\
&= \max_{j} \{ \delta_t(j) \, a_{ji} \} \, b_i(O_{t+1})
\end{aligned}
\tag{11.11}
$$

The key step in developing the recurrence relation for $\delta_{t+1}(i)$ is to note that we can make use of the solutions to the previous subproblems at time step t.

In particular, we can compute the most probable state sequence that accounts for the first $t + 1$ observations and ends in state i by maximizing over the K previous solutions [i.e., $\delta_t(j)$] *and* the appropriate transition probability (a_{ji}).

The recursion is initialized for each state i by computing the probability of the model occupying state i at the first time step and producing the first observation value O_1 from that particular state, that is,

$$\delta_1(i) = \pi_i \, b_i(O_1) \tag{11.12}$$

Equation (11.11) can then be used to compute the value of $\delta_t(i)$ for each state i and for each time step from $t = 2$ to $t = T$. Following the final computation at $t = T$, we have

$$\delta_T(i) = \max_{s_1 s_2 \cdots s_{T-1}} \{p(s_1 s_2 \cdots s_T = i, O_1 O_2 \cdots O_T \mid \lambda)\} \tag{11.13}$$

The optimal value for the hidden state at the final time step is then computed as the particular state which maximizes (11.13)

$$s_T^* = \operatorname*{argmax}_i \left\{\delta_T(i)\right\} \tag{11.14}$$

Using this knowledge of the optimal state value at the final time step, we can then "work back" to uncover the optimal state value at the previous time step $t = T - 1$. This is given by the particular state argument which maximized $\delta_T(s_T^*)$ as part of its recursive computation. Based on this value, we can follow a similar procedure to uncover the optimal state value at time step $T - 2$. This general backtracking procedure can be performed successively to uncover the full optimal hidden state sequence S^*.

When computing (11.11) in practice, it is common to record the particular "maximizing" state which maximizes the value of $\delta_{t+1}(i)$:

$$\psi_{t+1}(i) = \operatorname*{argmax}_j \left\{\delta_t(j) \, a_{ji}\right\} \tag{11.15}$$

The back-tracking procedure to uncover the optimal state sequence can then be implemented as a look-up process using the stored ψ values:

$$s_t^* = \psi_{t+1}(s_{t+1}^*) \qquad t = T - 1, T - 2, \cdots, 1 \tag{11.16}$$

Pseudo-code for the Viterbi procedure is shown in Listing 1. Note that in practice, the implementation of the Viterbi algorithm requires the use of a simple "scaling" procedure to ensure that the $\delta_t(i)$ values do not under- or overflow [10].

11.6.5   Learning in HMMs

The learning problem in hidden Markov models is concerned with determining the optimal model parameters given a particular training data set. If the data set consists of both the observation sequences and the corresponding hidden state sequences (which generated the observation sequences), then the HMM parameter

---

Listing 1 Viterbi algorithm

//Initialization:
for $i = 1$ to K
  $\delta_1(i) = \pi_i b_i(O_1)$
  $\psi_1(i) = 0$
end

//Recursion:
for $t = 2$ to T
  //Compute delta at time t for each state i
  //and record "maximizing" predecessor state
  for $i = 1$ to K
    $\delta_t(i) = \max_{1 \leq j \leq K}\{\delta_{t-1}(j)a_{ji}b_i(O_t)\}$
    $\psi_t(i) = \operatorname*{argmax}_{1 \leq j \leq K}\{\delta_{t-1}(j)a_{ji}\}$
  end
end

//Termination:
$P^* = \max_{1 \leq i \leq K}\{\delta_T(i)\}$
$s_T^* = \operatorname*{argmax}_{1 \leq i \leq K}\{\delta_T(i)\}$
//Backtracking:
for $t = T - 1$ to 1
  $s_t^* = \psi_{t+1}(s_{t+1}^*)$
end

---

estimation problem can be viewed as a *supervised* learning problem. Conversely, if the data set consists of *only* the observation sequences, then the problem is one of *unsupervised* learning. We now consider each of these two cases in turn.

11.6.5.1 Supervised Learning

In the *supervised* learning case, we can make use of both the observation sequences and the corresponding hidden state sequences to derive simple estimates for the model parameters. In particular, we can estimate the initial state distribution by evaluating the fraction of the hidden state sequences which commence in each of the given model states at the first time step. More precisely, denoting the total number of hidden state sequences which commence in state i at the first time step by $n_{\text{init}}(i)$, then we have the following estimator for the ith element of the initial state distribution:

$$\pi_i = \frac{n_{\text{init}}(i)}{\sum_{k=1}^{K} n_{\text{init}}(k)} \tag{11.17}$$

In a similar manner, we can estimate the transition matrix by evaluating the fraction of particular state transitions over all the hidden state sequences. More precisely, denoting the total number of transitions from state i to state j over all the hidden state sequences by $n_{\text{trans}}(i, j)$, then we have the following estimator for the (i, j)th element of the transition matrix:

$$a_{ij} = \frac{n_{\text{trans}}(i, j)}{\sum_{k=1}^{K} n_{\text{trans}}(i, k)} \tag{11.18}$$

The exact estimator for the parameters of the observation models depends on the specific functional form chosen for these models. However, the general estimation procedure for the observation models is straightforward. For each state i, we simply "extract" all the observations which correspond to that particular state (i.e., those that were "generated" by that state) and then fit the observation model to this data in a standard manner.

11.6.5.2   Unsupervised Learning

In the *unsupervised* learning case, we are provided with a data set of observation sequences *only* (i.e., we do not have access to the corresponding hidden state sequences). This makes the learning procedure much more difficult compared with the supervised case previously described.

Given the data set of observation sequences $\mathbf{O} = \{O_1, O_2, \ldots, O_N\}$, the unsupervised learning problem is typically cast in a maximum likelihood framework. More precisely, we seek the model parameters λ^* which maximize the probability of the data; that is,

$$\lambda^* = \underset{\lambda}{\mathrm{argmax}}\{p(\mathbf{O} \mid \lambda)\} \tag{11.19}$$

Fortunately, there exists a particularly effective approach to solving (11.19) for hidden Markov models (and many other types of statistical models). This approach is known as the EM algorithm,[4] and is a general method for unsupervised learning in the presence of "missing" or incomplete data [23].

We now discuss the application of hidden Markov models to the particular problem of ECG segmentation.

11.7   Hidden Markov Models for ECG Segmentation

This section presents a detailed analysis of the use of hidden Markov models for *segmenting* ECG signals. The general aim of any signal segmentation method is to "partition" a given signal into consecutive regions of interest. In the context of the ECG then, the role of segmentation is to determine as accurately as possible the onset and offset boundaries of the various waveform features (e.g., P wave, QRS complex, T wave, and so forth), such that the ECG interval measurements may be computed automatically.

In Section 11.7.1, we discuss the different types of hidden Markov model architecture which can be used for ECG segmentation. Following this, we discuss the two different forms of segmentations which can occur when a trained HMM is used to segment ECG signals in practice. The performance of HMMs for ECG segmentation is then considered in more detail. In particular, we examine a number of different state observation models, as well as the use of ECG signal normalization techniques.

---

4.   In the context of hidden Markov models, the EM algorithm is often referred to as the *Baum-Welch algorithm*.

11.7.1 Overview

The first step in applying hidden Markov models to the task of ECG segmentation is to associate each state in the model with a particular region of the ECG. As discussed previously in Section 11.6.5, this can either be achieved in a supervised manner (i.e., using expert measurements) or an unsupervised manner (i.e., using the EM algorithm). Although the former approach requires each ECG waveform in the training data set to be associated with expert measurements of the waveform feature boundaries (i.e., the P_{on}, Q, T_{off} points, and so forth), the resulting models generally produce more accurate segmentation results compared with their unsupervised counterparts.

Figure 11.5 shows a variety of different HMM architectures for ECG interval analysis. A simple way of associating each HMM state with a region of the ECG is to use individual hidden states to represent the P wave, QRS complex, JT interval and baseline regions of the ECG, as shown in Figure 11.5(a). In practice, it is advantageous to partition the single baseline state into multiple baseline states [9], one of which is used to model the baseline region between the end of the P wave and the start of the QRS complex (termed "baseline 1"), and another which is used to model the baseline region following the end of the T wave (termed "baseline 2"). This model architecture, which is shown in Figure 11.5(b), will be used throughout the rest of this chapter.[5]

Following the choice of model architecture, the next step in training an HMM is to decide upon the specific type of observation model which will be used to capture the statistical characteristics of the signal samples from each hidden state. Common choices for the observation models in an HMM are the Gaussian density, the Gaussian mixture model (GMM), and the autoregressive (AR) model. Section 11.7.4 discusses the different types of observation models in the context of ECG segmentation.

Before training a hidden Markov model for ECG segmentation, it is beneficial to consider the use of preprocessing techniques for ECG signal normalization.

11.7.2 ECG Signal Normalization

In many pattern recognition tasks it is advantageous to normalize the raw input data prior to any subsequent modeling [24]. A particularly simple and effective form of signal normalization is a linear rescaling of the signal sample values. In the case of the ECG, this procedure can help to normalize the dynamic range of the signal and to stabilize the baseline sections.

A useful form of signal normalization is given by *range normalization*, which linearly scales the signal samples such that the maximum sample value is set to $+1$ and the minimum sample value to -1. This can be achieved in a simple two-step process. First, the signal samples are "amplitude shifted" such that the minimum and maximum sample values are equidistant from zero. Next, the signal samples are linearly scaled by dividing by the new maximum sample value. These two steps

---

5. Note that it is also possible to use an "optional" U wave state (following the T wave) to model any U waves that may be present in the data, as shown in Figure 11.5(c).

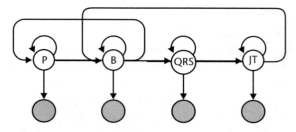

(a) HMM for ECG waveform segmentation (*common* baseline state)

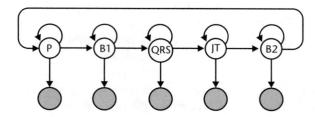

(b) HMM for ECG waveform segmenation (*separate* baseline states)

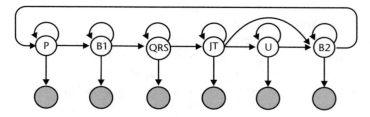

(c) HMM for ECG waveform segmentation (*with* U wave state)

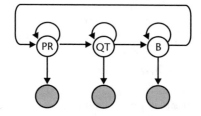
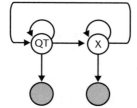

(d) HMM for PR and QT interval segmentation   (e) HMM for QT interval segmentation

Figure 11.5   (a–e) Hidden Markov model architectures for ECG interval analysis.

can be stated mathematically as

$$x'_n = x_n - \left(\frac{x_{min} + x_{max}}{2} \right) \tag{11.20}$$

and

$$y_n = \frac{x'_n}{x'_{max}} \tag{11.21}$$

where x_{min} and x_{max} are the minimum and maximum values in the original signal, respectively. The range normalization procedure can be made more robust to the presence of artefact or "spikes" in the ECG signal by computing the median of the minimum and maximum signal values over a number of different signal segments. Specifically, the ECG signal is divided evenly into a number of contiguous segments, and the minimum and maximum signal values within each segment are computed. The ECG signal is then range normalized (i.e., scaled) to the median of the minimum and maximum values over the given segments.

11.7.3 Types of Model Segmentations

Before considering in detail the results for HMMs applied to the task of ECG segmentation, it is advantageous to consider first the different types of ECG segmentations that can occur in practice. In particular, we can identify two distinct forms of model segmentations when a trained HMM is used to segment a given 10-second ECG signal:

- *Single-beat segmentations*: Here the model correctly infers only one heartbeat where there is only one beat present in a particular region of the ECG signal.
- *Double-beat segmentations*: Here the model incorrectly infers two or more heartbeats where there is only one beat present in a particular region of the ECG signal.

Figure 11.6(a, b) shows examples of single-beat and double-beat segmentations, respectively. In the example of the double-beat segmentation, the model incorrectly infers *two* separate beats in the ECG signal shown. The first beat correctly locates the QRS complex but incorrectly locates the end of the T wave (in the region of baseline prior to the T wave). The second beat then "locates" another QRS complex (of duration one sample) around the onset of the T wave, but correctly locates the end of the T wave in the ECG signal. The specific reason for the occurrence of double-beat segmentations and a method to alleviate this problem are covered in Section 11.9.

In the case of a single-beat segmentation, the segmentation errors can be evaluated by simply computing the discrepancy between each individual automated annotation (e.g., T_{off}) and the corresponding expert analyst annotation. In the case of a double-beat segmentation, however, it is not possible to associate uniquely each expert annotation with a corresponding automated annotation. Given this, it is therefore not meaningful to attempt to evaluate a measure of annotation "error" for double-beat segmentations. Thus, a more informative approach is simply to report the percentage of single-beat segmentations for a given ECG data set, along with the segmentation errors for the single-beat segmentations only.

11.7.4 Performance Evaluation

The technique of *cross-validation* [24] was used to evaluate the performance of a hidden Markov model for automated ECG segmentation. In particular, five-fold cross-validation was used. In the first stage, the data set of annotated ECG

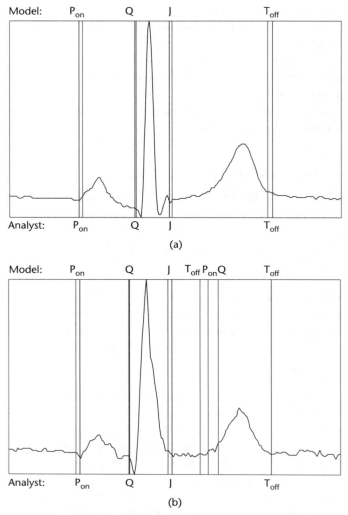

Figure 11.6　Examples of the two different types of HMM segmentations which can occur in practice: (a) single- and (b) double-beat segmentation.

waveforms was partitioned into five subsets of approximately equal size (in terms of the number of annotated ECG waveforms within each subset). For each "fold" of the cross-validation procedure, a model was trained in a supervised manner using all the annotated ECG waveforms from four of the five subsets. The trained model was then tested on the data from the remaining subset. This procedure was repeated for each of the five possible test subsets. Prior to performing cross-validation, the complete data set of annotated ECG waveforms was randomly permuted in order to remove any possible ordering which could affect the results.

As previously stated, for each fold of cross-validation a model was trained in a supervised manner. The transition matrix was estimated from the training waveform annotations using the supervised estimator given in (11.18). For Gaussian observation models, the mean and variance of the full set of signal samples were computed for each model state. For Gaussian mixture models, a combined MDL and EM algorithm was used to compute the optimal number of mixture components and the associated parameter values [25]. For autoregressive[6] or AR models, the Burg algorithm [26] was used to infer the model parameters and the optimal model order was computed using an MDL criterion.

Following the model training for each fold of cross-validation, the trained HMM was then used to segment each 10-second ECG signal in the test set. The segmentation was performed by using the Viterbi algorithm to infer the most probable underlying sequence of hidden states for the given signal. Note that the full 10-second ECG signal was processed, as opposed to just the manually annotated ECG beat, in order to more closely match the way an automated system would be used for ECG interval analysis in practice.

Next, for each ECG, the model annotations corresponding to the particular *beat* which had been manually annotated were then extracted. In the case of a single-beat segmentation, the *absolute* differences between the model annotations and the associated expert analyst annotations were computed. In the case of a double-beat segmentation, no annotation errors were computed. Once the cross-validation procedure was complete, the five sets of annotation "errors" were then averaged to produce the final results.

Table 11.1 shows the cross-validation results for HMMs trained on the raw ECG signal data. In particular, the table shows the percentage of single-beat segmentations and the annotation errors for different types of HMM observation models and with/without range normalization, for ECG leads II and V2.

The results for each lead demonstrate the utility of normalizing the ECG signals (prior to training and testing) with the range normalization method. In each case, the percentage of single-beat segmentations produced by an HMM (with a Gaussian observation model) is considerably increased when range normalization is employed. For lead V2, it is notable that the annotation errors (evaluated on the single-beat segmentations only) for the model with range normalization are greater than those for the model with no normalization. This is most likely to be due to the fact that the latter model produces double-beat segmentations for those waveforms that naturally give rise to larger annotation errors (and hence these waveforms are excluded from the annotation error computations for this model).

The most important aspect of the results is the considerable performance improvement gained by using autoregressive observation models as opposed to Gaussian or Gaussian mixture models. The use of AR observation models enables each HMM state to capture the statistical dependencies between successive groups of observations. In the case of the ECG, this allows the HMM to take account of the shape of each of the ECG waveform features. Thus, as expected, these models lead to a significant performance improvement (in terms of both the percentage of single-beat segmentations and the magnitude of the annotation errors) compared with models which assume the observations within each state are i.i.d.

---

6. In *autoregressive* modeling, the signal sample at time t is considered to be a linear combination of a number of previous signal samples plus an additive noise term. Specifically, an AR model of order m is given by $x_t = \sum_{i=1}^{m} c_i x_{t-i} + \epsilon_t$, where c_i are the AR model coefficients and ϵ_t can be viewed as a random residual noise term at each time step.

Table 11.1 Five-Fold Cross-Validation Results for HMMs Trained on the *Raw* ECG Signal Data from Leads II and V2

Hidden Markov Model Specification	*Lead II* *% of Single-Beat Segmentations*	*Mean Absolute Errors (ms)*			
		P_{on}	Q	J	T_{off}
Standard HMM Gaussian observation model No normalization	5.7%	175.3	108.0	99.0	243.7
Standard HMM Gaussian observation model Range normalization	69.8%	485.0	35.8	73.8	338.4
Standard HMM GMM observation model Range normalization	57.5%	272.9	48.7	75.6	326.1
Standard HMM AR observation model Range normalization	71.7%	49.2	10.3	12.5	52.8
Hidden Markov Model Specification	*Lead V2* *% of Single-Beat Segmentations*	*Mean Absolute Errors (ms)*			
		P_{on}	Q	J	T_{off}
Standard HMM Gaussian observation model No normalization	33.6%	211.5	14.5	20.7	31.5
Standard HMM Gaussian observation model Range normalization	77.9%	293.1	49.2	50.7	278.5
Standard HMM GMM observation model Range normalization	57.4%	255.2	49.9	65.0	249.5
Standard HMM AR observation model Range normalization	87.7%	43.4	5.4	7.6	32.4

Despite the advantages offered by AR observation models, the mean annotation errors for the associated HMMs are still considerably larger than the inter-analyst variability present in the data set annotations. In particular, the T wave offset annotation errors for leads II and V2 are 52.8 ms and 32.4 ms, respectively. This "level of accuracy" is not sufficient to enable the trained model to be used as an effective means for automated ECG interval analysis in practice.

The fundamental problem with developing HMMs based on the raw ECG signal data is that the state observation models must be flexible enough to capture the statistical characteristics governing the overall shape of each of the ECG waveform features. Although AR observation models provide a first step in this direction, these models are not ideally suited to representing the waveform features of the ECG. In particular, it is unlikely that a single AR model can successfully represent the statistical dependencies across whole waveform features for a range of ECGs.

Thus, it may be advantageous to utilize multiple AR models (each with a separate model order) to represent the different regions of each ECG waveform feature.

An alternative approach to overcoming the i.i.d. assumption within each HMM state is to encode information from "neighboring" signal samples into the representation of the signal itself. More precisely, each individual signal sample is transformed to a vector of transform coefficients which captures (approximately) the shape of the signal within a given region of the sample itself. This new representation can then be used as the basis for training a hidden Markov model, using any of the standard observation models previously described. We now consider the utility of this approach for automated ECG interval analysis.

11.8 Wavelet Encoding of the ECG

11.8.1 Wavelet Transforms

Wavelets are a class of functions that possess compact support and form a basis for all finite energy signals. They are able to capture the nonstationary spectral characteristics of a signal by decomposing it over a set of atoms which are localized in both time and frequency. These atoms are generated by scaling and translating a single mother wavelet.

The most popular wavelet transform algorithm is the discrete wavelet transform (DWT), which uses the set of dyadic scales (i.e., those based on powers of two) and translates of the mother wavelet to form an orthonormal basis for signal analysis. The DWT is therefore most suited to applications such as data compression where a compact description of a signal is required. An alternative transform is derived by allowing the translation parameter to vary continuously, whilst restricting the scale parameter to a dyadic scale (thus, the set of time-frequency atoms now forms a frame). This leads to the undecimated wavelet transform (UWT),[7] which for a signal $s \in L^2(\mathbb{R})$, is given by

$$w_v(\tau) = \frac{1}{\sqrt{v}} \int_{-\infty}^{+\infty} s(t) \, \psi^* \left(\frac{t - \tau}{v} \right) dt \qquad v = 2^k, k \in \mathbb{Z}, \tau \in \mathbb{R} \quad (11.22)$$

where $w_v(\tau)$ are the UWT coefficients at scale v and shift τ, and ψ^* is the complex conjugate of the mother wavelet.

In practice the UWT for a signal of length N can be computed in O using an efficient filter bank structure [27]. Figure 11.7 shows a schematic illustration of the UWT filter bank algorithm, where h and g represent the *lowpass* and *highpass* "conjugate mirror filters" for each level of the UWT decomposition.

The UWT is particularly well suited to ECG interval analysis as it provides a time-frequency description of the ECG signal on a sample-by-sample basis. In addition, the UWT coefficients are translation-invariant (unlike the DWT coefficients), which is important for pattern recognition applications.

---

7. The undecimated wavelet transform is also known as the stationary wavelet transform and the translation-invariant wavelet transform.

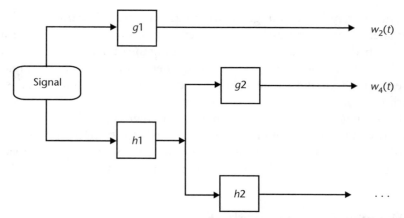

Figure 11.7 Filter bank for the undecimated wavelet transform. At each level k of the transform, the operators g and h correspond to the highpass and lowpass conjugate mirror filters at that particular level.

11.8.2   HMMs with Wavelet-Encoded ECG

In our experiments we found that the Coiflet wavelet with two vanishing moments resulted in the best overall segmentation performance. Figure 11.8 shows the squared magnitude responses for the lowpass, bandpass, and highpass filters associated with this wavelet (which is commonly known as the *coif1* wavelet).

In order to use the UWT for ECG encoding, the UWT wavelet coefficients from levels 1 to 7 were used to form a seven-dimensional encoding for each ECG signal. Table 11.2 shows the five-fold cross-validation results for HMMs trained on ECG waveforms from leads II and V2 which had been encoded in this manner (using range normalization prior to the encoding).

The results presented in Table 11.2 clearly demonstrate the considerable performance improvement of HMMs trained with the UWT encoding (albeit at the expense of a relatively low percentage of single-beat segmentations), compared with similar models trained using the raw ECG time series. In particular, the Q and T_{off} single-beat segmentation errors of 5.5 ms and 12.4 ms for lead II, and 3.3 ms and 9.5 ms for lead V2, are significantly better than the corresponding errors for the HMM with an autoregressive observation model.

Despite the performance improvement gained from the use of wavelet methods with hidden Markov models, the models still suffer from the problem of double-beat segmentations. In the following section we consider a modification to the HMM architecture in order to overcome this problem. In particular, we make use of the knowledge that the double-beat segmentations are characterized by the model inferring a number of states with a duration that is much shorter than the minimum state duration observed with real ECG signals. This observation leads on to the subject of duration constraints for hidden Markov models.

11.9   Duration Modeling for Robust Segmentations

A significant limitation of the standard HMM is the manner in which it models state durations. For a given state i with self-transition coefficient a_{ii}, the probability mass

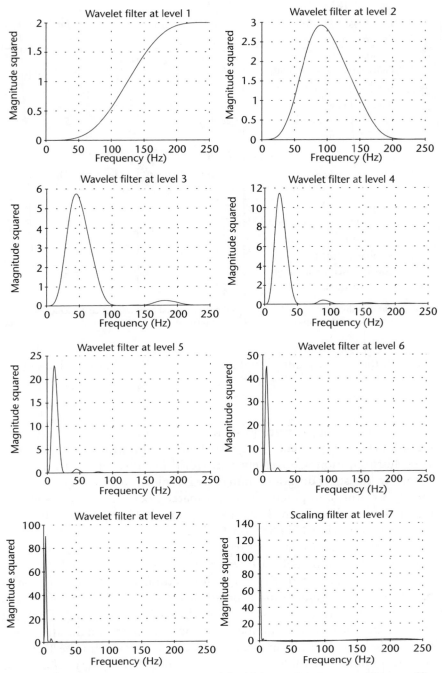

Figure 11.8   Squared magnitude responses of the highpass, bandpass, and lowpass filters associated with the *coifl* wavelet (and associated scaling function) over a range of different levels of the undecimated wavelet transform.

Table 11.2 Five-Fold Cross-Validation Results for HMMs Trained on the Wavelet-Encoded ECG Signal Data from Leads II and V2

Hidden Markov Model Specification	*Lead II*				
	% of Single-Beat Segmentations	*Mean Absolute Errors (ms)*			
		P_{on}	Q	J	T_{off}
Standard HMM Gaussian observation model UWT encoding	29.2%	26.1	3.7	5.0	26.8
Standard HMM GMM observation model UWT encoding	26.4%	12.9	5.5	9.6	12.4
Hidden Markov Model Specification	*Lead V2*				
	% of Single-Beat Segmentations	*Mean Absolute Errors (ms)*			
		P_{on}	Q	J	T_{off}
Standard HMM Gaussian obsevation model UWT encoding	73.0%	20.0	4.1	8.7	15.8
Standard HMM GMM observation model UWT encoding	59.0%	9.9	3.3	5.9	9.5

The encodings are derived from the seven-dimensional *coifl* wavelet coefficients resulting from a level 7 UWT decomposition of each ECG signal. In each case range normalization was used prior to the encoding.

function for the state duration d is a geometric distribution, given by

$$p_i(d) = (a_{ii})^{d-1}(1 - a_{ii}) \tag{11.23}$$

For the waveform features of the ECG signal, this geometric distribution is inappropriate. In particular, the distribution naturally favors state sequences of a very short duration. Conversely, real-world ECG waveform features do not occur for arbitrarily short durations, and there is typically a minimum duration for each of the ECG features. In practice this "mismatch" between the statistical properties of the model and those of the ECG results in unreliable "double-beat" segmentations, as discussed previously in Section 11.7.3.

Unfortunately, double-beat segmentations can significantly impact upon the reliability of the automated QT interval measurements produced by the model. Thus, in order to make use of the model for automated QT interval analysis, the robustness of the segmentation process must be improved. This can be achieved by incorporating duration constraints into the HMM architecture. Each duration constraint takes the form of a number specifying the minimum duration for a particular state in the model. For example, the duration constraint for the T wave state is simply the minimum possible duration (in samples) for a T wave. Such values can be estimated in practice by examining the durations of the waveform features for a large number of annotated ECG waveforms.

Once the duration constraints have been chosen, they are incorporated into the model in the following manner: For each state k with a minimum duration of $d_{min}(k)$, we augment the model with $d_{min}(k) - 1$ additional states directly preceding

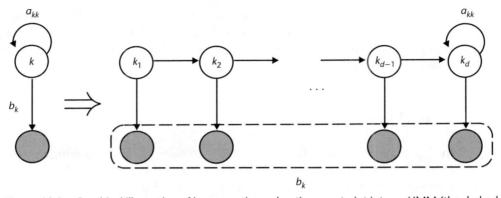

Figure 11.9 Graphical illustration of incorporating a duration constraint into an HMM (the dashed box indicates *tied* observation distributions).

Table 11.3 Five-Fold Cross-Validation Results for HMMs with Built-In Duration Constraints Trained on the Wavelet Encoded ECG Signal Data from Leads II and V2

Lead II					
Hidden Markov Model Specification	*% of Single-Beat Segmentations*	*Mean Absolute Errors (ms)*			
		P_{on}	Q	J	T_{off}
Duration-constrained HMM GMM observation model UWT encoding	100.0%	8.3	3.5	7.2	12.7
Lead V2					
Hidden Markov Model Specification	*% of Single-Beat Segmentations*	*Mean Absolute Errors (ms)*			
		Pon	Q	J	T_{off}
Duration-constrained HMM GMM observation model UWT encoding	100.0%	9.7	3.9	5.5	11.4

the original state k. Each additional state has a self-transition probability of zero, and a probability of one of transitioning to the state to its right. Thus, taken together, these states form a simple left-right Markov chain, where each state in the chain is only occupied for at most one time sample (during any run through the chain).

The most important feature of this chain is that the parameters of the observation density for each state are identical to the corresponding parameters of the original state k (this is known as "tying"). Thus the observations associated with the d_{min} states identified with a particular waveform feature are governed by a single set of parameters (which is shared by all d_{min} states). The overall procedure for incorporating duration constraints into the HMM architecture is illustrated graphically in Figure 11.9.

Table 11.3 shows the five-fold cross-validation results for a hidden Markov model with built-in duration constraints. For each fold of the cross-validation procedure, the minimum state duration $d_{min}(k)$ was calculated as 80% of the minimum duration present in the annotated training data for each particular state. The set of duration constraints were then incorporated into the HMM architecture and the resulting model was trained in a supervised fashion.

The results demonstrate that the duration constrained HMM eliminates the problem of double-beat segmentations. In addition, the annotation errors for leads II are of a comparable standard to the best results presented for the single-beat segmentations only in the previous section.

11.10   Conclusions

In this chapter we have focused on the two core issues in utilizing a probabilistic modeling approach for the task of automated ECG interval analysis: the choice of representation for the ECG signal and the choice of model for the segmentation. We have demonstrated that wavelet methods, and in particular the undecimated wavelet transform, can be used to generate an encoding of the ECG which is tuned to the unique spectral characteristics of the ECG waveform features. With this representation the performance of the models on new unseen ECG waveforms is significantly better than similar models trained on the raw time series data. We have also shown that the robustness of the segmentation process can be improved through the use of state duration constraints with hidden Markov models. With these models the robustness of the resulting segmentations is considerably improved.

A key advantage of probabilistic modeling over traditional techniques for ECG segmentation is the ability of the model to generate a statistical confidence measure in its analysis of a given ECG waveform. As discussed previously in Section 11.3, current automated ECG interval analysis systems are unable to differentiate between normal ECG waveforms (for which the automated annotations are generally reliable) and abnormal or unusual ECG waveforms (for which the automated annotations are frequently unreliable). By utilizing a confidence-based approach to automated ECG interval analysis, however, we can automatically highlight those waveforms which are least suitable to analysis by machine (and thus most in need of analysis by a human expert). This strategy therefore provides an effective way to combine the twin advantages of manual and automated ECG interval analysis [3].

References

[1]   Morganroth, J., and H. M. Pyper, "The Use of Electrocardiograms in Clinical Drug Development: Part 1," *Clinical Research Focus*, Vol. 12, No. 5, 2001, pp. 17–23.

[2]   Houghton, A. R., and D. Gray, *Making Sense of the ECG*, London, U.K.: Arnold, 1997.

[3]   Hughes, N. P., and L. Tarassenko, "Automated QT Interval Analysis with Confidence Measures," *Computers in Cardiology*, Vol. 31, 2004.

[4]   Jané, R., et al., "Evaluation of an Automatic Threshold Based Detector of Waveform Limits in Holter ECG with QT Database," *Computers in Cardiology*, IEEE Press, 1997, pp. 295–298.

[5]   Pan, J., and W. J. Tompkins, "A Real-Time QRS Detection Algorithm," *IEEE Trans. Biomed. Eng.*, Vol. 32, No. 3, 1985, pp. 230–236.

[6]   Lepeschkin, E., and B. Surawicz, "The Measurement of the Q-T Interval of the Electrocardiogram," *Circulation*, Vol. VI, September 1952, pp. 378–388.

[7]   Xue, Q., and S. Reddy, "Algorithms for Computerized QT Analysis," *Journal of Electrocardiology*, Supplement, Vol. 30, 1998, pp. 181–186.

[8]   Malik, M., "Errors and Misconceptions in ECG Measurement Used for the Detection of Drug Induced QT Interval Prolongation," *Journal of Electrocardiology*, Supplement, Vol. 37, 2004, pp. 25–33.

[9]   Hughes, N. P., "Probabilistic Models for Automated ECG Interval Analysis," Ph.D. dissertation, University of Oxford, 2006.

[10]   Rabiner, L. R., "A Tutorial on Hidden Markov Models and Selected Applications in Speech Recognition," *Proc. of the IEEE*, Vol. 77, No. 2, 1989, pp. 257–286.

[11]   Coast, D. A., et al., "An Approach to Cardiac Arrhythmia Analysis Using Hidden Markov Models," *IEEE Trans. Biomed. Eng.*, Vol. 37, No. 9, 1990, pp. 826–835.

[12]   Koski, A., "Modeling ECG Signals with Hidden Markov Models," *Artificial Intelligence in Medicine*, Vol. 8, 1996, pp. 453–471.

[13]   Gershenfeld, N., *The Nature of Mathematical Modeling*, Cambridge, U.K.: Cambridge University Press, 1999.

[14]   Murphy, K. P., "Dynamic Bayesian Networks: Representation, Inference and Learning," Ph.D. dissertation, University of California, Berkeley, 2002.

[15]   Roweis, S., and Z. Ghahramani, "A Unifying Review of Linear Gaussian Models," *Neural Computation*, Vol. 11, 1999, pp. 305–345.

[16]   Roweis, S., "Lecture Notes on Machine Learning, Fall 2004," http://www.cs.toronto.edu/roweis/csc2515/.

[17]   Nabney, I. T., *Netlab: Algorithms for Pattern Recognition*, London, U.K.: Springer, 2002.

[18]   Jordan, M. I., "Graphical Models," *Statistical Science*, Special Issue on Bayesian Statistics, Vol. 19, 2004, pp. 140–155.

[19]   Brand, M., *Coupled Hidden Markov Models for Modeling Interactive Processes*, Technical Report 405, MIT Media Lab, 1997.

[20]   Ghahramani, Z., and M. I. Jordan, "Factorial Hidden Markov Models," *Machine Learning*, Vol. 29, 1997, pp. 245–273.

[21]   Viterbi, A. J., "Error Bounds for Convolutional Codes and An Asymptotically Optimal Decoding Algorithm," *IEEE Trans. on Information Theory*, Vol. IT–13, April 1967, pp. 260–269.

[22]   Forney, G. D., "The Viterbi Algorithm," *Proc. of the IEEE*, Vol. 61, March 1973, pp. 268–278.

[23]   Dempster, A. P., N. M. Laird, and D. B. Rubin, "Maximum Likelihood from Incomplete Data Via the EM Algorithm," *Journal of the Royal Statistical Society Series B*, Vol. 39, No. 1, 1977, pp. 1–38.

[24]   Bishop, C. M., *Neural Networks for Pattern Recognition*, Oxford, U.K.: Oxford University Press, 1995.

[25]   Figueiredo, M. A. T., and A. K. Jain, "Unsupervised Learning of Finite Mixture Models," *IEEE Trans. on Pattern Analysis and Machine Intelligence*, Vol. 24, No. 3, 2002, pp. 381–396.

[26]   Hayes, M. H., *Statistical Digital Signal Processing and Modeling*, New York: Wiley, 1996.

[27]   Mallat, S., *A Wavelet Tour of Signal Processing*, 2nd ed., London, U.K.: Academic Press, 1999.

CHAPTER 12

Supervised Learning Methods for ECG Classification/Neural Networks and SVM Approaches

Stanislaw Osowski, Linh Tran Hoai, and Tomasz Markiewicz

12.1 Introduction

The application of artificial intelligence (AI) methods has become an important trend in ECG for the recognition and classification of different arrhythmia types. By arrhythmia we mean any disturbance in the regular rhythmic activity of the heart (amplitude, duration, and the shape of rhythm). From the diagnostic point of view of arrhythmia, the most important information is contained in the QRS complex, a sharp biphasic or triphasic wave of about 1-mV amplitude, and duration of approximately 80 to 100 ms.

Many solutions have been proposed for developing automated systems to recognize and classify the ECG on a real-time basis [1–6]. Depending on the type of the applied signal processing approach and its actual implementation, we can identify statistical and syntactic methods [7]. Nowadays the implementation of predictive models through the use of AI methods, especially neural networks, has become an important approach. Many solutions based on this approach have been proposed. Some of the best known techniques are the multilayer perceptron (MLP) [2], self-organizing maps (SOM) [1, 3], learning vector quantization (LVQ) [1], linear discriminant systems [6], fuzzy or neuro-fuzzy systems [8], support vector machines (SVM) [5], and the combinations of different neural-based solutions, so-called hybrid systems [4].

A typical heartbeat recognition system based on neural network classifiers usually builds (trains) different models, exploiting either different classifier network structures or different preprocessing methods of the data, and then the best one is chosen, while the rest are discarded. However, each method of data processing might be sensitive to artifacts and outliers. Hence, a consensus of experts, integrating available information into one final pattern recognition system, is expected to produce a classifier of the highest quality, that is of the least possible classification errors.

In this chapter we will discuss different solutions for ECG classification based on the application of supervised learning networks, including neural networks and SVM. Two different preprocessing methods for generation of features are illustrated: higher-order statistics (HOS) and Hermite characterization of QRS complex of the registered ECG waveform. To achieve better performance of the recognition system, we propose the combination of multiple classifiers by a weighted voting principle. This technique will be illustrated using SVM-based classifiers. In this example the weights of the integrating matrix are adjusted according to the results of individual classifier's performance on the learning data. The proposed solutions are verified on the MIT-BIH Arrhythmia Database [9] heartbeat recognition problems.

12.2 Generation of Features

The recognition and classification of patterns, including ECG signals, requires the generation of features [7] that accurately characterize these patterns in order to enable their type or class differentiation.

Such features represent the patterns in such a way that the differences of morphology of the ECG waveforms are suppressed for the same type (class) of heartbeats, and enhanced for waveforms belonging to different types of beats. This is a very important capability, since we observe great morphological variations in signals belonging to different clinical classes. This is, for example, observed in ECG waveforms contained in the MIT-BIH Arrhythmia Database [9]. In this database there are ECG waveforms of 12 types of abnormal beats: left bundle branch block (L), right bundle branch block (R), atrial premature beat (A), aberrated atrial premature beat (a), nodal (junctional) premature beat (J), ventricular premature beat (V), fusion of ventricular and normal beat (F), ventricular flutter wave (I), nodal (junctional) escape beat (j), ventricular escape beat (E), supraventricular premature beat (S), and fusion of paced and normal beat (f), and the waveforms corresponding to the normal sinus rhythm (N). Exemplary waveforms of ECG from one patient [9], corresponding to the normal sinus rhythm (N), and three types of abnormal rhythms (L, R, and V), are presented in Figure 12.1. The vertical axis y is measured in μV and the horizontal axis x in points (at 360-Hz sampling rate one point corresponds to approximately 2.8 ms).

It is clear that there is a great variety of morphologies among the heartbeats belonging to one class, even for the same patient. Moreover, beats belonging to different classes are morphologically similar to each other (look, for example, at the L-type rhythms and some V-type rhythms). They occupy a similar range of values and frequencies; thus, it is difficult to recognize one from the other on the basis of only time or frequency representations. Different feature extraction techniques have been applied. Traditional representations include features describing the morphology of the QRS complex, such as RR intervals, width of the QRS complex [1, 3, 4, 6], wave interval and wave shape features [6]. Some authors have processed features resulting from Fourier [2] or wavelet transformations [10] of the ECG. Clustering of the ECG data, using methods such as self-organizing maps [3] or learning vector quantization [1], as well as internal features resulting from the neural preprocessing stages [1] have been also exploited. Other important feature extraction methods generate statistical descriptors [5] or orthogonal polynomial representations [3, 8]. None of these methods is of course perfect and fully satisfactory. In this chapter we will illustrate supervised classification applications that rely on the processing of features originating from the description of the QRS complex by using the higher-order statistics and Hermite basis functions expansion.

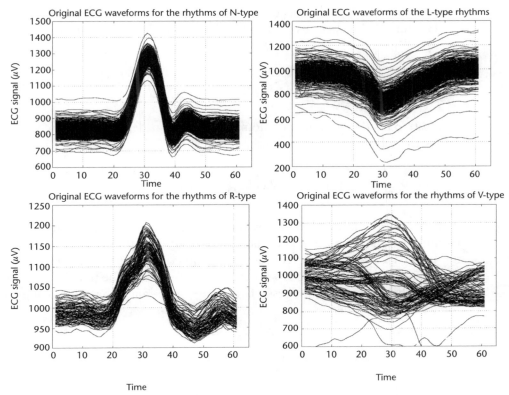

Figure 12.1 The exemplary waveforms of four types of heartbeats. (*From:* [4]. © 2004 IEEE. Reprinted with permission.)

The HOS description exploits the fact that the variance of cumulant functions is usually lower than the variance of the original signals. On the other hand, the Hermite expansion takes advantage of the similarity of the individual Hermite functions and different fragments of QRS complex of the ECG waveform.

12.2.1 Hermite Basis Function Expansion

In the Hermite basis function expansion method, the QRS complex is represented by a series of Hermite functions. This approach successfully exploits existing similarities between the shapes of Hermite basis functions and QRS complexes of the ECG waveforms under analysis. Moreover, this characterization includes a width parameter, which provides good representation of beats with large differences in QRS duration. Let us denote the QRS complex of the ECG curve by $x(t)$. Its expansion into Hermite series may be written in the following way:

$$\mathbf{x}(t) = \sum_{n=0}^{N-1} c_n \phi_n(t, \sigma) \tag{12.1}$$

where c_n are the expansion coefficients, σ is the width parameter, and $\phi_n(t, \sigma)$ are the Hermite basis functions of the nth order defined as follows [3]:

$$\phi_n(t, \sigma) = \frac{1}{\sqrt{\sigma 2^n n! \sqrt{\pi}}} e^{-t^2/2\sigma^2} H_n(t/\sigma) \qquad (12.2)$$

and $H_n(t/\sigma)$ is the Hermite polynomial of the nth order. The Hermite polynomials satisfy the following recurrence relation:

$$H_n(x) = 2x H_{n-1}(x) - 2(n-1) H_{n-2}(x) \qquad (12.3)$$

with $H_o(x) = 1$ and $H_1(x) = 2x$, for $n = 2, 3, \dots$. The higher the order of the Hermite polynomial, the higher its frequency of changes in the time domain, and the better its capability to reconstruct the quick changes of the ECG signal. The coefficients c_n of Hermite basis functions expansion may be treated as the features used in the recognition process. They may be obtained by minimizing the sum squared error, defined as

$$E = \sum_i \left[x(t_i) - \sum_{n=0}^{N-1} c_n \phi_n(t_i, \sigma) \right]^2 \qquad (12.4)$$

This error function represents the set of linear equations with respect to the coefficients c_n. They have been solved by using singular value decomposition (SVD) and the pseudo-inverse technique [11]. In numerical calculations, we have represented the QRS segment of the ECG signal by 91 data points around the R peak (45 points before and 45 after). A data sampling rate equal to 360 Hz generates a window of 250 ms, which is long enough to cover a typical QRS complex. The data have been additionally expanded by adding 45 zeros to each end of the QRS segment. This additional information is added to reinforce the idea that beats do not not exist outside the QRS complex. Subtracting the mean level of the first and the last points normalizes the ECG signals. The width σ was chosen proportional to the width of the QRS complex. These modified QRS complexes of the ECG have been decomposed onto a linear combination of Hermite basis functions. Empirical analyses have shown that 15 Hermite coefficients allow a satisfactory good reconstruction of the QRS curve in terms of the representation of the most important details of the curve [3]. Figure 12.2 depicts a representation of an exemplary normalized QRS complex by using 15 Hermite basis functions. The horizontal axis of the figure is measured in points identically as in Figure 12.1.

These coefficients, together with two classical signal features—the instantaneous RR interval length of the beat (the time span between two consecutive R points) and the average RR interval of 10 preceding beats, form the 17-element feature vector $\mathbf{x}$ applied to the input of the classifiers. These two features are usually considered for better representation of the actually processed waveform segment on the background of the average length of the last processed segments.

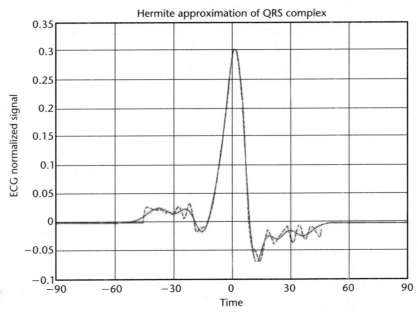

Figure 12.2   The approximation of the QRS complex by 15 Hermite basis functions. (*From:* [8]. © 2004 IEEE. Reprinted with permission.)

12.2.2   HOS Features of the ECG

Another important approach to ECG feature generation is the application of statistical descriptions of the QRS curves. Three types of statistics have been applied: the second-, third-, and fourth-order cumulants. The cumulants are the coefficients of the Taylor expansion around $s = 0$ of the cumulant generating function of variable x, defined as $\phi_x(s) = ln\{E[e^{sx}]\}$, where E means the expectation operator [12].

They can be also expressed in terms of the well-known statistical moments as their linear or nonlinear combinations. For a zero mean stationary process $x(t)$, the second- and third-order cumulants are equal to their corresponding moments

$$c_{2x}(\tau_1) = m_{2x}(\tau_1) \tag{12.5}$$

$$c_{3x}(\tau_1, \tau_2) = m_{3x}(\tau_1, \tau_2) \tag{12.6}$$

The nth-order moment of $x(k)$, $m_{nx}(\tau_1, \tau_2, \ldots, \tau_{n-1})$, is formally defined [12] as the coefficient in the Taylor expansion around $s = 0$ of the moment generating function $\varphi_x(s)$, where $\varphi_x(s) = E[e^{sx}]$. Equivalently, each nth-order statistical moment can be calculated by taking an expectation over the process multiplied by $(n-1)$ lagged versions of itself. The expression of the fourth-order cumulants is a bit more complex [12]:

$$c_{4x}(\tau_1, \tau_2, \tau_3) = m_{4x}(\tau_1, \tau_2, \tau_3) - m_{2x}(\tau_1)m_{2x}(\tau_3 - \tau_2) \tag{12.7}$$
$$-m_{2x}(\tau_2)m_{2x}(\tau_3 - \tau_1) - m_{2x}(\tau_3)m_{2x}(\tau_2 - \tau_1)$$

In these expressions c_{nx} means the nth-order cumulant and m_{nx} is the nth-order statistical moment of the process $x(k)$, while τ_1, τ_2, τ_3 are the time lags.

Table 12.1 The Variance of the Chosen Heart Rhythms of the MIT-BIH AD and Their Cumulants Characterizations

Rhythm Type	Original QRS Signal	Second-Order Cumulants	Third-Order Cumulants	Fourth-Order Cumulants
N	0.74E-2	0.31E-2	0.28E-2	0.24E-2
L	1.46E-2	0.60E-2	1.03E-2	0.51E-2
R	1.49E-2	0.94E-2	1.06E-2	0.55E-2
A	1.47E-2	0.67E-2	0.85E-2	0.38E-2
V	1.64E-2	0.68E-2	0.71E-2	0.54E-2
I	1.72E-2	0.52E-2	0.34E-2	0.24E-2
E	0.59E-2	0.42E-2	0.40E-2	0.60E-2

We have chosen the values of the cumulants of the second, third, and fourth orders at five points distributed evenly within the QRS length (for the third- and fourth-order cumulants the diagonal slices have been applied) as the features used for the heart rhythm recognition application examples. We have chosen a five-point representation to achieve a feature coding scheme (number of features) comparable with the Hermite representation. For a 91-element vector representation of the QRS complex, the cumulants corresponding to the time lags of 15, 30, 45, 60, and 75 have been chosen. Additionally, we have added two temporal features: one corresponding to the instantaneous RR interval of the beat and the second representing the average RR interval duration of 10 preceding beats. In this way each beat has been represented by a 17-element feature vector, with the first 15 elements corresponding to the higher-order statistics of QRS complex (the second-, third-, and fourth-order cumulants, each represented by five values) and the last two are the temporal features of the actual QRS signal. The application of the cumulant characterization of QRS complexes reduces the relative spread of the ECG characteristics belonging to the same type of heart rhythm and in this way makes the classification relatively easier. This is well seen in the example of the variance of the signals corresponding to the normal (N) and abnormal (L, R, A, V, I, E) beats. Table 12.1 presents the values of variance for the chosen seven types of normalized heartbeats (the original QRS complex) and their cumulant characterizations for over 6,600 beats of the MIT-BIH AD [9].

It is evident that the variance of the cumulant characteristics has been significantly reduced with respect to the variance of the original signals. It means that the spreads of parameter values characterizing the ECG signals belonging to the same class are now smaller and this makes the recognition problem much easier. This phenomenon has been confirmed by many numerical experiments for all types of beats existing in MIT-BIH AD.

12.3   Supervised Neural Classifiers

The components of the input vector, $\mathbf{x}$, containing the features of the ECG pattern represent the input applied to the classifiers. Supervised learning neural classifiers are currently considered as some of the most effective classification approaches [7, 13, 14]. We will concentrate on the following models: the MLP, the hybrid fuzzy network, the neuro-fuzzy Takagi-Sugeno-Kang (TSK) network, and also the SVM, which may be treated as a subtype of neural systems [13]. All of them base their learning process on a set of learning pairs $(\mathbf{x}_i, \mathbf{d}_i)$, where $\mathbf{x}_i$ represents the vector of features and $\mathbf{d}_i$ is the vector of class codes.

12.3.1   Multilayer Perceptron

The MLP [13, 15] is one of the best known neural networks, and it can work either in classification or regression modes. A MLP network consists of many simple neuron-like processing units of sigmoidal activation function grouped together in layers. The activation functions used in MLP may be of different forms, including logistic $f(x) = 1/(1 + exp(-x))$, hyperbolical tangent, signum, or linear. The typical network contains one hidden layer followed by the output layer of neurons. Information is processed locally in each unit by computing the dot product between the corresponding input vector and the weight vector of the neuron. Before training, the weights are initialized randomly. Training the network to produce a desired output vector $\mathbf{d}_i$ when presented with an input vector $\mathbf{x}_i$ traditionally involves systematically changing the weights of all neurons until the network produces the desired output within a given tolerance (error). This is repeated over the entire training set. Thus, learning is reduced to a minimization procces of the error measure over the entire learning set, during a finite number of learning cycles to prevent overfitting [13].

The most effective learning methods rely on gradient models. Gradient vectors in a multilayer network are computed using the backpropagation algorithm [13]. In the gradient method of learning, the weight vectors $\mathbf{w}$ are adapted from cycle to cycle according to the information of gradient of the error function

$$\mathbf{w}(k + 1) = \mathbf{w}(\mathbf{k}) + \eta \mathbf{p}(\mathbf{k}) \qquad (12.8)$$

where η is the learning constant calculated at each cycle and $\mathbf{p}(k)$ is the direction vector of minimization in the kth cycle. Some of the most effective implementations of this learning algorithm are the Levenberg-Marquard and quasi-Newton Broyden-Fletcher-Goldfarb-Shanno (BFGS) variable metric methods [13], for which

$$\mathbf{p}(k) = -\mathbf{H}^{-1}(k)\mathbf{g}(k) \qquad (12.9)$$

with $\mathbf{H}(k)$, the approximated Hessian matrix, and $\mathbf{g}(k)$, the gradient vector of the error function in the kth learning cycle. After finishing the training phase, the obtained weights are "frozen" and ready for use in the reproduction mode (test mode), in which an input vector, $\mathbf{x}$, is processed by the network to generate the output neuron signals responsible for class recognition. Usually the neuron of the highest output signal is associated with the recognized class.

It should be observed that gradient approach to learning leads to the local minimum of the objective function. Usually it is not a serious problem, since the quality of solution can be assessed immediately on the basis of the value of the final objective function. If this value is not acceptable, the learning process may be repeated starting from different initialization of weights. In the extreme case the global optimization algorithms like simulated annealing or evolutionary algorithms could be applied [16].

Generalization is a fundamental property that should be sought in practical applications of neural classifiers [13]. It measures the ability of a network to recognize patterns outside the training set. If the number of weights of the network is too large and/or the number of training examples is too small, then there will be a vast number of networks which are consistent with a training data, but only a small set which accurately fits the true solution space. Hence, poor generalization is likely. A common sense rule is to minimize the number of free parameters (weights) in the network so that the likelihood of correct generalization is increased. But this must be done without reducing the size of the network to the point where the desired target cannot be met. Moreover, the number of learning cycles should be kept under control in order to avoid over-fitting the model to the training data.

Another possibility is the cross-validation technique, where the data are divided into training, validation, and testing sets. The validation set is used to check the generalization ability of the network learned on the training data. The size of the network corresponding to the minimum validation error is accepted as the optimal one.

12.3.2 Hybrid Fuzzy Network

The hybrid fuzzy network is a combination of a fuzzy self-organizing layer and the MLP connected in cascade as shown in Figure 12.3. It is a generalization of the so called Hecht-Nielsen counterpropagation network. Instead of using a Kohonen layer, this model applies a fuzzy self-organizing layer, and a MLP subnetwork (with one hidden and one output layers) is applied instead of implementing a Grossberg layer.

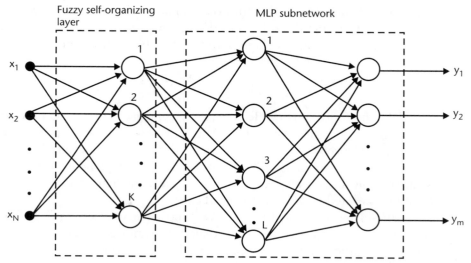

Figure 12.3   The general structure of the fuzzy hybrid network. (*From:* [4]. © 2004 IEEE. Reprinted with permission.)

The fuzzy self-organizing layer is responsible for the fuzzy clustering of the input data, in which the vector $\mathbf{x}$ is preclassified to all clusters with different membership grade. Each input vector, $\mathbf{x}_j$, then belongs to different clusters of the center $\mathbf{c}_i$ with a membership value $\mu_i(\mathbf{x}_j)$ defined by

$$\mu_i(\mathbf{x}_j) = \frac{1}{\sum_{k=1}^{K} (d_{ij}/d_{kj})^{\frac{2}{m-1}}} \tag{12.10}$$

where K is the number of clusters and d_{kj} is the distance between the jth input vector $\mathbf{x}_j$ and the kth center $\mathbf{c}_k$. The number of clusters is usually higher than the number of classes. It means that the class is associated with many clusters. Some of the best known fuzzy clustering algorithms are the c-means and the Gustafson-Kessel model [8, 15]. The application of fuzzy clustering allows a better penetration of the data space. In this model the localization of an input vector, $\mathbf{x}$, in the multidimensional space is more precise. This is essential for the implementation of heartbeat recognition systems, where the vectors associated with different classes occupy similar range of parameters.

The signals of the self-organizing neurons, representing the cluster membership grades $\mu_i(\mathbf{x}_j)$ form the input vector to the second subnetwork of MLP. The MLP is responsible for the final association between the input signals and the appropriate class (final classification). This subnetwork is trained after the first self-organizing layer has been obtained. The training algorithm is identical to that used for training a MLP alone.

12.3.3 TSK Neuro-Fuzzy Network

Another fuzzy approach to supervised classification consists of the application of the modified Takagi-Sugeno-Kang [8, 15] network models. It has been shown that the TSK neuro-fuzzy inference system can serve as a universal approximator of the data with arbitrary accuracy [15]. The TSK approximation function $y(\mathbf{x})$ can be simplified to [8]

$$y(\mathbf{x}) = \sum_{i=1}^{K} \mu_i(\mathbf{x}) \left[p_{i0} + \sum_{j=1}^{N} p_{ij} x_j \right] \tag{12.11}$$

where $\mu_i(\mathbf{x})$ is given by (12.10) and p_{ij} are the coefficients of the linear TSK functions $f_i(\mathbf{x}) = p_{i0} + \sum_{j=1}^{N} p_{ij} x_j$. The fuzzy neural network structure corresponding to this modified TSK system described by (12.11) is presented in Figure 12.4, in which $f_i(\mathbf{x})$ for $i = 1, 2, \ldots, K$, represent the linear TSK functions associated with each inference rule.

The parameters of the premise part (the membership values $\mu(\mathbf{x}_j)$) are selected very precisely using the Gustafson-Kessel self-organization algorithm [8, 15]. Afterwards they are frozen and do not take part in further adaptation. It means that when the input vector $\mathbf{x}$ is fed to the network, the membership values $\mu_i(\mathbf{x})$ are kept constant. The remaining parameters p_{ij} of the linear TSK functions can then be easily obtained by solving the appropriate set of linear equations following from

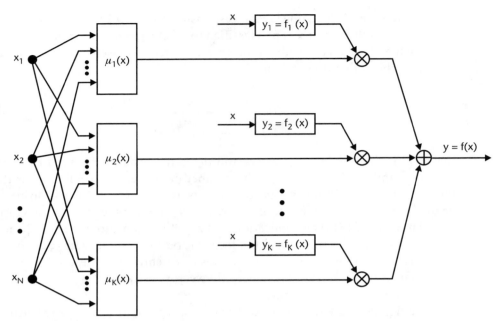

Figure 12.4 The fuzzy neural network structure corresponding to the modified TSK formula. (*From*: [8]. © 2004 IEEE. Reprinted with permission.)

equating the actual values of $y(\mathbf{x}_j)$ and the destination values d_j for $j = 1, 2, \ldots, p$. The determination of these variables can be done in one step by using the SVD algorithm and the pseudo-inverse technique [11].

12.3.4   Support Vector Machine Classifiers

The SVM solution of universal feedforward networks, pioneered by Vapnik [14], is already regarded as the most efficient tool for classification problems. It is characterized by a very good generalization performance. Unlike the classical neural network formulation of the learning problem, where the minimized error function is nonlinear with respect to the optimized variables of many potential minima, SVM leads to quadratic programming with linear constraints, and it is able to identify a well-defined global minimum. Basically, the SVM is a linear machine working in a high-dimensional feature space formed by the nonlinear mapping of the original N-dimensional input vector, $\mathbf{x}$, into a K-dimensional feature space ($K > N$) through the use of a function $\varphi(\mathbf{x})$. The equation of the hyperplane separating two different classes in the N-dimensional space is given by

$$y(\mathbf{x}) = \mathbf{w}^T \varphi(\mathbf{x}) + w_0 = \sum_{j=1}^{K} w_j \varphi_j(\mathbf{x}) + w_0 \tag{12.12}$$

where $\varphi(\mathbf{x}) = [\varphi_1(\mathbf{x}), \varphi_2(\mathbf{x}), \ldots, \varphi_K(\mathbf{x})]^T$, $\mathbf{w}$ is the weight vector of the network, $\mathbf{w} = [w_1, w_2, \ldots, w_K]^T$, and w_0 is the bias. When the condition $y(\mathbf{x}) > 0$ is fulfilled, the input vector, $\mathbf{x}$, is assigned to one class, and when $y(\mathbf{x}) < 0$, it is assigned to the other one. All mathematical operations during learning and testing modes are done in SVM using the so-called kernel functions $K(\mathbf{x}_i, \mathbf{x})$, satisfying the Mercer conditions [14]. The kernel function is defined as the inner product of the vector $\varphi(\mathbf{x})$, $K(\mathbf{x}_i, \mathbf{x}) = \varphi^T(\mathbf{x}_i)\varphi(\mathbf{x})$. Some of the best known kernels are linear, Gaussian, polynomial, and spline functions. The learning problem in a SVM is formulated as the task of separating training vectors $\mathbf{x}_i$ into two classes, described by the destination values either $d_i = 1$ or $d_i = -1$, with maximal separation margin. It is transformed to the so-called dual problem of maximization of the quadratic function $Q(\mathbf{x})$, defined as [14, 17, 18]

$$Q(\alpha) = \sum_{i=1}^{p} \alpha_i - 0.5 \sum_{i=1}^{p} \sum_{j=1}^{p} \alpha_i \alpha_j d_i d_j K(\mathbf{x}_i, \mathbf{x}_j) \qquad (12.13)$$

with the constraints

$$\sum_{i=1}^{p} \alpha_i d_i = 0$$

$$0 \leq \alpha_i \leq C$$

The variables α_i are the Lagrange multipliers, d_i refers to the destination values associated with the input vectors $\mathbf{x}_i$, C is the user-defined regularization constant, and p is the number of learning data pairs $(\mathbf{x}_i, d_i)$. The solution of the dual problem with respect to the Lagrange multipliers allows one to determine the optimal weight vector $\mathbf{w}_{opt}$ of the SVM network

$$\mathbf{w}_{opt} = \sum_{i=1}^{N_{sv}} \alpha_i d_i \varphi(\mathbf{x}_i) \qquad (12.14)$$

N_{sv} is the number of support vectors (the vectors $\mathbf{x}_i$ for which the Lagrange multipliers are different from zero). Substituting the solution of (12.14) into the relation (12.12) allows the expression of the output signal $y(\mathbf{x})$ of the SVM network as the function of kernels

$$y(\mathbf{x}) = \sum_{i=1}^{N_{sv}} \alpha_i d_i K(\mathbf{x}_i, \mathbf{x}) + w_0 \qquad (12.15)$$

The positive value of $y(\mathbf{x})$ is associated with 1 (membership in the target class) and the negative one with -1 (membership in the opposite class).

A critical parameter of the SVM is the regularization constant, C. It controls the trade-off between the width of the separation margin, affecting the complexity of the machine and the number of nonseparable points in the learning phase of the network. A small value of C results in a wider margin of separation at the cost of accepting more unseparated learning points. A higher value of C generates a lower number of classification errors of the learning data set, narrow separation margins and less support vectors. Too high values of C may result in the loss of generalization ability of the trained network. For the normalized input signals of the values in the range $(-1, 1)$ the regularization constant C is usually much bigger than 1 and empirically determined via the standard use of the validation test set.

An important advantage of the SVM approach is the transformation of the learning task to the quadratic programming problem. For this type of optimization there exist many very effective learning algorithms [18–20], leading in almost all cases to the global minimum of the cost function and to the best possible choice of the parameters of the network. Another advantage of the SVM models is its good generalization ability, which is highly independent of the number of learning samples.

Although the SVM separates data into two classes, the recognition of more classes is straightforward by applying either "one against one" or "one against all" methods [20]. The "one against one" approach is usually more effective. In this approach many local two-class recognition classifiers are independently trained, which allows the selection of a winning classifier. For M classes we have to train $M(M - 1)/2$ two-class SVM-based recognition systems. A simple integration approach consists of considering a majority vote across all trained classifiers to find the final winner at the presentation of an input vector, $\mathbf{x}$.

12.4   Integration of Multiple Classifiers

In a particular application, different classifiers may rely on either different feature sets or network structures, and therefore they may attain different degrees of success. This is because each method may be sensitive to artifacts and outliers in different ways. Usually, it is not possible to talk about the perfect classifier. Moreover, obtained models may not be as good as expected. Thus, there is a need to combine different solutions of classifiers into the ensemble of networks, so that a better result can be obtained. Combining multiple trained networks, instead of discarding them, may help to integrate the knowledge acquired by the component classifiers, which in turn may improve the accuracy of the classification task [21, 22].

There are many different methods of integration of individual classifiers. To the most known belong majority and weighted voting, application of the Bayes' rule, the Dempster-Shafer formalism, or Kullback-Leibler probability approach [23]. Most of these methods take into account the accuracy of performance of the individual classifiers for the learning data. A wide review of combining many classifiers into one ensemble network can be found in [23].

The integration approach presented in this chapter applies a weighted voting of the individual classifiers based on an integrating matrix, $\mathbf{W}$. Such a classifier integration framework is summarized in Figure 12.5.

It consists of M channels of individual classifiers combined into one classifying system through the integration mechanism introduced above. The input signals of the classification process form the vector $\mathbf{x}_{in}$. This vector is transformed into different feature vectors by the appropriate preprocessing blocks P_i $(i = 1, 2, \ldots, M)$. The features are packed into the vectors $\mathbf{x}_i$ treated as the inputs to the neural classifiers K_i. Each classifier has N outputs corresponding to the N classes under consideration. The output signals from each classifier form the N-dimensional vectors $\mathbf{y}_j$, for $j = 1, 2, \ldots, M$, containing the results of classification accomplished

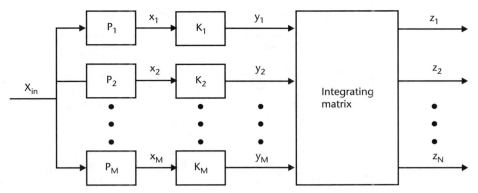

Figure 12.5   The general structure of the integrating system. (*From:* [5]. © 2004 IEEE. Reprinted with permission.)

by each classifier. They are linearly combined through the integrating matrix, $\mathbf{W} \in R^{N \times MN}$, to form one N-dimensional output vector $\mathbf{z}$. By introducing the notation $\mathbf{y} = \left[\mathbf{y}_1^T,\ \mathbf{y}_2^T, \ldots, \mathbf{y}_M^T \right]^T$, we can describe this vector as follows:

$$\mathbf{z} = \mathbf{W}\mathbf{y} \qquad (12.16)$$

The position of the highest value element of vector $\mathbf{z}$ indicates the membership of the input signal in the corresponding class.

The most important point in the weighted voting approach is how to adjust the values of elements of the matrix $\mathbf{W}$. We have used a method based on the minimization of the sum of squared errors of the final classification results of each classifier, measured on the learning data by using the pseudo-inverse technique and SVD [11]. After determining the matrix $\mathbf{W}$, its elements are kept constant and the classifier is ready for the online test mode operation (12.16).

12.5   Results of Numerical Experiments

This section illustrates classification experiments applied to ECG data from the MIT-BIH Arrhythmia Database [9], which corresponds to the normal sinus rhythm and different arrhythmias. Two types of experiments have been performed. In the first case six types of abnormal beats—L, R, A, V, E, I, and normal N—have been considered. All these seven rhythms have been observed in one patient [9]. So it may be regarded as an individual classification model specialized on a single patient.

In the second experiment we have considered all arrhythmias included in the MIT-BIH Arrhythmia Database. To the already mentioned beat types, we have added a, J, f, F, j, and S types, which represent a classification problem with a total of 13 types of beats. All of them coming from 52 patients. Due to the scarcity of data corresponding to some beat types, the distribution of data belonging to each beat type was modified. By limiting the number of some beat types, one may provide a minimal balance among the classes under consideration. As a result of such a data selection strategy, the total number of signals used for training the neural networks was equal to 6,690. The other 6,095 data points have been left for testing

Table 12.2 The Average Misclassification Rate for the Family of Seven Beat Types

Type of Classifier		Misclassification Rate	
		Learning Mode	Testing Mode
MLP	HER	4.85%	5.02%
	HOS	4.12%	4.40%
Hybrid	HER	3.54%	3.97%
	HOS	2.55%	3.94%
TSK	HER	3.98%	2.82%
	HOS	2.14%	3.20%
SVM	HER	2.24%	2.91%
	HOS	1.85%	3.10%

the classifiers only. An additional 1,500 data samples have been left for validation purposes (e.g., adjustment of the user-defined parameters of the trained networks—the parameters of the kernel function and regularization coefficient C of SVM, the number of hidden neurons in MLP, and so forth). The comparison of the classification methods will be made on the basis of the misclassification rate for the individual beat type in the learning and testing modes. For the purpose of simple comparison of all systems, we have calculated also the average of all mean errors in the learning and testing modes. Moreover, in order to obtain reliable results independently of the number of beats belonging to different classes, we have estimated the overall average of the mean errors calculated for each class.

The QRS complexes from each signal in the database were extracted and the features corresponding to HOS and Hermite expansion preprocessing were generated. Both preprocessing techniques generated 17 features. Different neural network types were assessed. Table 12.2 presents the average misclassification rate corresponding to different classifiers: MLP, hybrid neural network (Hybrid), modified TSK neuro-fuzzy network (TSK), and SVM combined with two types of preprocessing: Hermite function expansion (HER) and HOS.

As this table shows, for a small number of classes the best results correspond to the application of SVM and TSK classifiers. The MLP alone seems to be the worst solution. Increasing the number of classes significantly changed the results. Now the unbeatable is the SVM classifier working in "one against one" mode. This type of classifier was found to be extremely insensitive to the number of classes. The MLP or fuzzy classifiers applied to the same data set have produced misclassification errors much higher than SVM (approximately two times higher). Hence, from now on we will concentrate on the best models (i.e., SVM-based classification systems).

All SVM networks have been trained using the Platt algorithm [19]. We have used Gaussian radial kernels $K(\mathbf{x}, \mathbf{x}_i) = exp\left(-\gamma \parallel \mathbf{x} - \mathbf{x}_i \parallel^2\right)$ of the value $\gamma = 2$. The optimal value of the parameter C used in the experiments was found to be $C = 100$. These values have been selected after a series of numerical experiments on the learning and validation data, which produced the best generalization ability. As a result of such a learning procedure, we have SVM networks with a different number of hidden units (support vectors) changing from network to network.

The next step in the design of the optimal heartbeat recognition system is the integration of the individual classifiers. We have integrated SVM classifiers based

Table 12.3 The Comparison of the Average Misclassification Rate of Testing Different SVM Solutions for the Recognition of 13 Types of the Heartbeats

Classification Method	Number of Learning Errors	Average Rate of Learning Errors	Number of Testing Error	Average Rate of Testing Errors
HER	103	3.02%	172	5.23%
HOS	173	5.19%	216	6.28%
Integration	74	1.83%	159	4.09%

on two different preprocessing procedures: Hermite expansion and higher-order statistics representation of the data. Table 12.3 presents the summary of the average results of classification for 13 different heartbeats obtained by applying two individual classifiers and by our expert system integrating the outcomes of these classifiers (based on the two feature extraction methods). The average relative errors given in the table have been calculated in the same way as it was done in the previous examples (the simple mean of the relative errors of the recognition for each beat class). Thanks to such definition of mean, the average misclassification rates shown in Table 12.3 are practically independent on the number of beats, belonging to different classes that have taken part in the experiments. The results are given for individual classifiers named after the preprocessing methods (HOS, HER) and for integration of individual results of the classifiers.

It is evident that the best results have been obtained from the weighted voting strategy. Observe that by calculating the relative error in a different way, as the ratio of all misclassified cases $(74 + 159)$ to the total number of beats (12,785 beats used in learning and testing), we obtain a final misclassification rate of 1.83%. Table 12.4 presents the detailed classification results for all 13 heartbeat types when integrating the results from both SVM classifiers built with Hermite and HOS features.

Table 12.4 The Detailed Results of Different Heartbeat Type Recognition at Application of Integration of Both SVM Classifiers

Beat Type	Number of Learning Beats	Total Number of Errors	Average Relative Error	Number of Testing Beats	Total Number of Errors	Average Relative Error
L	700	7	1.00%	500	17	3.40%
R	600	2	0.33%	400	4	1.00%
A	484	20	4.13%	418	29	6.94%
V	1,272	14	1.10%	1,237	23	1.86%
I	272	5	1.84%	200	6	3.00%
E	55	0	0	50	2	4.00%
N	2,000	12	0.6%	2,000	44	2.20%
a	67	2	2.99%	64	4	6.25%
f	200	1	0.50%	200	3	1.5%
F	371	3	0.81%	370	10	2.70%
j	117	3	2.56%	105	10	9.52%
J	40	3	7.50%	39	4	10.25%
S	512	2	0.39%	512	3	0.58%
Total	6,690	74	1.83%	6,095	159	4.09%

By comparing the performance of the final expert classifier on individual beat types, we can identify some differences in terms of predictive quality. The worst results were generally observed for the models built on the smallest data sets. Hence, by increasing the number of training inputs above a predefined level (e.g., over 500), one should significantly increase the overall accuracy of classification.

The distribution of errors within different beat types is also very important from a practical point of view. Table 12.5 presents the classification results on the testing data in the form of a confusion matrix divided into the different beat types. The diagonal entries of this matrix represent correct classifications for a beat type, and the off-diagonal refer to misclassifications. Columns represent how the beats from a particular class have been classified. A row indicates which beats have been categorized into the beat type encoded by this row. The results of Table 12.5 allow one to analyze which classes confused the classifying system. In practice the most dangerous case is when an ill patient is diagnosed as a healthy one (false negative diagnosed patient). To deal with such situations, we have introduced the parameter DUV (dangerous uncertainty value), defined as the ratio of the number of all false negative diagnosed patients to the total number of misclassifications. Table 12.6 presents the values of this parameter for the individual SVM classifiers and for the integrated system. In relation to the integration approach there is an evident improvement of the classification quality, both in learning and the testing modes. Especially high relative improvement of this quality parameter is observed for the testing data. However, we should take into account that the total testing misclassification rate is almost 2.5 times higher than in the learning mode. Hence, the percentage of false negative diagnosed patients in both modes remains approximately at the same level.

It is also interesting to compare our results to the best results, published in the literature. Lagerholm et al. [3] have presented a recognition system for all beat types available in the MIT-BIH Arrhythmia Database based on an integrative classification procedure. Representations of misclassification ratio were obtained using different techniques. The confusion matrix method produced relevant results. For all 13 beat types, an average error rate, calculated as the average of the mean misclassification errors of all classes, of 7.12% was obtained. The error rate calculated as the simple ratio of the number of all misclassifications to the total number of rhythms was 1.5%.

The mixed expert approach (MEA) presented in [1] is similar in principle to our method. It implements the so-called Global Expert (GE), Local Expert (LE), and the mixture of them (MEA). The experts are built using SOM and LVQ methods and have been applied to classify four beat types included in the MIT-BIH Arrhythmia Database. The average misclassification rate obtained by MEA (6%) significanlty improved the results produced by the GE approach. Even better results were obtained by applying the LE method, which showed an average error around 4%.

Other authors [6] have recently proposed a new method for beat recognition based on the analysis of ECG morphology and heartbeat intervals, which reported good classification results for five beat classes recommended by the ANSI/AAMI EC57 standard. The average misclassification ratio obtained was around 5% using a very large database that contained almost 50,000 beats.

Table 12.5 The Confusion Matrix of the Integrated Classifying System for 13 Types of Rhythms of Testing Data

	A	a	f	E	F	j	I	J	L	N	R	S	V	Total
A	389	0	1	0	1	5	1	0	1	19	0	0	3	420
a	2	60	0	0	2	0	0	0	0	1	0	0	4	69
f	0	0	197	0	1	0	0	1	9	7	0	0	0	215
E	0	0	0	48	0	0	0	0	1	0	0	0	0	49
F	0	0	0	0	360	0	0	0	2	5	1	0	8	376
j	7	0	0	0	0	95	0	0	0	2	0	0	0	104
I	0	0	0	0	0	1	194	0	1	0	0	3	0	201
J	1	0	0	0	0	0	0	35	0	2	0	0	2	38
L	2	0	1	0	0	0	0	0	483	1	0	0	5	492
N	9	3	0	0	1	2	0	2	2	1,956	1	0	0	1,976
R	4	0	0	2	0	0	0	1	0	1	396	0	1	405
S	1	0	0	0	0	2	5	0	0	0	2	509	0	519
V	3	1	1	0	5	0	0	0	1	6	0	0	1,214	1,231
Total	418	64	200	50	370	105	200	39	500	2,000	400	512	1,237	6,095

Table 12.6 The Comparison of DUV Values for Different SVM-Based Classifiers

| Quality | Learning Data | | | Testing Data | | |
Measure	HOS	HER	Integration	HOS	HER	Integration
DUV	31.79%	38.83%	27.03%	18.52%	23.84%	12.58%

This comparison indicates that the supervised integrative method explained in this chapter is an effective and efficient approach to ECG beat classification. However, it should be noted that in these applications different numbers of beats and beat types belonging to different patients have been recognized. Thus, it is difficult to compare results in a fair, objective way.

12.6　Conclusions

The classification models implemented on the MIT-BIH Arrhythmia Database indicate that the supervised neural network and SVM approaches establish a good foundation for reliable heartbeat recognition on the basis of the ECG waveform. It is also important to stress the ability of the neural-based classifiers to deal with artifacts and outliers that may be observed in the ECG waveforms. Different preprocessing methods, cooperating with SVM-based classifiers and integrated into one expert system can significantly improve the overall accuracy of the heartbeat recognition process. Experimental results from the recognition of 13 types of beats have shown that instead of designing one single, high-performance classifier, we may build several classifiers exhibiting different advantages and disadvantages regarding predictive quality. The appropriate combination of these individual classifiers is able to produce a classification system of a significantly higher quality.

Future trends in ECG classification methods should include the development of other preprocessing procedures, which should offer more robust feature extraction capabilities. Furthermore, they should be less sensitive to different types of artifacts and outliers that may be present in the registered waveforms. On one hand, such new trends may include the application of a wavelet decomposition or deeper analyses of the morphology characterization of QRS complex for the generation of highly stable features. On the other hand, hierarchical classification and integration of many classifiers may further contribute to the improvement of the quality of the automatic classification of the heartbeats.

Acknowledgments

This work has been supported by Polish Ministry of Scientific Research and Information Technology.

References

[1]　Hu, G. M., S. Palreddy, and W, Tompkins, "Patient Adaptable ECG Beat Classifier Using a Mixture of Experts Approach," *IEEE Trans. Biomed. Eng.*, Vol. 44, 1997, pp. 891–900.

[2]   Minami, K., H. Nakajima, and T. Yoyoshima, "Real Time Discrimination of the Ventricular Tachyarrhythmia with Fourier-Transform Neural Network," *IEEE Trans. Biomed. Eng.*, Vol. 46, 1999, pp. 179–185.

[3]   Lagerholm, M., et al., "Clustering ECG Complexes Using Hermite Functions and Self-Organizing Maps," *IEEE Trans. Biomed. Eng.*, Vol. 47, 2000, pp. 839–847.

[4]   Osowski, S., and L. Tran Hoai, "ECG Beat Recognition Using Fuzzy Hybrid Neural Network," *IEEE Trans. Biomed. Eng.*, Vol. 48, 2001, pp. 1265–1271.

[5]   Osowski, S., L. Tran Hoai, and T. Markiewicz, "Support Vector Machine Based Expert System for Reliable Heart Beat Recognition," *IEEE Trans. Biomed. Eng.*, Vol. 51, 2004, pp. 582–589.

[6]   de Chazal, P., M. O'Dwyer, and R. B. Reilly, "Automatic Classification of Heartbeats Using ECG Morphology and Heartbeat Interval Features," *IEEE Trans. Biomed. Eng.*, Vol. 51, 2004, pp. 1196–1206.

[7]   Schalkoff, R., *Pattern Recognition: Statistical, Structural, and Neural Approaches*, New York: Wiley, 1992.

[8]   Osowski, S., and L. Tran Hoai, "On-Line Heart Beat Recognition Using Hermite Polynomials and Neuro-Fuzzy Network," *IEEE Trans. Instrum. and Measur.*, Vol. 52, 2003, pp. 1224–1231.

[9]   Mark, R., and G. Moody, *MIT-BIH Arrhythmia Database Directory*, Cambridge, MA: MIT Press, 1988.

[10]   Senhadji, L., et al., "Comparing Wavelet Transforms for Recognizing Cardiac Patterns," *IEEE Eng. in Medicine and Biology*, March/April 1995, pp. 167–173.

[11]   Golub, G., and C. Van Loan, *Matrix Computations*, New York: Academic Press, 1991.

[12]   Nikias, C., and A. Petropulu, *Higher-Order Spectra Analysis*, Englewood Cliffs, NJ: Prentice-Hall, 1993.

[13]   Haykin, S., *Neural Networks: A Comprehensive Foundation*, Englewood Cliffs, NJ: Prentice-Hall, 1999.

[14]   Vapnik, V., *Statistical Learning Theory*, New York: Wiley, 1998.

[15]   Jang, J. S., C. T. Sun, and E. Mizutani, *Neuro-Fuzzy and Soft Computing*, Englewood Cliffs, NJ: Prentice-Hall, 1997.

[16]   Hassoun, M. H., *Fundamentals of Artificial Neural Networks*, Cambridge, MA: MIT Press, 1995.

[17]   Smola, A., and B. Scholkopf, *A Tutorial on Support Vector Regression*, NeuroColt Technical Report NV2-TR-1998-030, Royal Holloway College, University of London, U.K., 1998.

[18]   Burges, C., "A Tutorial on Support Vector Machines for Pattern Recognition," in U. Fayyad, (ed.), *Knowledge Discovery and Data Mining*, Amsterdam: Kluwer, 2000, pp. 1–43.

[19]   Platt, J., "Fast Training of SVM Using Sequential Optimization," in B. Scholkopf, C. Burges, and A. Smola, (eds.), *Advances in Kernel Methods: Support Vector Learning*, Cambridge, MA: MIT Press, 1998, pp. 185–208.

[20]   Hsu, C. W., and C. J. Lin, "A Comparison Methods for Multi Class Support Vector Machines," *IEEE Trans. Neural Networks*, Vol. 13, 2002, pp. 415–425.

[21]   Hashem, S., "Optimal Linear Combinations of Neural Networks," *Neural Networks*, Vol. 10, 1997, pp. 599–614.

[22]   Xu, L., A. Krzyzak, and C. Y. Suen, "Methods of Combining Multiple Classifiers and Their Applications to Handwriting Recognition," *IEEE Trans. Systems, Man and Cybernetics*, Vol. 22, 1991, pp. 418–434.

[23]   Kuncheva, L., *Combining Pattern Classifiers: Methods and Algorithms*, New York: Wiley, 2004.

CHAPTER 13

An Introduction to Unsupervised Learning for ECG Classification

Haiying Wang and Francisco Azuaje

13.1 Introduction

The classification of the electrocardiogram into different categories of beat types and rhythms, representing one or more underlying pathologies, is essentially a pattern recognition task. Over the past three decades computational techniques have proliferated in this field of pattern recognition. This expansion is partly due to the capability of such techniques to process large amounts of high-dimensional and noisy data in the absence of complete physiological models to assist human experts in decision making. Unsupervised learning-based approaches play a crucial role in exploratory visualization-driven ECG data analysis. These approaches are useful for the detection of relevant trends, patterns, and outliers, which are not always amenable to expert labeling, as well as for the identification of complex relationships between subjects and clinical conditions.

This chapter offers an introduction to unsupervised learning-based approaches and their application to electrocardiogram classification with emphasis on recent advances in clustering-based techniques. The application of self-adaptive neural network-based approaches for supporting biomedical pattern discovery and visualization are described. It concludes with an outlook on future trends and problems to be addressed.

13.2 Basic Concepts and Methodologies

An ECG classification application typically aims to assign a given ECG recording to a physiological outcome, condition, or category based on a set of descriptive measurements. A typical computerized ECG classification process consists of several stages [1] that are illustrated in Figure 13.1.

The ECG is initially preprocessed to remove noise, detect beats, extract features, and remove abnormal or artifactual features that may disproportionally influence a classifier. This preprocessing stage aims to encode relevant information in the form of feature vectors, which represent the inputs to the classification stage. Successful classification is achieved by finding patterns in the ECG signal that effectively discriminate between the diagnostic categories or classes under investigation.

A wide range of algorithms have been proposed for ECG classification. Relevant methods include Bayesian approaches [2], statistical methods [3], expert

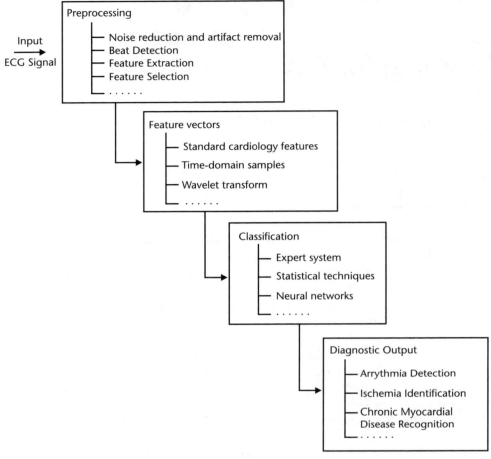

Figure 13.1   An architecture for computerized ECG classification.

systems [4], Markov models [5], and artificial neural networks (ANNs) [6], which have significantly contributed to the advancement of computerized ECG analysis. In terms of machine learning strategies, these techniques may be categorized into two main approaches: *supervised* and *unsupervised*. Based on the assumption that a data set represents distinct classes or groups known a priori, a trained supervised classification system assigns unseen data items (signals) to one of the classes learned. *Feedforward neural networks* [7] and *support vector machines* [8] are included in this approach. Supervised classification techniques are discussed in Chapter 12.

This chapter presents an overview of unsupervised learning-based methods for ECG classification. The remainder of this chapter is organized as follows. Section 13.3 introduces relevant techniques and their applications to ECG classification together with advances in clustering-based techniques. The application of self-adaptive neural networks (SANN)–based approaches to ECG pattern discovery and visualization is described in Section 13.4. The chapter concludes with a discussion of the limitations and future opportunities of unsupervised-based learning for ECG classification.

13.3 Unsupervised Learning Techniques and Their Applications in ECG Classification

Unsupervised classification, also known as *clustering analysis*, typically aims to group a given collection of patterns (i.e., signals or cases) into meaningful clusters without explicitly incorporating prior information about the classification of the patterns. There is no explicit teaching mechanism to oversee the learning process. Rather, the system must "learn" by discovering relevant similarity relationships between patterns. The main outcome of such approaches is a collection of clusters, which refer to a group of data vectors with numerically close values of a specified similarity metric. A cluster may be linked to significant classes such as disease or risk groups. In an ECG context, examples of clusters include groups of signals exhibiting recurrent QRS complexes and/or novel ST segments.

In this chapter, the term *pattern*, represents a single p-element data vector, $x_{ij} = (x_{i1}, x_{i2}, \ldots, x_{ip})$, to be processed by the clustering algorithm. The individual scalar components, $x_{ij}(j \in [1, p])$, of a pattern x_i are called *features*. Thus, given a set of patterns, $X = x_1, x_2, \ldots, x_n \in R^p$ in p-space, and based on a measure of distance or similarity, a clustering algorithm Q partitions X into a set of clusters $Q_i, i = 1, 2, \ldots, c$, where c is the total number of clusters and n is the size of the input data set. A typical clustering-based classification process is depicted in Figure 13.2, which may be implemented by the following steps [9]:

- *Pattern representation.* It refers to the definition of the number of available patterns, and the number, type, and scale of the features available to the clustering algorithm. Feature extraction and selection are fundamental components of this task. Chapter 9 of this book reviews feature extraction techniques.
- *Selection of distance or similarity measures.* The definition of a similarity measure between pairs of patterns is essential to implement a clustering algorithm. Some clustering algorithms may be implemented by applying different distance metrics. Other techniques are tailored to specific types of distance functions. Approaches to measuring distance or similarity have been extensively studied [9, 10]. The best known similarity measure is the Euclidean distance, $E = \sum_p (x_{ip}^2 - x_{kp}^2)^{\frac{1}{2}}$. The smaller the distance, the greater the similarity. The computation of distances between pairs of patterns consisting of different types of features may not be a trivial task and the selection of a distance measure is therefore data- and application-dependent [11]. In the case of time series data, it has been shown that traditional distance functions

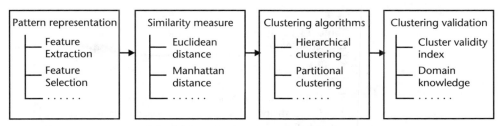

Figure 13.2 An overview of the basic steps constituting a clustering process.

(e.g., Euclidean distance) may fail to adequately capture notions of similarity [12]. Therefore, several techniques are also available for this type of data [12].

- *Selection of clustering algorithms.* Different clustering algorithms have different merits and limitations, which may depend on the statistical nature of the data under study, the problem domain, and user requirements [13]. There is no clear consensus as to whether one can identify the "best" algorithm for a particular problem since different algorithms may unveil various aspects of given data. Traditional examples of these algorithms include different types of hierarchical clustering, *k*-means, and the *Kohonen Self-Organizing Map* (SOM), which will be discussed later.

- *Cluster validation.* The validation or assessment of the clustering results is a fundamental task in clustering analysis [14, 15]. Given the putative clusters generated by an algorithm, it is essential to assist users in answering questions such as: What is the significance of this partition in terms of the number of clusters and cluster assignments? Are these clusters meaningful? This task becomes more complex in the absence of objective knowledge-driven criteria to interpret the quality of the clusters [15]. Relevant cluster validity and interpretation methods are introduced in the next sections.

13.3.1 Hierarchical Clustering

This method constructs a hierarchy of clusters by either repeatedly merging two smaller clusters into a larger one or splitting a larger cluster into smaller ones. There are two major approaches under this category: *agglomerative* and *divisive* methods. The agglomerative approach, which is summarized in Table 13.1, generates clusters in a bottom-up fashion until all patterns belong to the same cluster. Different algorithms may be implemented depending on the way similarity is measured between clusters, such as *single linkage*, *average linkage*, and *complete linkage* methods. The divisive method splits up a data set into smaller clusters in a top-down fashion until each cluster contains only one pattern.

A hierarchical clustering can be visualized using dendrograms where each step in the clustering process is illustrated by a join of the tree [16], as demonstrated in Figure 13.3. Such structures depict the sequence of successive mergers or divisions that occur in a clustering process. It may reveal basic relationships between all the patterns. However, for a given data set, the hierarchical cluster structure may not be unique. It depends on the criterion used to decide where and how to create branches in the dendrogram [16, 17].

Table 13.1 Traditional Agglomerative Hierarchical Clustering Algorithm

1: Initialize: Assign each pattern to its own cluster
2: **Repeat**
3:     Compute distances between all clusters
4:     Merge the two clusters that are closest to each other
5: **Until** all patterns belong to one cluster

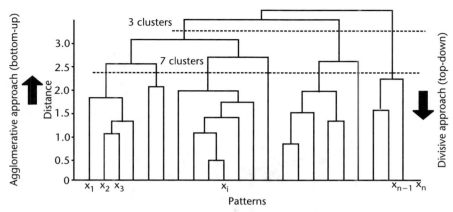

Figure 13.3   An illustration of a dendrogram produced by a hierarchical clustering. A partitioning can be obtained by cutting the dendrogram at a certain level, for example, at the level where it is possible to identify three clusters.

13.3.2   *k*-Means Clustering

The k-means method partitions a data set into k clusters such that all patterns in a given subset are closest to the same cluster centroid. First, it randomly selects k patterns to represent the initial clusters. Based on the selected features, all remaining patterns are assigned to their closest centroid. The algorithm then computes the new centroids by taking the mean of all the patterns belonging to the same cluster. The operation is iterated until there are no changes in the values of the centroids and hence class assignments for a particular cluster (Table 13.2). An illustration of the traditional k-means method is given in Figure 13.4.

A k-means clustering algorithm performs well when the clusters are clearly separated. However, the algorithm is extremely sensitive to noise and the selection of initial centroids. For example, a centroid may be trapped in a local optimal value if an inappropriate selection of initial centroids has been made [18]. In addition, it requires users to specify a priori the number of clusters in the data, which might be difficult to estimate in some applications.

13.3.3   SOM

The SOM neural network [19], introduced by Kohonen, is one of the best known unsupervised learning neural networks. It defines a mapping from a M-dimensional input space onto a lower-dimensional output space (usually a one- or two-dimensional

Table 13.2   Basic *k*-Means Clustering Algorithm

1: Initialize: determine the number of clusters
randomly select k patterns as initial centroids
2: **Repeat**
3:     Assign each pattern to the closest centroid to form k clusters
4:     Recalculate the centroid of each cluster
5: **Until** there is no change in the centroids

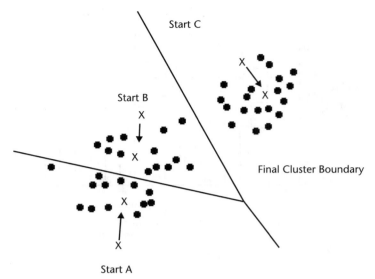

Figure 13.4   An illustration of *k*-means clustering. Dots are input patterns. A, B, and C stand for the initial selection of centroids. Arrows represent the direction of the movement of such centroids during the clustering process.

grid) that preserves original, key similarity relations between patterns. Such a model is characterized by the formation of a topographic map of the input patterns, in which the spatial locations of the *neurons* in the map reflect the similarity between groups of patterns, as illustrated in Figure 13.5.

The traditional SOM algorithm is summarized in Table 13.3. The reader is referred to [19] for a detailed description of SOM learning dynamics. The relative simplicity of this algorithm is one of its key advantages. It does not require the definition of a cost or energy function, and therefore, no complex mathematical

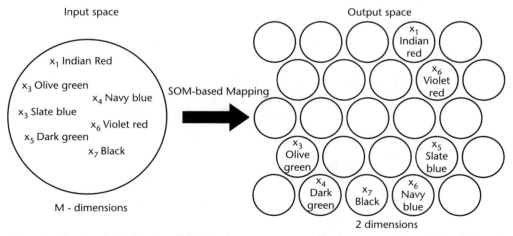

Figure 13.5   An illustration of SOM map. x_1 to x_7 are a set of color patterns encoded in their red, green, and blue (RGB) values. Once trained, the SOM is able to group similar patterns together. The red patterns, for example, are grouped on the top right of the map.

Table 13.3 The Traditional SOM Algorithm

1: Initialization: Determine network topology
                      Choose random weight value for each Kohonen neuron
                      Set the time parameter $t = 0$
2: **Repeat**
3:      Select an input pattern i_k from the training set
4:      Find the winning neuron at time t whose weight, w_j, is closest to i_k
5:      Update the weights of the winning neuron and its neighbours
6:      Increase the time parameter t: $t = t + 1$
7: **Until** network converges or
           computational bounds such as predefined learning cycles are exceeded

operations such as derivatives and matrix inversions are needed. In contrast to the rigid structure of hierarchical clustering and the lack of structure of k-means clustering, a SOM reflects similarity relationships between patterns and clusters by adapting its neurons, which are used to represent prototypical patterns [20]. Such adaptation and cluster representation mechanisms offer the basis for cluster visualization platforms. However, the predetermination of a static map representation contributes to its inability to implement automatic cluster boundary detection.

There are a number of techniques to enhance SOM-based data visualization, which have been extensively reviewed elsewhere [21]. Some of the best known are based on the construction of distance matrices, such as a unified distance matrix (U-matrix) [22]. A U-matrix encodes the distance between adjacent neurons, which is represented on the map by a color scheme. An example is illustrated in Figure 13.6.

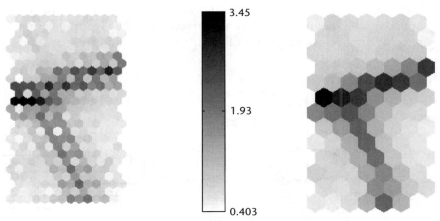

Figure 13.6 SOM-based data visualization for the Iris data set produced with the SOM-toolbox [23]. The U-matrix representation and a map based on the median distance matrix are shown on the right and left panels, respectively. The hexagons represent the corresponding map neurons. A dark coloring between the neurons corresponds to a large distance. A light coloring signifies that the input patterns are close to each other in the input space. Thus, light areas can be thought of as clusters and dark areas as cluster boundaries. These maps highlight three clusters in the data set.

13.3.4   Application of Unsupervised Learning in ECG Classification

The previous sections indicate that unsupervised learning is suitable to support ECG classification. Moreover, clustering-based analysis may be useful to detect relevant relationships between patterns. For example, recent studies have applied SOMs to analyse ECG signals from patients suffering from depression [24] and to classify spatiotemporal information from *body surface potential mapping* (BSPM) [25]. The results obtained in the former study indicate that an unsupervised learning approach is able to differentiate clinically meaningful subgroups with and without depression based on ECG information. Other successful applications include the unsupervised classification of ECG beats encoded with *Hermite basis functions* [26], which have shown to exhibit a low degree of misclassification. Thus, interactive and user-friendly frameworks for ECG analysis can be implemented, which may allow users to gain better insights into the class structure and key relationships between diagnostic features in a data set [27].

Hierarchical clustering has also provided the basis for the implementation of systems for the analysis of large amounts of ECG data. In one such study sponsored by the American Heart Association (AHA) [28], the data were accurately organized into clinically relevant groups without any prior knowledge. These types of tools may be particularly useful in exploratory analyses or when the distribution of the data is unknown. Figure 13.7 shows a typical hierarchical tree obtained from the ECG data set in the AHA study. Based on the pattern distributions over these clusters, one can see that the two clusters (A and B) at the first level of the tree correspond to Classes Normal and Abnormal, respectively, while the two subclusters at the second level of the hierarchy are associated to Class V (premature ventricular contraction) and Class R (R on T ventricular premature beat), respectively. Other interesting applications of hierarchical and *k*-means clustering methods for ECG classification are illustrated in [29, 30].

Although traditional unsupervised learning methods are useful to address different classification problems, they exhibit several limitations that limit their applicability. For example, the SOM topology needs to be specified by the user. Such a fixed, nonadaptable architecture may negatively influence its application to more complex, dynamic classification problems. The SOM indicates the similarities between

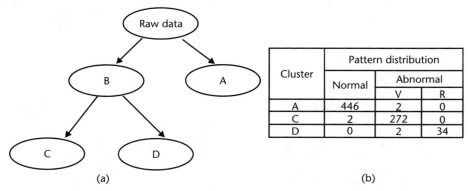

Cluster	Pattern distribution		
	Normal	Abnormal	
		V	R
A	446	2	0
C	2	272	0
D	0	2	34

(a)   (b)

Figure 13.7   The application of hierarchical clustering for ECG classification: (a) tree structure extracted by clustering; and (b) pattern distributions over the clusters [28].

input vectors in terms of the distances between the corresponding neurons. But it does not explicitly represent cluster boundaries. Manually detecting the clusters and their boundaries on a SOM may be an unreliable and time-consuming task [31]. The k-means model does not impose a cluster structure on the data. It produces a relatively disorganized collection of clusters that may not clearly portray significant associations between patterns [20]. Different versions of hierarchical clustering are conceptually simple and easy to implement, but they exhibit limitations such as their inability to perform adjustments once a splitting or merging decision has been made. Advanced solutions that aim to address some of these limitations will be discussed in the next section.

13.3.5 Advances in Clustering-Based Techniques

Significant advances include more adaptive techniques, semisupervised clustering, and various hybrid approaches based on the combination of several clustering methods.

13.3.5.1 Clustering Based on Supervised Learning Techniques

Traditional clustering ignores prior classification knowledge of the data under investigation. Recent advances in clustering-based biomedical pattern discovery have demonstrated how supervised classification techniques, such as supervised neural networks, can be used to support automatic clustering or class discovery [14]. These approaches are sometimes referred to as semisupervised clustering. Relevant examples include the *simplified fuzzy ARTMAP* (SFAM) [32, 33] and *supervised network self-organized map* (sNet-SOM) [34].

A SFAM is a simplified form of the *fuzzy ARTMAP neural network* based on Adaptive Resonance Theory (ART), which has been extensively studied for supervised, incremental pattern recognition tasks. The SFAM aims to reduce the computational costs and architectural complexity of the fuzzy ARTMAP model [32]. In simple terms a SFAM comprises two layers: the input and output layers (illustrated in Figure 13.8). In the binary input the input vector is first processed by the complement coder where the input vector is stretched to double its size by adding its complement as well [32]. The $(d \times n)$ weight matrix, W, encodes the relationship between the output neurons and the input layer. The category layer holds the names of the m categories that the network has to learn. Unlike traditional supervised back-propagation neural networks, the SFAM implements a self-organizing adaptation of its learning architecture. The assignment of output neurons to categories is dynamically assessed by the network. Moreover, the model requires one single parameter, ρ, or vigilance parameter, to be specified and can perform a training task with one pass through the data set (one learning epoch). In the SFAM model, when the selected output neuron does not represent the same category corresponding to the given input sample, a mechanism called *match tracking* is triggered. This mechanism gradually increases the vigilance level and forces a search for another category suitable to be associated with the desired output. Further information about the learning algorithm of the SFAM can be found in [32, 33]. Its application and useful aspects for decision making support have been demonstrated in different domains

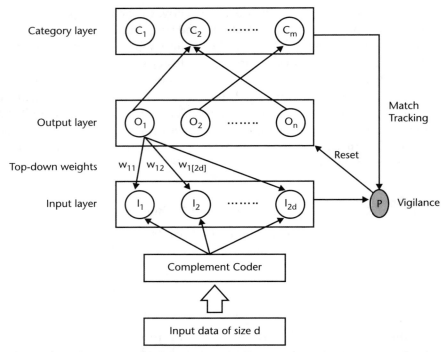

Figure 13.8 Architecture of a SFAM network. Based on a mechanism of match tracking, a SFAM mode adjusts a vigilance level to decide when new output neurons should be generated to learn the categories.

such as prognosis of coronary care patients and acute myocardial infarction diagnosis [35].

The sNet-SOM model [34] is an adaptation of the original SOM, which considers class information for the determination of the winning neurons during the learning process. The learning process is achieved by minimizing a heterogeneous measure, E, defined as follows:

$$E = \left(\sum_{i=1}^{k} (\zeta_i^l + R_{su} H_i) + \varphi \right) \tag{13.1}$$

where k is the number of output neurons. The ζ_i^l is associated with an unsupervised classification error corresponding to pattern i. This error promotes the separation of patterns that are different according to a similarity metric, even if they have the same class label. The entropy measure, H_i, considers the available a priori classification information to force patterns with similar labels to belong to the same clusters. The term φ punishes any increases in the model complexity and R_{su} is a supervised/unsupervised ratio, where $R_{su} = 0$ represents a pure unsupervised model. Thus, the sNet-SOM adaptively determines the number of clusters, but at the same time its learning process is able to exploit class information available. It has been demonstrated that the incorporation of a priori knowledge into the sNet-SOM model further facilitates the data clustering without losing key exploratory analysis capabilities exhibited by traditional unsupervised learning approaches [34].

13.3.5.2   Hybrid Systems

The term *hybrid system* has been traditionally used to describe any approach that involves more than one methodology. A hybrid system approach mainly aims to combine the strengths of different methodologies to improve the quality of the results or to overcome possible dependencies on a particular algorithm. Therefore, one key problem is how to combine different methods in a meaningful and reliable way. Several integration frameworks have been extensively studied [36, 37], including the strategies illustrated in Figure 13.9. Such strategies may be implemented by: (a) using an output originating from one method as the input to another method; (b) modifying the output of one method to produce the input to another method; (c) building two methods independently and combining their outputs; and (d) using one methodology to adapt the learning process of another one. These generic strategies may be applied to both supervised and unsupervised learning systems.

Hybrid models have supported the development of different ECG classification applications. For example, the combination of a variation of the SOM model, known as the *classification partition SOM* (CP-SOM), with supervised models, such as *radial basis function* and SVM, have improved predictive performance in the detection of ischemic episodes [38]. This hybrid approach is summarized in Figure 13.10. In this two-stage analysis system, the SOM is first used to offer a global, computationally efficient view of relatively unambiguous regions in the data. A supervised learning system is then applied to assist in the classification of ambiguous cases.

In another interesting example, three ANN-related algorithms [the SOM, LVQ, and the mixture-of-experts (MOE) method] [39] were combined to implement an ECG beat classification system. In comparison to a single-model system, this hybrid learning model significantly improved the beat classification accuracy. Given the fact

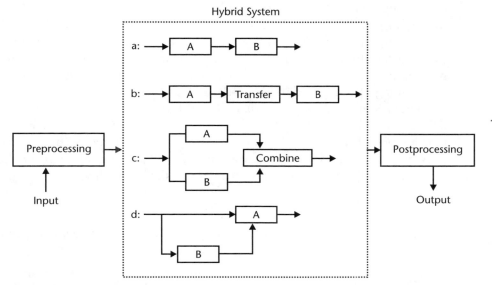

Figure 13.9   Basic strategies for combining two classification approaches. A and B represent individual clustering methods; a, b, c, and d stand for basic hybrid learning strategies.

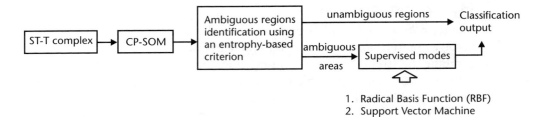

Figure 13.10 The combination of a SOM-based model with supervised learning schemes for the problem of ischemia detection.

that different approaches offer complementary advantages for pattern classification, it is widely accepted that the combination of several methods may outperform systems based on a single classification algorithm.

13.3.5.3   SANN-Based Clustering

Several SANNs have been proposed to address some of the limitations exhibited by the original SOM. SANNs represent a family of self-adaptive, incremental learning versions of the SOM. Their learning process generally begins with a set of simple maps on which new neurons are conditionally added based on heuristic criteria. For instance, these criteria take into account information about the relative winning frequency of a neuron or an accumulated optimization error. A key advantage of these models is that it allows the shape and size of the network to be determined during the learning process. Thus, the resulting map can show relevant relationships in the data in a more meaningful and user-friendly fashion. For example, due to the ability to separate neurons into disconnected areas, the *growing cell structures* (GCS) [40] and *incremental grid growing* (IGG) neural network [41] may explicitly represent cluster boundaries. Based on the combination of the SOM and the GCS principles, the *self-organizing tree algorithm* (SOTA) [42] is another relevant example of unsupervised, self-adaptive classification. An interesting feature in the SOTA is that the map neurons are arranged following a binary tree topology that allows the implementation of hierarchical clustering. Other relevant applications to biomedical data mining can be found in [43, 44].

The *growing self-organizing map* (GSOM) is another example of SANNs, which has been successfully applied to perform pattern discovery and visualization in various biomedical domains [45, 46]. It has illustrated alternative approaches to improving unsupervised ECG classification and exploratory analyses by incorporating different graphical display and statistical tools. This method is discussed in more detail in the next section.

13.3.6   Evaluation of Unsupervised Classification Models: Cluster Validity and Significance

In the development of medical decision-support systems, the evaluation of results is extremely important since the system's output may have direct health and economic implications [36]. In unsupervised learning-based applications, it is not always possible to predefine all the existing classes or to assign each input sample to a particular clinical outcome. Furthermore, different algorithms or even the same algorithm using different learning parameters may produce different clustering results. Therefore, it is fundamental to implement cluster validity and evaluation methodologies to assess the quality of the resulting partitions.

Techniques such as the GSOM provide effective visualization tools for approximating the cluster structure of the underlying data set. Interactive, visualization systems may facilitate the verification of the results with relatively little effort. However, cluster validation and interpretation solely based on visual inspection may sometimes only provide a rough, subjective description of the clustering results. Ideally, unbiased statistical evaluation criteria should be available to assist the user in addressing two fundamental questions: (1) *How many relevant clusters are actually present in the data?* and (2) *How reliable is a partitioning?* One such evaluation strategy is the application of *cluster validity indices*.

Cluster validity indices aim to provide a quantitative indication of the quality of a resulting partitioning based on the following factors [47]: (a) *compactness*, the members of each cluster should be as close to each other as possible; and (b) *separation*, the clusters themselves should be widely spaced. Thus, from a collection of available clustering results, the best partition is the one that generates the optimal validity index value.

Several validity indices are available, such as *Dunn's validity index* [48] and the *Silhouette index* [49]. However, it has been shown that different cluster validation indices might generate inconsistent predictions across different algorithms. Moreover, their performance may be sensitive to the type of data and class distribution under analysis [50, 51]. To address this limitation, it has been suggested that one should apply several validation indices and conduct a voting strategy to confidently estimate the quality of a clustering result [52]. For example, one can implement an evaluation framework using validity indices such as the generalized Dunn's index [48, 52], $V_{ij}(U)$, defined as

$$V_{ij} = \min_{1 \le s \le c} \left\{ \min_{1 \le t \le c, s \ne t} \left\{ \frac{\delta_i(X_s, X_t)}{\max_{1 \le k \le c}\{\Delta_j(X_k)\}} \right\} \right\} \qquad (13.2)$$

where $\delta_i(X_s, X_t)$ represents the ith intercluster distance between clusters X_s and X_t, $\Delta_j(X_k)$ represents the jth intracluster distance of cluster X_k, and c is the number of clusters. Hence, appropriate definitions for intercluster distances, δ, and intracluster distances, Δ, may lead to validity indices suitable to different types of clusters. Thus, using combinations of several intercluster distances, δ_i, (e.g., complete linkage defined as the distance between the most distant pair of patterns, one from each cluster) and intracluster distances, Δ_j, (e.g., centroid distance defined as the average distance of all members from one cluster to the corresponding cluster center) multiple Dunn's validity indices may be obtained. Based on a voting strategy, a more robust validity framework may be established to assess the quality of the obtained clusters. Such a clustering evaluation strategy can help the users not only to estimate the optimal number of clusters but also to assess the partitioning generated. This represents a more rigorous mechanism to justify the selection of a particular clustering outcome for further examination. For example, based on the same methodology, a robust framework for supporting quantitatively assessing the quality of classification outcomes and automatically identifying relevant partitions were implemented in [46].

Other clustering evaluation techniques include different procedures to test the statistical significance of a cluster in terms of it class distribution [53]. For example, one can apply *hypergeometric distribution* function to quantitatively assess the degree of class (e.g., signal category, disease) enrichment or over-representation in a given cluster. For each class, the probability (*p*-value) of observing k class members within a given cluster by chance is calculated as

$$p = 1 - \sum_{i=0}^{k-1} \frac{\binom{K}{i}\binom{N-K}{n-i}}{\binom{N}{n}} \tag{13.3}$$

where k is the number of class members in the query cluster of size n, N is the size of the whole data set, and K is the number of class members in the whole data set. If this probability is sufficiently low for a given class, one may say that such a class is significantly represented in the cluster; otherwise, the distribution of the class over a given cluster could happen by chance. The application of this technique can be found in many clustering-based approaches to improving biomedical pattern discovery. For example, it can be used to determine the statistical significance of functional enrichment for clustering outcomes [54].

An alternative approach to cluster validation may be based on resampling and cross-validation techniques to stimulate perturbations of the original data set, which are used to assess the stability of the clustering results with respect to sampling variability [55]. The underlying assumption is that the most reliable results are those ones that exhibit more stability with respect to the stimulated perturbations.

13.4   GSOM-Based Approaches to ECG Cluster Discovery and Visualization

13.4.1   The GSOM

The GSOM, originally reported in [56], preserves key data processing principles implemented by the SOM. However, the GSOM incorporates methods for the incremental adaptation of the network structure. The GSOM learning process, which typically starts with the generation of a network composed by four neurons, includes three stages: *initialization*, *growing*, and *smoothing* phases. Two learning parameters have to be predefined by the user: the initial learning rate, $LR(0)$, and a network *spread factor*, *SF*.

Once the network has been initialized, each input sample, x_i, is presented. Like other SANNs, the GSOM follows the basic principle of the SOM learning process. Each input presentation involves two basic operations: (1) determination of the winning neuron for each input sample using a distance measure (e.g., Euclidean distance); and (2) adaptation of the weight vectors w_j of the winning neurons and their neighborhoods as follows:

$$w_j(t+1) = \begin{cases} w_j(t) + LR_t \times (x_i - w_j(t)), & j \in N_c(t) \\ w_j(t), & \text{otherwise} \end{cases} \quad (13.4)$$

where t refers to the current learning iteration, $LR(t)$ is the learning rate at time t, and $N_c(t)$ is the neighborhood of the winning neuron c at time t. During the learning process, a cumulative quantization error (E) is calculated for each winning neuron using the following formula:

$$E_i(t+1) = E_i(t) + \sqrt{\sum_{k=1}^{D}(x_k - m_{i,k})^2} \quad (13.5)$$

where $m_{i,k}$ is the kth feature of the ith winning neuron, x_k represents the kth feature of the input vector, x, and $E_i(t)$ represents the quantization error at time t.

In the growing phase, the network keeps track of the highest error value and periodically compares it with the *growth threshold* (GT), which can be calculated with the predefined *SF* value. When $E_i > GT$, new neurons are grown in all free neighboring positions if neuron i is a boundary neuron; otherwise the error will be distributed to its neighboring neurons. Figure 13.11 summarizes the GSOM learning process. The smoothing phase, which follows the growing phase, aims to fine-tune quantization errors, especially in the neurons grown at the latter stages. The reader is referred to [46, 56] for a detailed description of the learning dynamics of the GSOM.

Due to its dynamic, self-evolving architecture, the GSOM exhibits several interesting properties for ECG cluster discovery and visualization:

- The network structure is automatically derived from the data. There is no need to predetermine the size and structure of the output maps.
- The GSOM keeps a regular, two dimensional grid structure at all times. The resulting map reveals trends hidden in the data by its shape and attracts attention to relevant areas by branching out. This provides the basis for user-friendly pattern visualization and interpretation platforms.
- In some SANNs, such as GCS and IGG, the connectivity of the map is constantly changing as connections or neurons are added and deleted. But once a connection is removed inappropriately, the map will have no chance of recovery. This makes them more sensitive to the initial parameter settings [41, 57]. The GSOM does not produce isolated clusters based on the separation of network neurons into disconnected areas. Such an approach requires less parameters in comparison to IGG and GCS. The impact of learning parameters on the GSOM performance were empirically studied in [45, 46].
- The user can provide a spread factor, $SF \in [0, 1]$, to specify the spread amount of the GSOM. This provides a straightforward way to control the expansion of the networks. Thus, based on the selection of different values of SF, hierarchical and multiresolution clustering may be implemented.

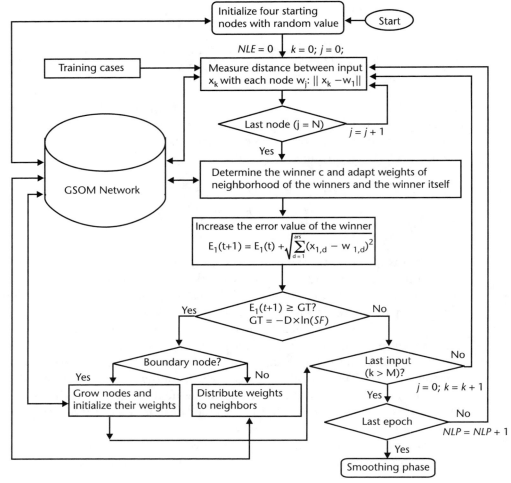

Figure 13.11 The GSOM learning algorithm. *NLE*: number of learning epochs; *N*: number of existing neurons; *M*: number of training cases; *j*: neuron index; *k*: case index; $E_i(t)$: accumulative quantization error of neuron *i* at time *t*; *D*: dimensionality of input data; *GT*: growth threshold; *SF*: spread factor.

- The GSOM can represent a data set with a lesser number of neurons than the SOM, resulting in faster computing processing. Having fewer neurons at the early stage and initializing the weight of new neurons to match their neighborhood further reduce the processing time.

13.4.2 Application of GSOM-Based Techniques to Support ECG Classification

This section introduces the application of GSOM-based approaches to supporting ECG classification. The GSOM model is tested on two real data sets to illustrate its data visualization and classification capabilities.

The first application is an ECG beat data set obtained from the MIT/BIH Arrhythmia database [58]. Based on a set of descriptive measurements for each beat, the goal is to decide whether a beat is a *ventricular ectopic beat* (Class V) or a *normal beat* (Class N). It has been suggested that the RR intervals between the previous beat, the processing beat, and the next beat may be significantly different in premature beats [59]. In view of this, data are extracted as one feature vector represented by nine temporal parameters for each of the beats in all selected records. The first four features are temporal parameters relating to RR intervals between four consecutive beats. The next two features are the cross-correlation of normalized beat templates of the current beat with the previous and subsequent beats, respectively. The last three features are based on the calculation of percent durations of the waveform above three predetermined thresholds, which are 0.2, 0.5, and 0.8, respectively. A detailed description of this data set can be found at the Web site of the Computer-Aided Engineering Center of the University of Wisconsin-Madison [60]. Each class in the data set is represented by a number: $N \rightarrow 1$ and $V \rightarrow 2$. In this example, a total of 5,000 beats (3,000 Class N samples and 2,000 Class V samples) have been randomly chosen to implement and test the model.

The second data set is a sleep apnea data set, which was designed to detect the presence or absence of apnea events from ECG signals, each one with a duration of 1 minute. A total of 35 records obtained from the *2000 Computers in Cardiology Challenge* [58] were analyzed. Each record contains a single ECG signal during approximately 8 hours. Each subject's ECG signal was converted into a sequence of beat intervals, which may be associated with prolonged cycles of sleep apnea. The *Hilbert transformation*, an analytical technique for transforming a time series into corresponding values of instantaneous amplitudes and frequencies [61], was used to derive the relevant features from the filtered RR interval time series [62]. Previous research has shown that by using the Hilbert transformation of the RR interval time series, it is possible to detect obstructive sleep apnea from single-lead ECG with a high degree of accuracy [62]. The corresponding software is freely available at PhysioNet [58]. The results reported in this example are based on the analysis of 2,000 episodes, 1,000 of which are normal episodes.

Unless indicated otherwise, the parameters for the GSOM-based results reported in this chapter are as follows: $SF = 0.001$, $N_0 = 6$ for the ECG beat data set and $N_0 = 4$ for sleep apnea data set, initial learning rate, $LR(0), = 0.5$ and the maximum NLE (growing phase) $= 5$, NLE (smoothing phase) $= 10$.

13.4.2.1 Cluster Visualization and Discovery

The resulting GSOM maps for the ECG beat and sleep apnea data sets are shown in Figures 13.12(a) and 13.13(a), respectively. The numbers shown on the map neurons represent the order in which they were created during the growth phase. Based on a majority voting strategy, where the class with the highest frequency renders its name to the corresponding output neuron, the corresponding label maps are given in Figures 13.12(b) and 13.13(b), respectively. The class labels for each neuron are represented as integer numbers. As a way of comparison, the SOM maps produced for these two data sets using the *SOM toolbox* (an implementation of the SOM in the Matlab 5 environment) [23] are depicted in Figures 13.14 and 13.15. The SOM Toolbox automatically selects the map size for each data set. In this example: 23×16 neurons for the ECG beat data set, and 28×8 neurons for the sleep apnea data set. The U-matrices are shown in Figures 13.14(a) and 13.15(a).

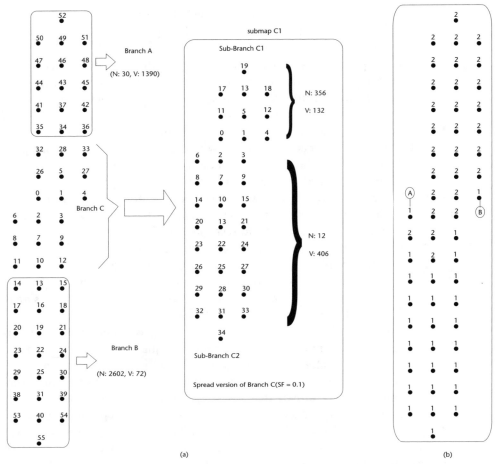

Figure 13.12 GSOM-based data visualization for a ECG beat data set: (a) resulting map with $SF = 0.001$; and (b) label map. The numbers shown on the map represent the class label for each node. Only a majority class renders its name to the node. In case of a draw, the first class encountered is used as a label.

Shades of gray indicate the distances between adjacent neurons as illustrated in the middle scale bar. The corresponding label maps based on a majority voting strategy are depicted in Figures 13.14(b) and 13.15(b).

The SOM manages to group similar patterns together. However, in Figure 13.14(b), neuron A, which is associated with Class 2, lies far away from other Class 2 neurons, and it is surrounded by Class 1 neurons. Moreover, a neuron B, labeled as Class 1, is clustered into the Class 2 area. In Figure 13.15(b), several Class 2 neurons, such as neurons A and B, are grouped together with Class 1 neurons. The boundaries between the class regions are ambiguous. The U-matrix, generally regarded as an enhanced visualization technique for SOM map, fails to offer a user-friendly visualization of the cluster structure in this problem [Figure 13.14(a)]. The U-matrix shown in Figure 13.14 provides information about the cluster structure in the underlying data set. But in this and other examples it could be difficult to directly link a U-matrix graph with its corresponding label map.

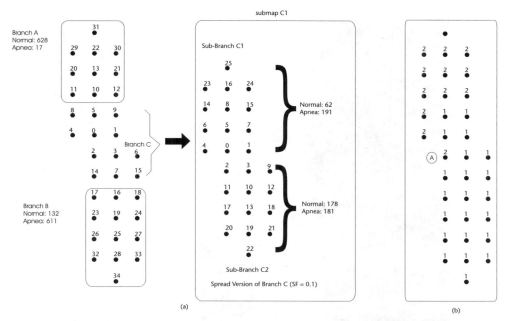

Figure 13.13 GSOM-based data visualization for sleep apnea data set: (a) resulting map with $SF =$ 0.001; and (b) label map. The numbers shown on the map represent the class label for each node. Only a majority class renders its name to the node. In case of a draw, the first class encountered is used as a label.

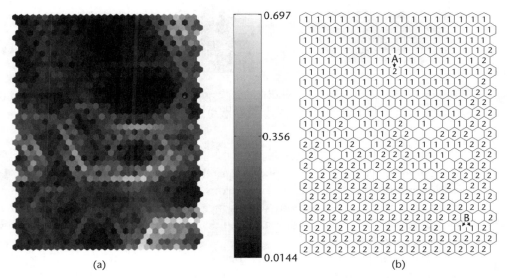

Figure 13.14 SOM-based data visualization for ECG beat data set: (a) U-matrix; and (b) label map. The numbers represent the classes assigned to a node ($1 \rightarrow N$ and $2 \rightarrow V$).

The GSOM model provided meaningful, user-friendly representations of the clustering outcomes [see, for example, label maps in Figures 13.12(b) and 13.13(b)]. At the borders of the cluster regions, some neurons, such as neurons A and B, are incorrectly grouped with other class neurons. These regions, however, can be

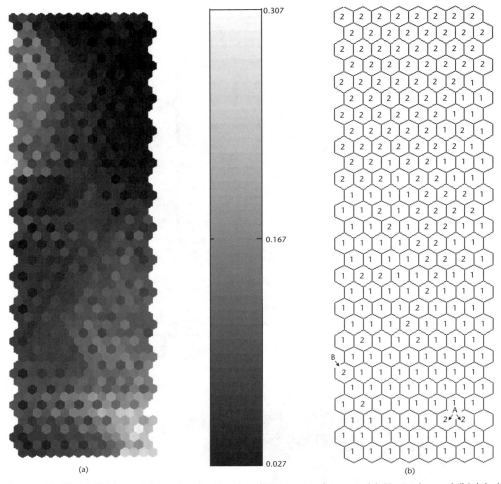

Figure 13.15 SOM-based data visualization for sleep apnea data set: (a) U-matrix; and (b) label map. "1" stands for Class Normal and "2" represents Class Apnea.

further analyzed by applying the GSOM algorithm with a higher *SF* value. Moreover, due to its self-adaptive properties, the GSOM is able to model the data set with a relatively small number of neurons. The GSOM model required 56 and 35 neurons for the ECG beat and sleep apnea data sets, respectively. The SOM Toolbox automatically selected 468 and 224 neurons, respectively, to represent the same classification problem.

After completing a learning process, the GSOM can develop into different shapes to reveal the patterns hidden in the data. Such visualization capabilities may highlight relevant trends and associations in a more meaningful way. For instance, in Figure 13.12(a), the GSOM has branched out in two main directions. An analysis of the pattern distribution over each branch [see the summary of the distribution of patterns beside each branch in Figure 13.12(a)] confirms that there is a dominant class. Thus, 98% of the patterns in Branch A are Class V patterns, and 97% of the patterns in Branch B belongs to Class N. Using these figures, one may assume that Branch A is linked to Class V, and Branch B is associated with

Class N. Likewise, in Figure 13.13(a), 97% of the samples in Branch A are Class Normal patterns, and 82% of the samples in Branch B belong to Class Apnea.

Since the *SF* controls the map spread, one may also implement multiresolution and hierarchical clustering on areas of interest. Previous research has shown that the GSOM may reveal significant clusters by its shape even with a low *SF* value. A finer analysis, based on a larger *SF* value, can be applied to critical areas, such as those areas categorized as ambiguous. Figure 13.12(a) highlights the main clusters in the data when using a $SF = 0.001$. For those areas where it is difficult to differentiate between clusters [such as Branch C in Figure 13.12(a)], a higher *SF* value may be applied (e.g., $SF = 0.1$). Thus, a more understandable map was obtained (submap C1). This submap has clearly been dispersed in two directions (Sub-Branches C1 and C2). A similar analysis is carried out on the sleep apnea data set, as illustrated in Figure 13.13(a). Interestingly, as can be seen from the pattern distribution in Sub-Branch C2, there is no dominant class in this branch. This might suggest that the apnea patterns assigned to the Sub-Branch C2 may be related to Normal patterns. In these cases a closer examination with expert support is required.

13.4.2.2   Cluster Assessment Based on Validity Indices

Cluster validity techniques may be applied to automatically detect relevant partitions. For example, they can be used to identify significant relationships between branches A and B and subbranches C1 and C2 shown on Figures 13.12(a) and 13.13(a). Based on the combinations of six intercluster distances, i, (single linkage, complete linkage, average linkage, centroid linkage, combination average linkage with centroid linkage, and Hausdorff metric [63]) and four intracluster distances, j, (standard diameter, average distance, centroid distance, and nearest neighbor distance), Table 13.4 lists 24 Dunn's-based validity indices for various partitions, which may be identified in the GSOM maps illustrated in Figures 13.12(a) and 13.13(a). Bold entries correspond to the optimal validation index values across three partitions. Such values indicate the optimal number of clusters estimated for each application. In the case of the ECG beat classification, 18 indices, including the average index value, favour the partition $c = 2$, which is further examined in column two, as the best partition for this data set. The first cluster of this partition is represented by branches A and C2. The second cluster comprises branches B and C1. This coincides with the pattern distributions over these areas. Similarly, for the sleep apnea data set, 21 indices suggest the partition shown in column 5 as the best choice for this data set. The description of these partitions is shown in Tables 13.5 and 13.6.

13.5   Final Remarks

Clearly, one cannot expect to do justice to all relevant unsupervised classification methodologies and applications in a single chapter. Nevertheless, key design and application principles of unsupervised learning-based analysis for ECG classification have been discussed. Emphasis has been placed on advances in clustering-based approaches for exploratory visualization and classification. In contrast to supervised learning, traditional unsupervised learning aims to find relevant clusters, categories

Table 13.4 Validity Indices for ECG Beat and Sleep Apnea Data Sets Based on the Resulting GSOM Maps in Figures 13.12 and 13.13

V_{ij}	ECG Beat Data Set			Sleep Apnea Data Set		
	$c = 2$ (A + C1, B + C2)	$c = 2$ (A + C2, B + C1)	$c = 3$ (A,B, C1 + C2)	$c = 2$ (A + C1, B + C2)	$c = 2$ (A + C2, B + C1)	$c = 3$ (A,B, C1 + C2)
V_{11}	0.01	**0.02**	0.01	**0.02**	0.02	0.02
V_{12}	0.05	**0.06**	0.04	0.04	0.05	0.06
V_{13}	0.03	**0.04**	0.03	0.03	0.04	0.04
V_{14}	0.47	**0.54**	0.42	0.51	0.44	0.47
V_{21}	1.08	**1.24**	1.01	1.26	1.31	1.16
V_{22}	**4.55**	4.22	3.27	3.25	3.71	3.46
V_{23}	**3.16**	2.97	2.24	2.17	2.56	2.41
V_{24}	**45.51**	39.27	32.94	36.75	31.92	25.94
V_{31}	0.29	**0.36**	0.32	0.49	0.57	0.39
V_{32}	**1.24**	1.23	1.04	1.27	1.63	1.15
V_{33}	**0.86**	**0.86**	0.72	0.85	1.12	0.80
V_{34}	**12.45**	11.40	10.52	14.35	13.97	8.62
V_{41}	0.19	**0.25**	0.21	0.37	0.50	0.29
V_{42}	0.81	**0.87**	0.69	0.97	1.42	0.88
V_{43}	0.56	**0.61**	0.47	0.65	0.98	0.61
V_{44}	**8.11**	8.07	6.99	10.95	12.19	6.58
V_{51}	0.24	**0.30**	0.26	0.43	0.54	0.34
V_{52}	**1.04**	**1.04**	0.83	1.11	1.52	1.02
V_{53}	0.72	**0.73**	0.57	0.75	1.05	1.02
V_{54}	**10.37**	9.63	8.39	12.60	13.07	7.61
V_{61}	0.14	**0.60**	0.06	0.62	0.76	0.72
V_{62}	0.58	**2.03**	0.19	1.60	2.15	2.14
V_{63}	0.40	**1.43**	0.13	1.07	1.48	1.49
V_{64}	5.80	**18.87**	1.94	18.11	18.50	16.01
Average	4.11	**4.44**	3.05	4.59	4.65	3.46

or associations in the absence of prior class knowledge during the learning process. One may define it as a *knowledge discovery task*, which has proven to play a fundamental role in biomedical decision support and research. In the case of ECG classification, unsupervised models have been applied to several problems such as ischemia detection [38], arrhythmia classification [26], and to pattern visualization [28, 46].

SANN-based approaches, such as the GSOM introduced in Section 13.4, have demonstrated advantages over traditional models for supporting ECG cluster discovery and visualization. Instead of using a static grid representation or long lists

Table 13.5 Clustering Description ($c = 2$) of the Second Partition for ECG Beat Data Set Using GSOM

Cluster	Class V	Class N
Branch A + Subbranch C2	1796	42
Branch B + Subbranch C1	204	2958

Table 13.6 Clustering Description ($c = 2$) of the Second Partition for Sleep Apnea Data Set Using GSOM

Cluster	Class V	Class N
Branch A + Subbranch C2	198	791
Branch B + Subbranch C1	802	209

of numbers to describe partitions, the GSOM is able to reflect relevant groups in the data by its incrementally generated topology. Such structure provides the basis for user-friendly visualization platforms to support the detection of relevant patterns. By introducing a spread factor, multiresolution and hierarchical clustering may also be implemented. Although the data sets analyzed in this chapter only contain two classes, results published elsewhere [46] have demonstrated the GSOM model's ability to support multiple-class prediction problems in related biomedical domains.

SANN-based clustering techniques also exhibit important limitations. Potentially irrelevant neurons or connections are commonly found and removed by models such as the GCS and IGG during a learning process. This advantage, however, may be achieved at the expense of robustness. It has been shown that IGG and GCS are susceptible to variations in initial parameter settings [41, 57] in comparison to the original SOM. Moreover, in the case of the GSOM there are no deletion steps involved in its learning process. Instead of calculating the exact position of the new neurons, the GSOM generates new neurons in all free neighboring position. Unfortunately, such an approach will inevitably generate dummy neurons, which sometimes can severely degrade the visualization ability of GSOM models. Thus, additional research on the incorporation of pruning algorithms into the GSOM growing process is needed.

It is worth noting that for the same data set and clustering model different results may be obtained for different parameter settings. There is no standard to determine a priori the optimal input parameters, such as the learning rate in the SOM and the spread factor in the GSOM. Techniques for the automatic and dynamic determination of optimum combinations of learning parameters also deserve further investigations.

Given the diversity of unsupervised learning algorithms available and the inexistence of universal clustering solutions for ECG classification, it is important to understand critical factors that may influence the choice of appropriate clustering techniques. Thus, it is crucial to be aware of key factors that may influence the selection of clustering algorithms, such as the statistical nature of the problem domain under study and constraints defined by the user and the clustering options available [14]. A single clustering algorithm may not always perform well for different types of data sets. Therefore, the application of more than one clustering model is recommended to facilitate the generation of more meaningful and reliable results [13, 14].

An advanced generation of unsupervised learning systems for ECG classification should also offer improvements in connection to information representation and the assessment of classification results. Ideally, an ECG classification platform should be capable of processing multiple information sources. In today's distributed healthcare environment, ECG data are commonly stored and analyzed using different formats and software tools. Thus, there is a need to develop cross-platform solutions to support data analysis tasks and applications [64]. A relevant solution consists of applying *eXtensible Markup Language* (XML) for representing ECG information. *ecgML* [65], a markup language for ECG data acquisition and analysis, has been designed to illustrate the advantages offered by XML for supporting data exchange between different ECG data acquisition and analysis devices. Such representation approaches may facilitate data mining using heterogeneous software platforms. The data and metadata contained in an ecgML record may be useful to support both supervised and unsupervised ECG classification applications. It is also crucial to expand our understanding of how to evaluate the quality of unsupervised classification models. This chapter introduced two useful cluster assessment approaches: cluster validity indices and class representation significance tests. Even when such strategies may provide users with measures of confidence or reliability, it is also important to consider domain-specific constraints and assumptions, as well as human expert support [36]. In comparison to supervised classification, the evaluation of outcomes in clustering-based analysis may be a more complex task. It is expected that more tools for unsupervised classification validation and interpretation will be available. One basic evaluation principle consists of using the resulting clusters to classify samples (e.g., sections of signals) unseen during the learning process [66]. Thus, if a set of putative clusters reflects the true structure of the data, then a prediction model based on these clusters and tested on novel samples should perform well. A similar strategy was adopted in [26] to quantitatively assess the quality of clustering results. Other advances include the application of supervised learning to evaluate unsupervised learning outcomes [67], which are not discussed here due to space constraints.

Finally, it should be emphasized that unsupervised models may also be adapted to perform supervised classification applications. Based on the same principle of the *supervised SOM* model, for example, a supervised version of the GSOM algorithm has been proposed [45]. Nevertheless, performing supervised classification using methods based on unsupervised learning should not be seen as a fundamental goal. The strengths of unsupervised learning are found in exploratory, visualization-driven classification tasks such as the identification of relevant groups and outlier detection. Unsupervised (clustering-based) learning is particularly recommended to obtain an initial understanding of the data. Thus, these models may be applied as a first step to uncover relevant relationships between signals and groups of signals, which may assist in a meaningful and rigorous selection of further analytical steps, including supervised learning techniques [19, 56].

References

[1]　Nugent, C. D., J. A. Webb, and N. D. Black, "Feature and Classifier Fusion for 12-Lead ECG Classification," *Medical Informatics and the Internet in Medicine*, Vol. 25, No. 3, July–September 2000, pp. 225–235.

[2]　Gao, D., et al., "Arrhythmia Identification from ECG Signals with a Neural Network Classifier Based on a Bayesian Framework," *24th SGAI International Conference on Innovative Techniques and Applications of Artificial Intelligence*, 2004.

[3]   de Chazal, P., M. O'Dwyer, and R. B. Reilly, "Automatic Classification of Heartbeats Using ECG Morphology and Heartbeat Interval Features," *IEEE Trans. Biomed. Eng.*, Vol. 51, No. 7, 2004, pp. 1196–1206.

[4]   Georgeson, S., and H. Warner, "Expert System Diagnosis of Wide Complex Tachycardia," *Proc. of Computers in Cardiology 1992*, 1992, pp. 671–674.

[5]   Coast, D. A., et al., "An Approach to Cardiac Arrhythmia Analysis Using Hidden Markov Models," *IEEE Trans. Biomed. Eng.*, Vol. 37, No. 9, 1990, pp. 826–836.

[6]   Silipo, R., and C. Marchesi, "Artificial Neural Networks for Automatic ECG Analysis," *IEEE Trans. on Signal Processing*, Vol. 46, No. 5, 1998, pp. 1417–1425.

[7]   Bortolan, G., and J. L. Willems, "Diagnostic ECG Classification Based on Neural Networks," *Journal of Electrocardiology*, Vol. 26, No. Suppl: 1993, pp. 75–79.

[8]   Osowski, S., L. T. Hoai, and T. Markiewicz, "Support Vector Machine-Based Expert System for Reliable Heartbeat Recognition," *IEEE Trans. Biomed. Eng.*, Vol. 51, No. 4, 2004, pp. 582–589.

[9]   Jain, A. K., M. N. Murty, and P. J. Flynn, "Data Clustering: A Review," *ACM Computing Surveys*, Vol. 31, No. 3, 1999, pp. 264–323.

[10]   Su, M. S., and C. H. Chou, "A Modified Version of the k-Means Algorithm with a Distance Based on Cluster Symmetry," *IEEE Trans. on Pattern Analysis and Machine Intelligence*, Vol. 23, No. 6, 2001, pp. 674–680.

[11]   Jagadish, H. V., et al., "Similarity-Based Queries," *Proc. of the 14th ACM SIGACT-SIGMOD-SIGART Symposium on Principles of Database Systems (PODS'95)*, ACM Press, 1995, pp. 36–45.

[12]   Kalpakis, K., D. Gada, and V. Puttagunta, "Distance Measures for Effective Clustering of ARIMA Time-Series," *Proc. of the 2001 IEEE International Conference on Data Mining (ICDM'01)*, 2001, pp. 273–280.

[13]   Azuaje, F., "Clustering-Based Approaches to Discovering and Visualising Microarray Data Patterns," *Brief Bioinform.*, Vol. 4, No. 1, 2003, pp. 31–42.

[14]   Azuaje, F., and N. Bolshakova, "Clustering Genomic Expression Data: Design and Evaluation Principles," in D. Berrar, W. Dubitzky, and M. Granzow, (eds.), *Understanding and Using Microarray Analysis Techniques: A Practical Guide*, London, U.K.: Springer, 2002, pp. 230–245.

[15]   Monti, S., et al., "Consensus Clustering: A Resampling-Based Method for Class Discovery and Visualization of GENE Expression Microarray Data," *Machine Learning*, Vol. 52, No. 1–2, 2003, pp. 91–118.

[16]   Sommer, D., and M. Golz, "Clustering of EEG-Segments Using Hierarchical Agglmerative Methods and Self-Organizing Maps," *Proc. of Int. Conf. Artificial Intelligent Networks 2001*, 2001, pp. 642–649.

[17]   Ding, C., and X. He, "Cluster Merging and Splitting in Hierarchical Clustering Algorithms," *Proc. of 2002 IEEE International Conference on Data Mining (ICDM'02)*, 2002, pp. 139–146.

[18]   Maulik, U., and S. Bandyopadhyay, "Performance Evaluation of Some Clustering Algorithms and Validity Indices," *IEEE Trans. on Pattern Analysis and Machine Intelligence*, Vol. 24, No. 12, 2002, pp. 1650–1654.

[19]   Kohonen, T., *Self-Organizing Maps*, Berlin: Springer, 1995.

[20]   Tamayo, P., et al., "Interpreting Patterns of Gene Expression with Self-Organizing Maps: Methods and Application to Hematopoietic Differentiation," *Proc. of National Academy of Sciences of the United States of America*, Vol. 96, No. 6, 1999, pp. 2907–2912.

[21]   Vesanto, J., "SOM-Based Data Visualization Methods," *Intelligent Data Analysis*, Vol. 3, No. 2, 1999, pp. 111–126.

[22]   Ultsch, A., and H. P. Siemon, "Kohonen's Self Organizing Feature Maps for Exploratory Data Analysis," *Proc. of Int. Neural Network Conf. (INNC'90)*, 1990, pp. 305–308.

[23]   Vesanto, J., et al., "Self-Organizing Map in Matlab: The SOM Toolbox, *Proc. of the Matlab DSP Conference 1999*, 1999, pp. 35–40.

[24]   Gaetz, M., et al., "Self-Organizing Neural Network Analyses of Cardiac Data in Depression," *Neuropsychobiology*, Vol. 49, No. 1, 2004, pp. 30–37.

[25]   Simelius, K., et al., "Spatiotemporal Characterization of Paced Cardiac Activation with Body Surface Potential Mapping and Self-Organizing Maps," *Physiological Measurement*, Vol. 24, No. 3, 2003, pp. 805–816.

[26]   Lagerholm, M., et al., "Clustering ECG Complexes Using Hermite Functions and Self-Organizing Maps," *IEEE Trans. Biomed. Eng.*, Vol. 47, No. 7, 2000, pp. 838–848.

[27]   Bortolan, G., and W. Pedrycz, "An Interactive Framework for an Analysis of ECG Signals," *Artificial Intelligence in Medicine*, Vol. 24, No. 2, 2002, pp. 109–132.

[28]   Nishizawa, H., et al., "Hierarchical Clustering Method for Extraction of Knowledge from a Large Amount of Data," *Optical Review*, Vol. 6, No. 4, July-August 1999, pp. 302–307.

[29]   Maier, C., H. Dickhaus, and J. Gittinger, "Unsupervised Morphological Classification of QRS Complexes," *Proc. of Computers in Cardiology 1999*, 1999, pp. 683–686.

[30]   Boudaoud, S., et al., "Integrated Shape Averaging of the P-Wave Applied to AF Risk Detection," *Proc. of Computers in Cardiology 2003*, 2003, pp. 125–128.

[31]   Rauber, A., *Visualization in Unsupervised Neural Network*, M. S. thesis, Technische Universität Wien, Austria, 1996,

[32]   Kasuba, T., "Simplified Fuzzy ARTMAP," *AI Expert*, Vol. 8, 1993, pp. 19–25.

[33]   Rajasekaran, S., and G. A. V. Pai, "Image Recognition Using Simplified Fuzzy ARTMAP Augmented with a Moment Based Feature Extractor," *International Journal of Pattern Recognition and Artificial Intelligence*, Vol. 14, No. 8, 2000, pp. 1081–1095.

[34]   Mavroudi, S., S. Papadimitriou, and A. Bezerianos, "Gene Expression Data Analysis with a Dynamically Extended Self-Organized Map that Exploits Class Information," *Bioinformatics*, Vol. 18, No. 11, 2002, pp. 1446–1453.

[35]   Downs, J., et al., "Application of the Fuzzy ARTMAP Neural Network Model to Medical Pattern Classification Tasks," *Artificial Intelligence in Medicine*, Vol. 8, No. 4, 1996, pp. 403–428.

[36]   Hudson, D. L., and M. E. Cohen, *Neural Networks and Artificial Intelligence for Biomedical Engineering*, New York: IEEE Press, 2000.

[37]   Hudson, D. L., et al., "Medical Diagnosis and Treatment Plans from a Hybrid Expert System," in A. Kandel and G. Langholtz, (eds.), *Hybrid Architectures for Intelligent Systems*, Boca Raton, FL: CRC Press, 1992, pp. 330–344.

[38]   Papadimitriou, S., et al., "Ischemia Detection with a Self-Organizing Map Supplemented by Supervised Learning," *IEEE Trans. on Neural Networks*, Vo., 12, No. 3, 2001, pp. 503–515.

[39]   Hu, Y. H., S. Palreddy, and W. J. Tompkins, "A Patient-Adaptable ECG Beat Classifier Using a Mixture of Experts Approach," *IEEE Trans. Biomed. Eng.*, Vol. 44, No. 9, 1997, pp. 891–900.

[40]   Fritzke, B., "Growing Cell Structures—A Self-Organizing Network for Unsupervised and Supervised Learning," *Neural Networks*, Vol. 7, No. 9, 1994, pp. 1441–1460.

[41]   Blackmore, J., "Visualising High-Dimensional Structure with the Incremental Grid Growing Neural Network," *Proc. of 12th Intl. Conf. on Machine Learning*, 1995, pp. 55–63.

[42]   Dopazo, J., and J. M. Carazo, "Phylogenetic Reconstruction Using an Unsupervised Growing Neural Network That Adopts the Topology of a Phylogenetic Tree," *Journal of Molecular Evolution*, Vol. 44, No. 2, 1997, pp. 226–233.

[43]   Herrero, J., A. Valencia, and J. Dopazo, "A Hierarchical Unsupervised Growing Neural Network for Clustering Gene Expression Patterns," *Bioinformatics*, Vol. 17, No. 2, 2001, pp. 126–136.

[44] Wang, H. C., et al., "Self-Organizing Tree-Growing Network for the Classification of Protein Sequences," *Protein Science*, Vol. 7, No. 12, 1998, pp. 2613–2622.

[45] Wang, H., F. Azuaje, and N. Black, "Improving Biomolecular Pattern Discovery and Visualization with Hybrid Self-Adaptive Networks," *IEEE Trans. on Nanobioscience*, Vol. 1, No. 4, 2002, pp. 146–166.

[46] Wang, H., F. Azuaje, and N. Black, "An Integrative and Interactive Framework for Improving Biomedical Pattern Discovery and Visualization," *IEEE Trans. on Information Technology in Biomedicine*, Vol. 8, No. 1, 2004, pp. 16–27.

[47] Halkidi, M., Y. Batistakis, and M. Vazirgiannis, "On Clustering Validation Techniques," *Journal of Intelligent Information Systems*, Vol. 17, No. 2–3, 2001, pp. 107–145.

[48] Dunn, J. C., "A Fuzzy Relative of the ISODATA Process and Its Use in Detecting Compact Well-Separated Clusters," *J. Cybernetics*, Vol. 3, No. 3, 1973, pp. 95–104.

[49] Rousseeuw, P. J., "Silhouettes—A Graphical Aid to the Interpretation and Validation of Cluster-Analysis," *Journal of Computational and Applied Mathematics*, Vol. 20, 1987, pp. 53–65.

[50] Milligan, G. W., and M. C. Cooper, "An Examination of Procedures for Determining the Number of Clusters in a Data Set," *Psychometrika*, Vol. 50, No. 2, 1985, pp. 159–179.

[51] Halkidi, M., and M. Vazirgiannis, "Clustering Validity Assessment: Finding the Optimal Partitioning of a Data Set," *Proc. of IEEE International Conference on Data Mining (ICDM'01)*, 2001, pp. 187–194.

[52] Bezdek, J. C., and N. R. Pal, "Some New Indexes of Cluster Validity," *IEEE Trans. on Systems, Man and Cybernetics, Part B-Cybernetics*, Vol. 28, No. 3, 1998, pp. 301–315.

[53] Bock, H. H., "On Some Significance Tests in Cluster Analysis," *Journal of Classification*, Vol. 2, No. 1, 1985, pp. 77–108.

[54] Tavazoie, S., et al., "Systematic Determination of Genetic Network Architecture," *Nature Genetics*, Vol. 22, 1999, pp. 281–285.

[55] Levine, E., and E. Domany, "Resampling Method for Unsupervised Estimation of Cluster Validity," *Neural Computation*, Vol. 13, No. 11, 2001, pp. 2573–2593.

[56] Alahakoon, D., S. K. Halgamuge, and B. Srinivasan, "Dynamic Self-Organizing Maps with Controlled Growth for Knowledge Discovery," *IEEE Trans. on Neural Networks*, Vol. 11, No. 3, 2000, pp. 601–614.

[57] Kohle, M., and D. Merkl, "Visualising Similarities in High Dimensional Input Spaces with a Growing and Splitting Neural Network," *Proc. of Int. Conf. of Artificial Neural Networks (ICANN'96)*, 1996, pp. 581–586.

[58] Goldberger, A. L., et al., "PhysioBank, PhysioToolkit, and PhysioNet: Components of a New Research Resource for Complex Physiologic Signals," *Circulation*, Vol. 101, No. 23, 2000, pp. E215–E220.

[59] Lichstein, E., et al., "Characteristics of Ventricular Ectopic Beats in Patients with Ventricular Tachycardia: A 24-Hour Holter Monitor Study," *Chest*, Vol. 77, No. 6, 1980, pp. 731–735.

[60] Hu, Y. H., "ECG Beat Classification Data File, December 31, 2003," http://www.cae.wisc.edu/ece539/data/ecg/.

[61] Rosenblum, M. G., et al., "Scaling Behaviour of Heartbeat Intervals Obtained by Wavelet-Based Time-Series Analysis," *Nature*, Vol. 383, 1996, pp. 323–327.

[62] Mietus, J. E., et al., "Detection of Obstructive Sleep Apnea from Cardiac Interbeat Interval Time Series," *Proc. of Computers in Cardiology 2000*, 2000, pp. 753–756.

[63] Preparata, F. P., and M. I. Shamos, *Computational Geometry: An Introduction*, New York: Springer-Verlag, 1985.

[64] Varri, A., et al., "Standards for Biomedical Signal Databases," *IEEE Engineering in Medicine and Biology Magazine*, Vol. 20, No. 3, 2001, pp. 33–37.

[65]   Wang, H., et al., "A Markup Language for Electrocardiogram Data Acquisition and Analysis (ecgML)," *BMC Medical Informatics and Decision Making*, Vol. 3, No. 1, 2003, p. 4.

[66]   Golub, T. R., et al., "Molecular Classification of Cancer: Class Discovery and Class Prediction by Gene Expression Monitoring," *Science*, Vol. 286, No. 5439, 1999, pp. 531–537.

[67]   Roiger, R., and M. Geatz, *Data Mining: A Tutorial-Based Primer*, Reading, MA: Addison-Wesley, 2003.

About the Authors

Gari D. Clifford received a B.Sc. in physics and electronics from Exeter University, Devon, United Kingdom, an M.Sc. in mathematics and theoretical physics from Southampton University, Southampton, United Kingdom, and a Ph.D. in neural networks and biomedical engineering from Oxford University, Oxford, United Kingdom, in 1992, 1995, and 2003, respectively. He has worked in industry on the design and production of several C∈- and FDA-approved medical devices. Dr. Clifford is currently a research scientist in the Harvard-MIT Division of Health Sciences where he is the engineering manager of an R01 NIH-funded research program, "Integrating Data, Models, and Reasoning in Critical Care," and a major contributor to the well-known PhysioNet Research Resource. He has taught at Oxford, MIT, and Harvard and is currently an instructor in biomedical engineering at MIT. Dr. Clifford, a senior member of the IEEE, has authored and coauthored more than 40 publications in the field of biomedical engineering. Dr. Clifford is on the editorial boards of *BioMedical Engineering OnLine* and the *Journal of Biological Systems*. His research interests include multidimensional biomedical signal processing, linear and nonlinear time series analysis, relational database mining, decision support, and mathematical modeling of the ECG and the cardiovascular system.

Francisco Azuaje focuses his research on the areas at the intersection of computer science and life sciences. It comprises machine and statistical learning methods to support predictive data analysis and visualization in biomedical informatics and postgenome informatics. He has extensively published in journals, books, and conference proceedings in the areas of medical informatics, computational intelligence, and bioinformatics. He is a senior member of the IEEE. He has several editorial board memberships in journals relevant to biomedical informatics and bioinformatics. Dr. Azuaje has coedited two other books relevant to the areas of bioinformatics and systems biology.

Patrick E. McSharry received a B.A. in theoretical physics in 1993 and an M.Sc. in electronic and electrical engineering in 1995 from Trinity College, Dublin. He was awarded a Marie Curie Research Fellowship in 1995 and received a Ph.D. in mathematics, on time series analysis and forecasting, from the University of Oxford in 1999. He is currently a Royal Academy of Engineering/EPSRC research fellow at the University of Oxford, a research associate at St. Catherine's College, and a senior member of the IEEE. His research interests include biomedical engineering, complex dynamical systems, signal processing, systems biology, risk management, operations research, and forecasting.

Andrew T. Reisner received a B.S. in mechanical engineering and biological sciences from Stanford University, in 1992, and an M.D. from Harvard Medical School, in 1997, and trained in emergency medicine at the Harvard-affiliated Emergency Medicine Residency program. He is presently an attending physician at Massachusetts General Hospital in the Department of Emergency Medicine, an instructor at Harvard Medical School, and a visiting scientist at MIT. Dr. Reisner's research is oriented toward the intersection of diagnostic expert systems, medical sensor technology, and the clinical problem of circulatory shock.

Roger G. Mark is the Distinguished Professor of Health Sciences & Technology and Professor of Electrical Engineering at MIT. He is a coprincipal investigator of the Research Resource for Complex Physiologic Signals. Dr. Mark served as the codirector of the Harvard-MIT Division of Health Sciences & Technology from 1985 to 1996. Dr. Mark's research activities include physiological signal processing and database development, cardiovascular modeling, and intelligent patient monitoring. He led the group that developed the MIT-BIH Arrhythmia Database.

Franc Jager received a B.Sc. and an M.Sc. in electrical engineering from the University of Ljubljana in 1980 and 1984, respectively. In 1994, he received a Ph.D. in computer and information science from the University of Ljubljana. Between 1990 and 1991, he was a visiting scientist the MIT. Currently, he is a full professor in the Faculty of Computer and Information Science at the University of Ljubljana and is a research affiliate at MIT. In 1995 Dr. Jager established the Laboratory for Biomedical Computer Systems and Imaging at the University of Ljubljana. His research interests include biomedical signal processing, and medical imaging, and biomedical computer systems.

Matt B. Oefinger earned B.Sc. degrees from Southern Methodist University in electrical engineering, computer science, and applied mathematics, graduating summa cum laude in all areas. After working at Texas Instruments for a year, Mr. Oefinger matriculated at MIT, where he earned an M.Sc. in electrical engineering and continues doctoral work on automated ST segment analysis.

Nicholas P. Hughes is a postdoctoral research assistant in the Department of Engineering Science at the University of Oxford and is the W. W. Spooner Junior Research Fellow in Engineering at New College, Oxford. He holds an M.Eng. in engineering and computing science from St. Hugh's College, Oxford, and an M.Sc. by research in pattern analysis and neural networks from Aston University. His D.Phil. research concerned the development of probabilistic models for automated ECG interval analysis, with a particular focus on the accurate measurement and assessment of the QT interval for clinical drug trials. Dr. Hughes' postdoctoral research is focused on a number of problems at the interface of information engineering and the biomedical sciences. In particular, he is currently developing new techniques for assessing brain activity based on the integration of fMRI and EEG data.

Haiying Wang received a B.Eng. and an M.Sc. in optical electronics engineering from Zhejiang University, Hangzhou, China, in 1987 and 1989, respectively, and a Ph.D. from the University of Ulster, United Kingdom, in 2004. He is currently a postdoctoral research fellow in the faculty of engineering at the University of Ulster. His research focuses on artificial intelligence, machine learning, data mining, pattern discovery and visualization, neural networks, XML, and their applications in medical informatics and bioinformatics. He has published several publications in scientific journals, books, and conference proceedings relating to the areas at the intersection of computer science and life science.

Raquel Bailón received an M.Sc. in telecommunications engineering from the University of Zaragoza in 2001. In 2001 she started her Ph.D. degree studies at the Department of Electronic Engineering and Communications at University of Zaragoza with a grant supported by the Spanish government. Since 2003, she has been an assistant professor in the same department. Her main research activity lies in the field of biomedical signal processing, especially in the analysis of the electrocardiogram for diagnosis purposes.

Pablo Laguna received an M.S. and a Ph.D. in physics from the Science Faculty at the University of Zaragoza, Spain, in 1985 and 1990, respectively. His Ph.D. thesis was developed at the Biomedical Engineering Division of the Institute of Cybernetics (U.P.C.-C.S.I.C.) under the direction of Pere Caminal. He is a full professor of signal processing and communications in the department of electrical engineering at the Engineering School, and a researcher at the Aragón Institute for Engineering Research (I3A), both at University of Zaragoza, Spain. From 1992 to 2005 he was an associate professor at the same university and from 1987 to 1992 he worked as assistant professor of automatic control in the Department of Control Engineering at the Politecnic University of Catalonia (U.P.C.), Spain, and as a researcher at the Biomedical Engineering Division of the Institute of Cybernetics (U.P.C.-C.S.I.C.). His professional research interests are in signal processing, particularly applied to biomedical applications. He is the coauthor of *Bioelectrical Signal Processing in Cardiac and Neurological Applications* (Elsevier, 2005).

Leif Sörnmo received an M.S.E.E. and a Ph.D. in electrical engineering from Lund University, Lund, Sweden, in 1978 and 1984, respectively. He is presently a professor in the Signal Processing Group in the area of biomedical signal processing. He held a position at Department of Clinical Physiology, Lund University, from 1983 to 1995. His main research interests include statistical signal processing and modeling of biomedical signals. Current research projects include applications in atrial fibrillation, hemodialysis, high-resolution ECG analysis, power efficient signal processing in pacemakers, and detection of otoacoustic emissions. He is an author of *Bioelectrical Signal Processing in Cardiac and Neurological Applications* (Elsevier, 2005). Dr. Sörnmo was on the editorial board of *Computers in Biomedical Research* from 1997 to 2000. Since 2001, he has been an associate editor of *IEEE Transactions on Biomedical Engineering*. He is also on the editorial boards of *Journal of Electrocardiology* and *Medical and Biological Engineering & Computing*.

Sanjiv M. Narayan is the director of electrophysiology at the San Diego Veterans Affairs Medical Center, the codirector of the Electrophysiology Fellowship training program at the University of California, San Diego, and a member of the Whitaker Institute for Biomedical Engineering. Since 1996, Dr. Narayan has conducted research on normal and abnormal repolarization dynamics, their link with mechanical deformation of the heart and ventricular arrhythmias, and, via a grant from the National Institutes of Health, their relationship with T wave alternans. Dr. Narayan has also conducted studies that explore the contribution of repolarization abnormalities to the interface between atrial fibrillation and flutter, to better understand their pathophysiology and for improved ECG diagnosis. Dr. Narayan received his medical degree, master's degree in computer science, and doctoral degree in neuroscience from the University of Birmingham, England, and is a Fellow of the Royal College of Physicians of London. He pursued postdoctoral training in neuro-electrophysiology at the University of California, Los Angeles, was a fellow in medicine at Harvard Medical School, a tutor at the Harvard-MIT Division of Health Sciences and Technology, and a fellow in cardiology and cardiac electrophysiology at the Washington University School of Medicine, St. Louis, Missouri. He has authored more than 50 articles and book chapters and is board certified in internal medicine, cardiology, and clinical cardiac electrophysiology.

Stanislaw Osowski received an M.Sc., a Ph.D., and a Dr. Sc. from the Warsaw University of Technology, Warsaw, Poland, in 1972, 1975, and 1981, respectively, all in electrical engineering. Currently he is a professor of electrical engineering at the Institute of the Theory of Electrical Engineering, Measurement and Information Systems, Warsaw University of Technology. His research and teaching interest are in the areas of neural networks, optimization techniques, and their application in biomedical signal and image processing. He is the author or coauthor of more than 200 scientific papers and 10 books.

Linh Tran Hoai received an M.Sc., and a Ph.D. from Warsaw University of Technology, Warsaw, Poland, in 1997 and 2000, respectively, in computer science and electrical engineering. Currently he is employed in Electrical Engineering Department, Hanoi University of Technology, Vietnam. His research interests are in neural networks and computer aided circuit analysis and design. He is the author or coauthor of more than 40 scientific papers.

Tomasz Markiewicz received an M.Sc. and a Ph.D. in electrical engineering from the Warsaw University of Technology, Warsaw, Poland, in 2001 and 2006, respectively. Currently he is an assistant professor of electrical engineering at the Institute of the Theory of Electrical Engineering, Measurement and Information Systems, Warsaw University of Technology. His scientific interest is in neural networks and biomedical signal and image processing. He is the author or coauthor of more than 30 scientific papers.

Index

Recent Related Artech House Titles

Intelligent Systems Modeling and Decision Support in Bioengineering, Mahdi Mahfouf

Microfluidics for Biotechnology, Jean Berthier and Pascal Silberzan

Fundamentals and Applications of Microfluidics, Nam-Trung Nguyen and Steven T. Wereley

Text Mining for Biology and Biomedecine, Sophia Ananiadou and John McNaught, editors

An Intoduction to Micromechanical Systems Engineering, Second Edition, Nadim Maluf and Kirt Williams

MEMS Mechanical Sensors, Steve P. Beeby, Graham Ensel, Michael Kraft, and Neil M. White

Nanotechnology Applications and Markets, Lawrence Gasman

Nanoelectronics: Principles and Devices, Mircea Dragoman and Daniela Dragoman

For further information on these and other Artech House titles, including previously considered out-of-print books now available through our In-Print-Forever® (IPF®) program, contact:

Artech House
685 Canton Street
Norwood, MA 02062
Phone: 781-769-9750
Fax: 781-769-6334
e-mail: artech@artechhouse.com

Artech House
46 Gillingham Street
London SW1V 1AH UK
Phone: +44 (0)20 7596-8750
Fax: +44 (0)20 7630-0166
e-mail: artech-uk@artechhouse.com

Find us on the World Wide Web at: www.artechhouse.com